Orientation to

NURSING
IN THE
RURAL
COMMUNITY

This book is dedicated to
Jack
Andrea
my parents
my sisters and brothers
and
Q-tip, a little ghost-dog,
who rarely left my side through the many months of writing

Orientation to
NURSING
IN THE
RURAL
COMMUNITY

Angeline Bushy

Sage Publications
International Educational and Professional Publisher
Thousand Oaks ■ London ■ New Delhi

For information:

Sage Publications, Inc.
2455 Teller Road
Thousand Oaks, California 91320
E-mail: order@sagepub.com

Sage Publications Ltd.
6 Bonhill Street
London EC2A 4PU
United Kingdom

Sage Publications India Pvt. Ltd.
M-32 Market
Greater Kailash I
New Delhi 110 048 India

Printed in the United States of America

Library of Congress Cataloging-in-Publication Data

Bushy, Angeline.
  Orientation to nursing in the rural community / by Angeline Bushy.
       p. cm.
Includes bibliographical references and index.
ISBN 0-7619-1156-1 (cloth: alk. paper)
ISBN 0-7619-1157-X (pbk.: alk paper)
 1. Rural nursing. I. Title.
 RT120.R87 B87 2000
 610.73'43—dc21   00-008364

This book is printed on acid-free paper.

            03   04   05   06   7   6   5   4   3

Acquiring Editor: Rolf Janke
Editorial Assistant: Heidi Van Middlesworth
Production Editor: Sanford Robinson
Editorial Assistant: Nevair Kabakian
Designer/Typesetter: Marion Warren
Cover Designer: Michelle Lee

Contents

PREFACE

Since the publication of *Rural Nursing,* Volumes 1 and 2 (1991), the American health care system has changed dramatically. With the new paradigm, health care is less likely to be provided in acute care institutions and more likely to be delivered in a community-based facility. Health promotion and illness prevention are the buzzwords at the start of the new millennium. As the system evolves, outdated models are being redesigned, and new models of care delivery are emerging. Concomitantly, professional roles and responsibilities are being revisited. In turn, this affects the way nurses, physicians, and other health professionals practice in rural as well as urban settings. The purpose of this book is to examine the evolving health care delivery system and nursing role within the rural context.

Even though there have been significant changes in the health care system, in many cases the rural challenges remain the same as a decade ago. Rural nurses still must contend with factors that urban counterparts may not even be aware of. For instance, nurses and other kinds of caregivers in rural environments may need to provide cost-effective, quality services to a very sparse population living within a very large geographical area. Rural caregivers must be flexible and possess proficient generalist skills to creatively coordinate a continuum of care within the constraints of limited resources. Professionals in rural practice also must be able to establish, and sustain, peer support systems in regions that some would describe as geographically isolated. Those who live and work in rural communities often report that there is no clear separation between their professional roles and personal life. More often than not, urban-based health professionals are unaware of these and other practice-related issues. Nor are they knowledgeable about the rural lifestyle or the health care needs and preferences of residents in these communities. This book addresses that information deficit—not only for nurses in rural practice but for urban nurses who care for clients who live and work in rural catchment areas.

Citations on the topics of rural nursing and rural health care have increased phenomenally since the publication of *Rural Nursing.* Currently, most nursing journals include at least one article on some aspect of ruralness in each issue. Occasionally, some editors devote an entire issue to articles having a rural theme. The amount of research also has increased in the last decade as agendas of funding agencies have promoted the rural dimension. Likewise, nurses are being exposed to research-based presentations having a rural focus at regional, national, and international nursing conferences.

These combined efforts have produced greater awareness among educators of the need to expose students in the health professions to rural clients and rural environments. Many nursing educational programs are incorporating content on rural populations in their curricula. The need for information on the rural phenomenon will continue at both the undergraduate and graduate level, stemming from external political and professional mandates. This textbook is intended for individuals with little background on rural health care delivery systems. It can be used with various nursing audiences but is appropriate for other types of health professionals as well.

First and foremost, it is designed as the primary text for a graduate-level course. The content exposes students who are preparing for advanced roles (i.e., as nurse practitioners, nurse midwives, nurse administrators/managers, certified nurse anesthetists, and clinical specialists in acute and community practice settings) to the particulars of rural practice. Graduate students and faculty alike can use the book to examine current issues and future trends for professional nursing and health care delivery in rural environments from a global perspective. Second, the book can be used as a supplementary text for the traditional undergraduate community health nursing course with its in-depth perspectives on rural community-related issues. Third, it can be used for interdisciplinary (elective) courses that focus on rural health care delivery systems. Finally, it is my hope that practicing nurses who are working with rural clients, contemplating practice in a rural environment, or undertaking a research project having a rural focus will also use this book.

Orientation to Nursing in the Rural Community presents a wide range of rural topics. It is divided into three parts: "Foundations of Rural Nursing" (five chapters), "Special Populations" (seven chapters), and "National and Global Futuristic Perspectives" (six chapters).

To assist the student in learning, each chapter includes objectives, key terms, essential points to remember, an overview, discussion questions, suggested research activities, and an extensive reference list. The appendices include a list of useful hypertext links (URLs) for accessing other resources and up-to-date information on rural health care delivery, rural nursing, rural communities, and specific rural populations (Appendix A); maps of nonmetropolitan and frontier counties (Appendices B and C); a list of significant pieces of legislation that have affected rural health care delivery (Appendix D); and maps of health professional shortage areas and persistent poverty counties (Appendices E and F).

This edition celebrates what nurses in rural areas have accomplished over the centuries. Hopefully, it will also stimulate a vision of what can be accomplished by nurses within our global village as we continue to meet the health care needs of rural residents in new and creative ways.

ACKNOWLEDGMENTS

When preparing *Rural Nursing* (Vols. 1 and 2), I never imagined that one day I would be writing another book on the topic. Many things in rural practice seem to stay the same. Yet the need for an updated version of these edited texts became evident to me several years ago on the basis of feedback from practitioners, educators, students, and researchers across the nation. Their encouragement motivated me to write *Orientation to Nursing in the Rural Community,* which provides information on the changing health care delivery system and nursing practice within the rural context. However, many others also need to be recognized and thanked as this book is being published.

I gratefully acknowledge all of the rural nurses from across the nation with whom I have worked and spoken over the decades. Your ideas are integrated throughout this book. I appreciate, too, the authors who contributed the three chapters to this book. They willingly shared their expertise to provide an international perspective and develop an exemplar that can be used to develop interventions for rural populations.

My appreciation must extend to the Bert Fish Foundation. They established the Endowed Chair that I am honored to hold at the University of Central Florida School of Nursing. Their interest in the health care needs of the underserved encouraged me to learn and write about rural groups that I was not aware of when preparing the first editions of this text.

Thanks to my friends and colleagues, especially Dr. Elizabeth Stullenbarger, director of the University of Central Florida School of Nursing. Without their understanding and support, this book would never have reached completion.

I want to acknowledge Sage Publications, particularly Dan Ruth and Heidi Van Middlesworth, for their assistance and encouragement.

My family again deserves much credit for my accomplishments over the years. They have been very understanding and extremely tolerant when I leave family gatherings to work on book revisions and finish some writing that always should have been done "yesterday." I sincerely appreciate what you have all done, with and for me, during this entire process.

PART I

FOUNDATIONS OF RURAL NURSING

Part I of this book, "Foundations of Rural Nursing," provides the theoretical basis for nursing practice and research with rural clients. Chapter 1, "Nursing and Rural Health Care Delivery: Yesterday and Today," highlights relevant historical perspectives and cross-cutting issues that present in most discussions about rural health care delivery and nursing. These issues arise in the discussions throughout this book as well. This chapter concludes with an overview of the features of rural nursing. Chapter 2 presents the various definitions of *rural* and *urban* and examines their implications for nursing. Chapter 3 examines the current progress in the development of a theory for nursing in rural environments. Chapter 4 focuses on the community health assessment process, describing the process and emphasizing the role of nurses as partners with the community.

Part II concludes with Chapter 5, which presents a framework for developing nursing interventions for rural populations. Dr. Jeri Dunkin, a well-known expert in the field of rural nursing, applies the information that was presented in the preceding chapters. This chapter also establishes the basis for discussions in Part II which focuses on special populations, and Part III, which focuses on international and futuristic perspectives on rural nursing.

CHAPTER 1

Nursing and Rural Health Care Delivery

Yesterday and Today

KEY TERMS

➤ Health professional shortage areas (HPSAs)
➤ Frontier areas
➤ Cross-cutting rural issues
➤ Telehealth/telemedicine
➤ Population density

OBJECTIVES

After reading this chapter, you will be able to

➤ Discuss historical and sociopolitical trends in rural health care delivery.
➤ Elaborate on the contributions of Lillian Wald and Mary Breckenridge to rural nursing.
➤ Describe cross-cutting issues in discussions related to health care and nursing practice in rural communities.
➤ Analyze population trends and the subsequent impact on rural communities' economic, social, and cultural structures.
➤ Identify rural barriers to health care.

ESSENTIAL POINTS TO REMEMBER

➤ There is great diversity in the social, cultural, and economic structures and the overall health status of rural communities across the 50 states. Rural people are known for their creativity in the use of seemingly scarce resources to meet their health care needs.
➤ Health care resources include facilities, services, providers, technology, informal social structures, consumers' knowledge level, ability to access and pay for care, and reimbursement rates to providers for rendered services. These vary from one rural community to another.

> Several themes are present in most discussions related to rural health care and nursing practice in rural environments. These are highly interrelated; therefore, they cannot be viewed in isolation or addressed as separate entities.

OVERVIEW

The health and nursing care needs of rural Americans are numerous—not necessarily unique but somewhat different from the concerns of more densely populated communities. Nurses living and working in rural communities provide care and services to clients much as their urban counterparts do. However, the context of rural and urban environments differs, so nurses adapt services to fit with the demands and the needs of their clients who live in those settings. This chapter highlights the evolution of health care delivery in the rural environment, cross-cutting issues, and salient characteristics of rural nursing practice.

INCREASED AWARENESS

Until a decade ago, health care delivery in rural communities was virtually ignored by lawmakers, policy developers, educators of health professionals, students, and even major professional nursing organizations (Lee, 1998; National Rural Health Association, 1994). Philanthropic organizations, specifically the Robert Wood Johnson and Kellogg Foundations, were among the first to acknowledge these concerns and subsequently supported rural initiatives to address the inequities. A few innovative nursing schools located in states having a significant rural population also recognized the particular educational needs of nurses who lived and worked there. Consequently, opportunities were created to expose nursing students to practice in rural settings, with the hope that some eventually would return and work there. Not until the mid-1980s did the nursing profession as a whole notice rural consumers' disparate health status and access to care. Lack of awareness was due in part to the scarcity of written materials on the topic prior to 1990. Until then, few nursing textbooks included rural content, and only one journal was devoted to the topic: *Journal of Rural Health,* which originated in the mid-1980s.

Fortunately, the trend of rural obscurity seems to be changing. For example, in reviewing the literature of the last 5 years, it is unusual to find a nursing journal that does not include at least one article discussing some aspect of rural health care delivery or populations living in rural environments. Likewise, editors of major nursing textbooks, particularly publications targeting community health and advanced practice nurses, are including chapters on rural practice. In addition, most schools of nursing are incorporating rural content in their curricula, and many are providing clinical practice in rural settings. Some nurse scientists also are interested in studying health issues and nursing interventions that are most appropriate to the particular concerns of rural consumers (Bushy, 1991, 1999a, 1999b; Weinert & Long, 1991; Yawn, Bushy, & Yawn, 1994). These concerted efforts are providing glimpses into the somewhat unusual features of nursing practice with clients in rural environments. A better appreciation of that type of practice, however, requires some discussion of the evolution of the health care delivery system and formal nursing in rural America. Nursing must have an understanding of both of these entities, and this text will attempt to inform nurses about rural nursing practice and suggest potential areas of research on rural phenomena.

HISTORICAL PERSPECTIVES

Even though the topic of rural health only recently has caught the attention of the public, caring for the sick in an isolated and remote setting is not a new phenomenon. Illness has been around since the beginning of humankind, even among the earliest and most isolated cave dwellers. Archeological findings show that through the ages, to heal their sick, communities made do with the natural resources that were available to them. Often, their resources were sparse and their healers tended to be few. Our ancestors relied heavily on family members and the community in times of illness and crisis. Until recent years, the oral tradition was the usual way to transmit healing practices from one generation to another. In fact, similar self-care practices continue to be used today, as evidenced by the wide array of over-the-counter products to prevent diseases and treat symptoms. Across regions and cultures, even under the most harsh conditions, the sick were cared for, often by women of the community (Bigbee & Crowder, 1985).

Nursing in rural areas of the United States was influenced by, and intertwined with, the unique features of specific locales. For most of our nation's history, there have been regions known as "frontier." This term refers to large and mostly uninhabited regions, to be conquered by the bold and daring. With each decade, the frontier always seemed to extend a little further west—somewhere well beyond the home front. Even today, the term *frontier* continues to be used in reference to health care delivery systems (Health Resources Services Administration, 1997; Office of Rural Health Policy, 1994). In Chapter 2 of this text, definitions of *rural* are examined, along with the criteria for defining frontier regions, with their low population density and great distances between services and providers (see Appendices B and C). Self-reliance, hardiness, resourcefulness, and creativity in confronting life's challenges are attributed to early frontier residents. Along with informal social systems, these characteristics still play a critical role in the rural health care delivery system. The concept of hardiness as it fits with contemporary rural nursing practice is discussed in Chapter 3.

Nursing is filled with stories of the sacrifices and successes of those who provided care to families on the new frontier. In many places, education and health care delivery systems were established by congregations of religious groups. Because there were few doctors on the frontier and woefully few formally prepared nurses, care of the sick and injured usually fell to women, who were volunteer "nurses." The community depended on mothers, wives, and friends to provide midwifery services and to administer crude but helpful treatments, as well as to offer sympathetic "nursing" care. There was little time for keeping diaries in the busy days of frontier communities. The few that remain, however, substantiate that these dedicated women not only cared for their large families but were active in a variety of community roles, a characteristic of rural nursing that prevails to this day.

Adventurous women educated in the eastern states found their way to the westward frontier to care for the ill and injured, often in isolated camps and remote settlements. Organized efforts for a nationwide rural nursing service were initiated as early as 1908 by Lillian Wald. Her ideas came to fruition in 1912 with the establishment of the Rural Nursing Service. However, by the end of the first year, the name had already been changed to the Town and Country Nursing Service. Reportedly, the name change reflected the change in the focus of services from strictly rural populations to include cities of up to 25,000 people. Even at the start of this century, extremely high standards were required in the education and experience of rural nurses. High standards for nurses were staunchly maintained because Wald believed that rural work was the most varied, demanding, and independent. Thus, she recruited only the most capable and dedicated women (Bigbee & Crowder, 1985).

Several decades later, nursing services to rural Appalachian populations in Kentucky were significantly influenced by another nurse, Mary Breckenridge. She began the Frontier Nursing Service in 1925 and expanded the role of nurses in primary health care. Breckenridge expressed concern about the extremely limited preparation of midwives who were practicing in rural regions of the Appalachians. Her interviews with 53 practicing lay midwives revealed the use of archaic and potentially dangerous midwifery practices. None of the interviewees had any formal preparation or education for practice, and only 12 could read or write. Under Breckenridge's leadership, lay midwives were replaced by "frontier nurses" who were prepared in general nursing, public health, and midwifery. Typically, frontier nurses lived in pairs in log cabins centrally located in a settled district. The two women were responsible for providing health and midwifery services to approximately 200 families in an assigned 80-square-mile region. Subsequently, in 1932, she found that complications that occurred during pregnancy were lower among women cared for by frontier nurses than among the general population. After World War I and up to the beginning of World War II, Breckenridge's rural initiative resulted in dramatic improvement in the level of midwife practice in an underserved area of our nation. Essentially, Lillian Wald and Mary Breckenridge established a framework for nursing in rural environments that is still relevant as we enter the new millennium.

The period after World War II saw dramatic economic growth in the United States and major changes in the organization of the health care system and consumers' expectations of it. Appendix D highlights federal legislation that affected rural health care delivery systems. For instance, enactment of the Hill-Burton Act in 1948 brought about major changes in the way care was delivered in rural regions. Motivated by matching federal funds, community hospitals were built in small towns all across the nation during the 1950s and 1960s. In many cases, however, the small community was unable to recruit doctors and nurses to staff its local hospital. Consequently, access to health care for those rural residents was not much better than before the hospital was built. Eventually, with improved transportation and communication systems, many residents found that they had quicker access to health professionals in an urban center some distance from their home.

During the 1980s, many small and rural hospitals closed their doors due to very low patient census, increased external regulations, and financial failure. It became increasingly difficult to recruit and retain health professionals, especially nurses and physicians, to work in the rural hospitals that still were financially viable. By the end of that decade, the rural health care delivery system was in a crisis. Persistent shortages led to the development of federal and state initiatives to entice health professionals to practice in rural settings by offering stipends, scholarships, and work-forgiveness loans. Occasionally, federal, state, or local incentives attracted nurses or doctors, but more often the intended outcomes were not achieved.

The health care reform movement of the early 1990s included measures that attempted to address health status disparities in rural America. The new paradigm emphasized cost containment, disease prevention, access to primary health care in community-based settings, and reduced hospital stays. Patients were discharged from hospitals "quicker and sicker," but the national cost for health care still continued to escalate. In an effort to pass federal health care legislation in 1994, partisan debates focused on making primary care accessible to all, regardless of place of residence. However, there was no consensus among lawmakers or health care planners on the best way to achieve this ideal. This was partly because many policy makers, being urban, were not familiar with access barriers in rural communities. It is important to stress that there are regional variations: Not every rural resident experiences all of the barriers. Some people must contend with more obstacles than others. Nurses should become sensitive to the ramifications of these barriers and how they affect a family's care-seeking behaviors and the overall health status of a rural community. As in earlier times, nurses have an important role in the rural health care delivery system. Unfortunately, there is limited research and theory on which to base our practice. The core of nursing practice is essentially the same, whether the setting is rural or urban. However, rural nursing increasingly is perceived as having some rather unusual features that are consistent with those described by Lillian Wald and Mary Breckenridge several decades earlier.

CROSS-CUTTING ISSUES

In discussions of rural health care delivery and throughout this book, several common issues emerge (Table 1.1). These do not function in isolation; rather, they are highly interrelated dimensions of rural social, cultural, economic, and environmental factors. Each is affected by and affects all of the other issues in one way or another. Directly, and sometimes indirectly, these issues also affect nurses and nursing practice in rural environments—sometimes for better and sometimes for worse. Even though the issues do not exist in isolation, several of them have entire chapters devoted to them. Specifically, Chapter 2 focuses on definitions of *rural,* Chapter 4 focuses on partnership models, Chapter 12 addresses managed care, and Chapter 17 focuses on ethical issues.

TABLE 1.1 Cross-Cutting Issues in Rural Health Care Delivery and Nursing
Practice

➤ Imprecise definitions

➤ Incomplete and conflicting data on the health status of rural populations

➤ Fewer people living in a larger and more remote geographical area

➤ Inadequate public utilities, transportation, and communication infrastructures

➤ Managed health care, cost containment, and access to services

➤ Sparse resources

➤ Recruitment, retention, and education of health professionals

➤ Access to, and use of, biomedical, telecommunications, and information technology

➤ Quality assurance and the need for the rural perspective in policy making and health planning

➤ Partnerships

➤ Ethical issues

Imprecise and Conflicting Definitions of Terms

The problem of imprecise and sometimes conflicting definitions of terms such as *rural* is probably the most obvious and pervasive theme in discussions related to health care delivery and nursing practice in rural environments. The term *rural* is subjective and can mean many things to different people. As many have stated for concepts of art, beauty, and pornography, "I can't define it, but I know it when I see it." The multitude of terms used by various federal agencies confuses the matter further. Terms and definitions, along with current rural population trends, will be examined in greater detail in Chapter 2 of this text.

Incomplete and Conflicting Health Data

Along with imprecise definitions as to what constitutes ruralness, there is an incomplete picture on the health status of rural residents. Even less is known about the health care needs of the numerous minority groups who live in diverse rural regions across the 50 states. The information deficit partly is attributable to the manner in which national health surveys and the Bureau of the Census analyze and report findings from their very large data sets: that is, by county and by the major racial groups. Issues relevant to particular at-risk populations will be examined in depth in Part 2 of this book. Specifically, Chapter 6 addresses special rural populations; Chapter 7, cultural diversity; Chapter 8, behavioral health; Chapter 9, rural homelessness; Chapter 10, HIV/AIDS-infected persons and their families; and Chapter 11, occupational health issues.

Low Population Density

Another recurrent theme in discussions about rural health care is that of low population density: small numbers of people living in large and often remote regions. These demographic factors can be advantageous but can also pose challenges for some communities. For example, less congestion and an opportunity for solitude afford an optimum quality of life for some people, whereas others perceive this same situation as geographic, social, and cultural isolation. Living in a small town usually means knowing most of the people who live there. This characteristic may be viewed as a positive feature by one individual but for another may pose a threat to maintaining confidentiality and anonymity. Likewise, churches and schools often are centers for socialization, whereas the town itself is a center for trade and business. This feature may be rather restrictive for someone who is accustomed to having access to the array of business and recreational opportunities that exist in more populated metropolitan areas.

Adequacy of Community Infrastructures

Intertwined with low population density are difficulties in developing and sustaining a community's infrastructures, such as its sewage and water, other public utilities, transportation, health care providers, and communication systems. In turn, infrastructures, or the lack thereof, can affect residents' health status along with their access to services, including health-related services such as nursing services. From an economic perspective, low population often means that there are fewer people among whom to disperse the costs for capital investments and long-term support of public utilities or health care services. Hence, the cost per unit of a service, if it even is known, usually is higher than in a densely populated urban area.

Managed Health Care, Cost Containment, and Access to Services

Managed care, cost containment, and access to services are major issues in almost all discussions about health care, regardless of the setting. The rapid emergence of managed care organizations (MCOs) is associated with large conglomerates purchasing hospitals and buying out providers in rural as well as urban areas. The development of large systems is associated with an emphasis on stockholders' profit margins that often goes against the altruistic values into which health care providers in general, and nurses in particular, have been socialized. Profit sharing is even more problematic to rural people, with their scarce resources and long-standing cultural traditions of reciprocal informal support. Large health care systems are purchasing small community hospitals and rural extended-care facilities, and they may or may not include providers from the local community. Sometimes outreach or satellite services are provided to a rural community, often established to refer patients to urban-based tertiary medical centers. In some instances, such mergers improve access to care for rural consumers. In other cases, the MCOs' designated (preferred) primary care providers are located many miles from an enrollee's residence, occasionally in another county or state. Sometimes the MCO purchases a rural physician's clinic along with the local hospital. So long as they are revenue producing, the rural providers are retained. However, when they do not generate either an adequate number of referrals or sufficient profits, the doctor's office and hospital are closed. Hence, for some rural consumers (enrollees) the outcome is having even less access to care than before the MCO came to town. Managed care is examined more extensively in Chapter 12.

Health Care Resources

Rural communities are characterized not only by their health care needs but by their resources, how these are accessed, and when these are used. Resources, or the lack of these, is another recurrent theme in discussions about health care systems and nursing practice in rural settings. Health care resources generally include facilities, services, providers, technology, consumers' knowledge level, consumers' ability to access and pay for care, and the availability of informal social support (Winstead-Fry, Tiffany, & Shippee-Rice, 1992; Yawn et al., 1994). Cross-cutting issues specifically focusing on resources are the recruitment, retention, and education of health professionals and the access to and use of biomedical technology. It is important to emphasize that even though resources may seem scarce to outsiders, historically, rural communities have been known for their creative use of existing resources and ability to deal with challenges confronting them. In and of itself, this attribute must be considered as a potential resource and is the basis for establishing partnerships with rural communities—another recurrent theme in this text.

Recruitment, Retention, and Education of Health Professionals

Health professionals—nurses and physicians in particular—are critical resources, and their recruitment, retention, and education are much debated in discussions about rural health care delivery. To provide a comprehensive continuum of care with an array of services, a community must be able to recruit and retain physicians, nurses, and social workers, as well as physical, occupational, and dietary therapists. Rural areas historically have had fewer of all types of health professionals, but the various disciplines cannot be viewed as distinct entities. Rather, rural professionals in general, and nurses in particular, often are expected to function in multiple and expanded roles that may overlap with those of other allied health disciplines (Barger, 1996; Bushy, 1991, 1999a, 1999b; Pickard, 1996).

It cannot be overstated that the roles and scope of practice of health professionals in the various disciplines are highly interdependent. Metaphors such as the "domino effect" and the "missing link in a chain" are highly appropriate when discussing retention and recruitment issues. More specifically, for a nurse to be able to work in a rural community, there must first be a hospital or some other type of health care facility in which to practice. In turn, having a hospital usually means that there is at least one physician to admit patients. Physicians rely heavily on nurses to augment and enhance medical care and provide direct nursing care for hospitalized patients and clients using community-based services. A lack of nurses will directly affect a local physician's ability to practice, which will in turn indirectly affect the health of the community. Likewise, to offer a continuum of care, most social services and health-related agencies require the skills and support of physicians, nurses, and other types of health professionals. A missing link, in this case nurses, can affect the entire health care delivery system in that community. The absence of one element may lead to closure of the local hospital and restrict opportunities for nurses to practice in the community.

Federal workforce reports do not completely reflect the numbers and types of health professionals in rural areas either. More is known about the physician workforce than about nurses in rural areas. The two, however, are interrelated and reflect similar workforce trends. Overall averages tend to obscure the real differences between sections of the country having critical health professional shortages areas (HPSAs) and those areas having sufficient and in some cases even excessive numbers of providers (Appendix E). Since 1980, the overall numbers of nurses have increased in rural as well as urban areas. In rural communities, the gain is attributable to women over the age of 40 years who returned to nursing because of the economic recession in the agricultural industry. Federal initiatives have also supported reeducating agricultural workers, and a number of them have completed programs of nursing using those funds.

In the last decade, there has been an increase in the numbers of advanced practice nurses in rural areas. This trend is attributable to rural nurses' again seeking additional education, but this time as advanced practice registered nurses (APRNs)—particularly as nurse practitioners, nurse midwives, and nurse anesthetists. Still, overall, nurses in rural communities have fewer years of professional education. More precisely, a higher proportions of BSN- and MSN-prepared nurses work in urban-based health facilities than in rural settings. The inequitable distribution of nurses by years of education is partly attributable to institutions of higher learning because nursing educational programs tend to be located in more populated regions. Another factor may be that younger nurses choose to work in urban-based facilities because of the "glamor" or excitement sometimes associated with large medical centers. Consistent with the aging American population as a whole, the graying of the nursing workforce must be considered in future workforce projections. Even with the increase in the actual number of nurses (5% to 10%), anecdotal reports by administrators indicate that they still are a scarce commodity in some rural communities. Essentially, recruitment, retention, and education of health professionals are interrelated issues and must be addressed from a multidisciplinary perspective. The rural community and its health care providers must partner with educators of health professionals to secure an adequate number and an appropriate mix of caregivers.

Technology

This is a technologically driven era, so access to and use of biomedical, telecommunications, and information systems is a recurrent theme in discussions about health care delivery in urban as well as rural areas. Technology must therefore be considered in any appraisal of the resources in a community; it includes communication infrastructures, biomedical equipment, pharmacotherapeutics, and personnel who are proficient in these areas. It also includes telehealth (telemedicine), or the use of technology to deliver health-related education, diagnostic, and consultation services between two or more sites that are not physically proximate. Electronic communication technology is promising to support and sustain providers and consumers alike in remote or isolated rural regions. Technology, for example, makes it possible to transmit radiographic and pathologic images from one continent to another. It also makes possible the remote monitoring of patients: For example, it allows a home health nurse to watch a client located in a remote rural site change a dressing or even self-administer intravenous medications. Now nurse practitioners in rural practice can remain with a client during a video consult with a medical specialist located at an urban-based health science center. For rural clients, technology means having services in their community or even in their own home. For nurses in the rural environment, technology may be a vital link in pursing advanced and continuing educational offerings (Fuller, 1998; Granda, 1997).

Quality Assurance and Measurement of Health Outcomes

Closely associated with resources and having an adequate number and mix of health professionals is the issue of assessing, maintaining, and ensuring quality of rendered services. Small and rural health care facilities can be challenged to offer a span of high-quality services while at the same time containing or even reducing costs. Issues surrounding quality assurance and measurement of outcomes are pervasive, as are those of managed care, and thus they are discussed throughout this text. Logically, an emphasis on assessment of quality and measurement of outcomes implies a need for the input of the rural perspective in policy making and health planning. Nurses must develop the skills to inform policy makers about what is needed to offer high-quality services in an environment where resources and personnel are in short supply.

Public awareness about the inequities in health care delivery in rural regions is a rather recent occurrence. Many policy makers, health planners, and health professionals, including nurses, continue to have an idyllic perspective of ruralness and its associated lifestyle. Rural perspectives must therefore be included in discussions related to policy development, health planning, and nursing educational programs. Often this does not happen because health policy and planning meetings are usually held in a distant urban site. Rural community leaders in general, and rural nurses in particular, often remain unaware of these events. The problem is intensified by the lack of financial resources and the time to travel to meetings. Moreover, many small communities do not have commercial air transportation. In the last decade, the National Rural Health Association (NRHA) has become a recognized presence in the national policy arena, but there is an urgent need for grassroots efforts to present the rural perspective.

Partnerships

Rural citations in the last 5 years reiterate the importance of community and consumer involvement in developing, implementing, controlling, and evaluating health care. Coupled with efforts to downsize the federal government and decentralize power to the state and local levels is the need for communities to build partnerships to address their particular health care needs. Partnership models vary in how they are organized. Membership can comprise a variety of players, including government and private entities, nonprofit organizations, the faith community, health professionals, and local groups and leaders, all working together for the common good. Partnerships offer exciting opportunities to nursing in urban as well as rural environments; the topic is examined extensively in Chapter 4.

Ethical Issues

Changes in the health care delivery system and the exponential development of biotechnology have been accompanied by a barrage of new and unanticipated ethical questions. Hence, ethical issues are a pervasive theme in this text too. Although ethical issues emerge in all settings, urban and rural alike, there may be some unique features stemming from social, economic, cultural, demographic, and spiritual factors relevant to a particular setting. There are no quick or easy answers for ethical issues. Society as a whole and individuals must deal with issues such as the allocation of scarce resources, use of technology, and an individual's responsibility for his or her health (Chapter 17).

RURAL NURSING: THE BIG PICTURE

What do we know about nurses who practice in rural areas? Interestingly, a significant number who choose to work here tend to have rural roots (Barger, 1996; Hanson, 1997; Lee, 1998; Pickard, 1996). Many who grew up in a rural setting simply choose to return and practice in communities similar to those of their youth. In fact, a significant proportion of nurses in rural practice actually work in their community of origin and plan to continue living and raising families there. Most report that they need and want additional education to maintain and upgrade their nursing skills. However, for many this goal is nearly impossible due to extensive costs, great distances, family responsibilities, and work-related constraints.

What is the big picture for nurses and nursing practice in rural settings as we enter the new millennium? Based on word-of-mouth reports and the literature, there is a consensus that rural practice is different from urban practice and different from what most students have experienced in their nursing education. Living and working in a small town can be a different experience from living and working in a highly populated urban setting. Still, one could say, the more things change, the more they stay the same. For example, nursing in rural hospitals usually is less specialized and involves generalist skills. Moreover, rural nurses are likely to provide care to clients across a broad age range and with a variety of health problems. Nurses usually are well-known and highly regarded by the community. In many cases, nurses are acquainted, or even related, to clients in their care. Lack of anonymity characterizes rural practice, whereas the nurse in an urban area often is only one more person living and working in a city of many, perhaps several million, people. These contemporary features of rural practice are in many ways consistent with those described in the writings of Mary Breckenridge and Lillian Wald. However, the two nursing leaders probably were not aware of the fact that in large urban-based facilities nurses are more likely to specialize in a particular area of practice or in work with a certain age group—for example, oncology, obstetrics, or pediatric or geriatric nursing.

Health care reform is affecting nursing in all settings and will continue to do so. For instance, with managed care's shift to an emphasis on primary health care and away from illness interventions, there has been an increase in the demand for nurses who can function in expanded roles outside of hospitals. They are recognized by some policy developers and health planners as potential providers of high-quality and cost-effective primary health care in community-based settings.

Advanced practice nurses in particular can fill the professional void, especially in communities where medical services are limited or nonexistent. These changes in the delivery system have led to the implementation of more university-based educational programs that prepare nurses in advanced practice roles, specifically those of nurse practitioner, certified nurse midwife, certified nurse anesthetist, and clinical specialist. Nursing curricula also are beginning to reflect where services are delivered and are preparing graduates who can function outside of hospitals. However, the adage "One shoe does not fit every foot" also applies to nursing in rural communities. Consequently, nurse educators must ensure that educational programs and clinical experiences reflect the needs and expectations of diverse communities where their graduates eventually will practice. The content in Chapter 3 provides readers with the theoretical foundations for nursing in rural environments. In Chapter 5, Dunkin offers a framework that can be used by nurse scholars and practitioners to get a handle on some of the features of ruralness. Chapters 13, 14, 15, and 16 address national and global rural environments for the practice of nursing. Chapter 13 examines rural nursing in the United States; it is followed by Hegney's Australian perspective (Chapter 14) and Rennie, Baird-Crooks, Remus, and Engel's Canadian perspective (Chapter 15). Chapter 16 presents global commonalities of nursing practice in rural environments.

SUMMARY

How close are we to providing the necessary health care for rural residents? There is no simple answer to this complex and multifaceted question. Rural communities are extremely diverse, as are their health care resources and nursing care needs. It is unreasonable to assume that rural health care and nursing practice will look exactly like that in urban environments. Health concerns are influenced by multiple factors, including age, gender, race, occupation, culture, and social and economic factors, as well as by access to providers and services. In addition to assessing community resources, it is helpful for the nurse to complete a self-appraisal of his or her ability to deal with practice issues in a rural community; this text is designed to help achieve those goals. This chapter presented an overview of rural health care delivery systems and nursing practice in that setting and summarized cross-cutting issues in discussions about rural health care as these affect rural residents' access to health care. Essentially, it established the framework for the subsequent chapters in this text.

DISCUSSION QUESTIONS

➤ Obtain a regional or state map, and identify rural communities in your area. What are your perceptions about rural residency and rural residents? What experiences are your ideas based on? How do these fit with the concepts discussed in this chapter?

➤ Visit a rural hospital and a county health department. Ask about the role and scope of nurses in those health care facilities. How do they compare with nurses' role and scope in a larger urban-based facility? Ask local residents about the health care delivery system in their community. Compare their perceptions and remarks with those of classmates who visited other rural communities. What common themes emerge in these discussions? How do these fit with the cross-cutting issues listed in this chapter?

SUGGESTED RESEARCH ACTIVITIES

➤ Describe the historical evolution of the health care delivery system or a particular health care institution in a rural community of interest to you, such as a clinic, hospital, or school of nursing. Write a historical report of your findings.

➤ Explore the self-described role(s) of nurses in a rural health care facility (i.e., managed care organization, rural health clinic, migrant health center, nursing center, small hospital).

REFERENCES

Barger, S. (1996). Rural nurses: Here today and gone tomorrow. *Rural Clinician Quarterly, 6*(3), 3-4.

Bigbee, J., & Crowder, E. (1985). The Red Cross Rural Nursing Service: An innovation in public health delivery. *Public Health Nursing, 2*(2), 109-121.

Bushy, A. (Ed.). (1991). *Rural nursing* (2 vols.). Newbury Park, CA: Sage.

Bushy, A. (1999a). Community health nursing in rural areas. In C. Smith & F. Maurer (Eds.), *Community health nursing: Theory and practice* (2nd ed.). Philadelphia: W. B. Saunders.

Bushy, A. (1999b). Community health nursing in rural environments. In M. Stanhope & J. Lancaster (Eds.), *Community health nursing* (4th ed., pp. 315-333). St. Louis, MO: C. V. Mosby.

Fuller, K. (1998, January). The Telecommunication Act and universal service. *Rural Health Education Newsletter* (Western Michigan University), pp. 1, 3.

Granda, P. (1997). The brave new world of telemedicine. *RN, 25*(7), 59-62.

Hanson, M. (1997, September 24). Rural nurses scarce. *Bismarck Tribune,*, pp. 1, 12A.

Health Resources Services Administration. (1997). *Selected statistics on health professional shortage areas as of September 30, 1997.* Washington, DC: U.S. Department of Health and Human Services.

Lee, H. (1998). *Conceptual basis for rural nursing.* New York: Springer.

National Rural Health Association. (1994). *Health care in frontier America.* Kansas City, MO: Author.

Office of Rural Health Policy. (1994). *Seventh annual report on rural health: Recommendations to the Secretary of Health and Human Services.* Washington, DC: Author.

Pickard, M. (1996). Rural nursing: A decade in review. *Rural Clinician Quarterly, 6*(3), 1-3.

Weinert, C., & Long, K. (1991). The theory and research base for rural nursing practice. In A. Bushy (Ed.), *Rural nursing* (Vol. 1). Newbury Park, CA: Sage.

Winstead-Fry, P., Tiffany, J., & Shippee-Rice, R. (1992). *Rural health nursing: Stories of creativity, commitment, and connectedness.* New York: National League for Nursing.

Yawn, B., Bushy, A., & Yawn, R. (Eds.). (1994). *Exploring rural medicine.* Thousand Oaks, CA: Sage.

CHAPTER 2

Definitions of *Rural* and Their Implications

KEY TERMS

➤ Standard metropolitan statistical area (SMSA)
➤ Standard nonmetropolitan statistical area (non-SMSA)
➤ Urban/rural/frontier
➤ Farm/nonfarm residency
➤ Non-SMSA county types
➤ Outsourcing
➤ Working poor
➤ Outmigration/in-migration
➤ Rural-urban continuum

OBJECTIVES

After reading this chapter, you will be able to

➤ Compare and contrast common federal definitions that differentiate rural from urban regions.
➤ Characterize six U.S. Department of Agriculture rural county types based on a county's predominant industry.
➤ Discuss the relevance of a continuum versus dichotomous definitions for *rural/urban*.
➤ Analyze the implications for nursing of having multiple definitions of *rural* and *urban*.

ESSENTIAL POINTS TO REMEMBER

➤ Definitions put forth by the federal government for *rural* and *urban* are imprecise and sometimes conflicting. A continuum approach may be better suited for describing rural-urban residency, ranging from a very remote farmstead to a densely populated core inner city within a metropolitan area.

> ➤ The U.S. Department of Agriculture describes rural counties by their predominant economic base. This approach can provide insights about particular health issues and nursing care needs of a targeted population. Many rural counties have experienced persistent poverty for generations. About 40% of all rural families live at or below the national poverty level.

> ➤ There have been significant population shifts in the United States. Some rural areas have had an influx of relocating urban residents, whereas others have had a significant outmigration of working-age people. These demographic shifts are affecting the population mix, social structures, health status, and nursing care needs of rural communities.

OVERVIEW

America's rural communities are very diverse, and the definitions of rurality are equally diverse. Yet analyses of large national databases use the single category "nonmetropolitan" for rural areas and do not differentiate between regions having a population density of 5 or 100 persons per square mile; between regions 20 or 100 miles from a full-service hospital; or between regions 50 or 500 miles from a major urban-based tertiary medical center. In this chapter, commonly used federal definitions of *rural* and *urban* are discussed, along with the implications of varying definitions for nursing.

FEDERAL DEFINITIONS

Nearly everyone can come up with a definition of *rural,* but seldom will these definitions be in agreement. Some see the notion of "rural" as a subjective state of mind based on life experiences, whereas researchers attempt to use quantitative measures to define it. Governmental agencies—specifically, the Bureau of the Census, the Office of Management and the Budget (OMB), the U.S. Department of Health and Human Services (USDHHS), and the U.S. Department of Agriculture (USDA)—use a wide range of definitions to differentiate *rural* from *urban*. Three agencies incorporate a region's population density into their definitions, and the USDA defines six rural county types based on their predominant industries. Other rural experts suggest that a continuum better reflects gradations of rural-urban residency. In the literature related to rural nursing, all of the following definitions are used at one time or another. Essentially, imprecise definitions hinder theory development for rural nursing and limit the reliability and generalizability of research findings that focus on rural populations (Hewitt, 1992).

Bureau of the Census

One of the more often used set of definitions for *rural/urban* is offered by the Bureau of the Census, which defines urbanized areas (UAs) by population density (Office of Technology Assessment [OTA], 1992). Each UA includes a central city and the surrounding densely settled territory, which together have a population of 50,000 or more. Generally, the population density of a UA exceeds 1,000 people per square mile, and a UA may cover parts of several counties. The Bureau of the Census counts as urban all persons living in (or near) places (cities, towns, suburbs, villages) with a population of 2,500 or more. Areas with fewer inhabitants are classified as rural. Using this broad definition, it is estimated that of the total population, 67.1 million (25%) live in rural areas. Of the total U.S. land mass, more than 90% is defined as rural. Yet of all rural people, less than 5% live in towns of 2,500 or fewer. The Bureau of the Census uses yet another subcategory for "rural," that of "farm residency." Of the total rural population, less than 2% live on farms. In some instances, the Bureau of the Census definitions are inconsistent with those of another agency, the OMB.

Office of Management and the Budget

The OMB categorizes counties as metropolitan (metro/urban) or nonmetropolitan (non-metro/rural) (OTA, 1992). A standard metropolitan statistical area (SMSA) includes an urbanized area (as defined by the Bureau of the Census) that is economically and socially integrated, with at least 50,000 inhabitants. A subclassification of urban-metro is "core metropolitan," referring to densely populated areas of a county with 1 million or more residents. After the OMB identifies metro/urban counties, it defines *non-metro/rural* by exclusion. In other words, any county not listed as metropolitan (SMSA, urban) is therefore non-metro/rural (non-SMSA). Of the total U.S. population, about 55.9 million (23%) live in non-SMSA counties. Of the total land mass, 84% is classified as non-metro/rural (Appendix B). The remainder of the U.S. population resides in urban/metro areas, including suburbs and counties that are adjacent to very large cities (SMSAs). Periodically, the OMB reclassifies counties on the basis of census data and population estimates. Using current urban-to-rural migration trends, the OMB projects that after the year 2000 there will be an increase in the number of SMSAs (currently there are 813) along with a decrease in non-SMSAs (currently there are 2,276). Even in SMSA counties, there are pockets or clusters of rural areas (Comartie & Swanson, 1995). Some residents in these small towns do not have easy access to services that are located in a metropolitan area or in adjacent suburbs. Of the total rural population, about 43% live in an SMSA, and the remainder (57%) live in sparsely populated non-SMSA counties. Often the concerns of rural people living in more densely populated counties are not the same as those of rural residents who live in sparsely populated areas. Table 2.1 highlights select lifestyle features of rural and urban residency.

U.S. Department of Health and Human Services

In the 1980s, the USDHHS recognized the need for a different approach that considered population density in a geographical area for the purpose of health care planning. Hence, it added the designator *frontier area* (Ellison, 1986; OTA, 1992). More specifically, *urban* refers to areas having 100 or more persons per square mile; *rural* refers to ar-

TABLE 2.1 Selected Lifestyle Features of Rural-Urban Residency

Feature	Rural	Urban
Population density	Lower	Higher
Distances between places and services	Greater/further Fewer options	Closer More options to choose from
Social interactions	Residents often related or acquainted	Less familiarity among residents
	Interactions tend to be less formal, more face to face	Social interactions tend to be more formal
	Preference for interacting with local person	Wider array of designated places for socialization, business, and recreation
	Mistrust of outsiders	
	Difficult to maintain anonymity	
	Church and school are centers for socialization	
Occupations	Cyclical and seasonal work and recreational activities	More likely to be year round, with cyclical fluctuations in intensity and production
	More high-risk occupations (e.g., agriculture, mining, logging, fishing)	
	Higher proportion of occupation-related injuries without immediate access to health services	Workers in high-risk occupations probably have faster and better access to health care if injured
	Less available information technology	Greater access to information technology
Predominant industries	Fewer industries in a small community	Economic diversity
		More large employers/industries
	More family-owned, smaller enterprises	Wider array of places designated for business and trade interactions
	Town is center of trade	
Economic orientation	Based on extraction from land and nature (agriculture, mining, logging, fishing, tourism)	Varied—wider range of economic enterprises

NOTE: There are wide variations among and between rural and urban communities. These are general characteristics, and each community exhibits varying degrees of each particular trait.

eas with 7 to 99 persons per square mile; and *frontier* refers to areas with 6 or fewer persons per square mile (see Table 2.2 and Appendices B and C). The USDHHS definitions also include driving time to a health care facility and a hospital with a certain number of beds but do not consider the particulars of diverse rural communities.

TABLE 2.2 USDHHS Criteria: Urban, Rural, Frontier

Criteria	Frontier	Rural	Urban
Population density per square mile	6 or fewer persons	7 to 99 persons	100 or more persons
Hospital by numbers of beds	No hospital, or one with 25 beds or less	Small—25 to 100 beds; may have swing beds	Large facility or satellite; 100 or more beds
Driving time to facility in minutes	60 or more minutes, or severe geographic, seasonal, or climatic conditions	30 to 59 minutes	Less than 30 minutes

SOURCE: USDHHS (1997).

U.S. Department of Agriculture

The Economic Research Service of the USDA systematically collects and compiles information to describe changes and differences in rural economic patterns and population trends (USDA, 1995, 1997). As in urban areas, no single industry dominates the rural economy. There is no common pattern of population decline or growth, but there are regional similarities. The USDA's six non-SMSA county types are *farming dependent, manufacturing dependent, services dependent, retirement destination, federal lands,* and *persistent poverty.* The first three (farming, manufacturing, services) have a highly specialized economy, and residents who live here are for the most part dependent on that particular industry. The other county types are not characterized by such an economy but are of relevance to policy makers. Some regions have a dual classification such as services dependent and retirement destination or services dependent and federal lands, and persistent poverty can exist in any of the other county types. Characteristics of each county type are examined in the following paragraphs along with some of the health implications for residents (Table 2.3). To reiterate, geographical regions vary in terms of available resources and the ways these are used by a community. In turn, this affects the availability of jobs, salaries, unemployment rates, and, ultimately, the health status of families who live and work in a particular community. The USDA's work on rural county types is useful for nurses to identify real and potential occupational health and lifestyle risks, implement and evaluate health-promoting and nursing interventions, and refine a theory to guide nursing research and practice. It can also offer insights into common occupation-related health problems and potential environmental hazards for people who live in a given county type. Such information is useful for implementing nursing services and developing educational offerings that target the unique needs and interests of a targeted rural community. (Chapter 11 expands on rural occupational health risks.)

TABLE 2.3 Non-SMSA County Type: Population and Income

Non-SMSA County Type	No. of Counties	Population (% of Total Non-SMSAs)	Average per Capita Income	Median Family Income
Farming dependent	556	9.1%	$14,743	$24,394
Manufacturing dependent	506	31.0%	$13,081	$26,936
Services dependent	323	18.8%	$14,384	$27,677
Retirement destination	190	10.2%	$13,698	$26,657
Federal lands	270	10.7%	$13,807	$27,923
Persistent poverty	535	18.8%	$11,056	$20,731
All non-SMSA counties	2,276	100%	$13,580	$25,949
All SMSA counties	813	—	$16,399	$35,072

SOURCE: Adapted from USDA (1995, 1997).

Farming-Dependent Counties

At one time in the history of the United States, the majority of rural counties depended on farming as their principal source of income. Of all non-SMSA counties ($N = 2,276$), less than 25% are farming counties ($n = 556$), and most of these are concentrated in the Great Plains states. To be classified as such, 20% or more of income in this county type must be from agriculture. In some counties, however, the percentage of income from agriculture is as high as 90%. Even in farming-dependent counties, nonfarm industries are a major source of employment, providing nearly 80% of the local jobs. Often, nonfarm jobs are held by farmers and their families, who depend on the supplemental incomes to make ends meet. The decline in farming jobs is attributable to successes in the agriculture industry. Increases in productivity, for instance, are attributable to advances in technology, crop science, and management practices—all perpetuating loss of farming-related jobs. In other words, fewer people are needed to produce ever-increasing amounts of agricultural produce. In most of these communities, other industries have not replaced the lost farm jobs.

The remoteness of many farming-dependent counties and their inadequate transportation and communication infrastructures often are identified as barriers to local economic development and diversification. With few urban centers located near farming-dependent counties, these residents have restricted access to information, trade, finance, and health care services, which are essential to participate in, and compete in, the global market. With the development of communications technology, however, even the smallest and most remote community can be connected with the world.

Major population shifts continue to take place in these county types. Many younger, working-age people are leaving farming communities to seek employment elsewhere. The persistent outmigration from small towns is taking a heavy toll and disrupting traditional social structures. It is not unusual to hear longtime residents report, "What we do best here is raise and educate our children, who then go someplace else to find work." Those who remain behind—specifically, the elderly and the young—are the most vulnerable, but in many cases essential health-related and support services do not exist for them.

Generally, farming counties have a low average population density (11.8 persons per square mile) compared to other non-SMSA counties (36.3 persons per square mile). The average population in farming counties also is significantly lower (8,400) than in other non-SMSA counties (22,000). Even with the declining job market and population outmigration, the income in farming counties compares favorably with that in other non-SMSA counties. In light of recent population and economic trends, it has become difficult for some farming-dependent communities to support and maintain transportation systems, public utilities, and educational, health care, and social services that urban dwellers often take for granted.

Currently, the well-being of residents in farming-dependent counties hangs in the balance. Stabilizing the population, enhancing job opportunities, and improving access to health care services are concerns in many farming-dependent counties. If people continue to leave, the costs of sustaining the public infrastructure, health care, and education systems will increase even more. Moreover, it can be especially difficult to recruit and retain health care professionals, particularly nurses, in farming-dependent communities. Departure of the working-age and better educated population poses challenges to sustaining viable economic stability. Long term, this migration pattern has health-related implications for residents in farming-dependent counties and could be a phenomenon of interest to nurse researchers.

Manufacturing-Dependent Counties

Manufacturing is replacing agriculture as the predominant economic industry in rural America. Of all non-SMSA counties ($N = 2,276$), manufacturing-dependent counties rank second ($n = 506$). These counties are home to nearly one third of all rural people. They are concentrated in the Southeast, and many of them are adjacent to or within an SMSA. Hence, residents of these rural county types tend to experience more of an urban influence. Compared to other non-SMSAs, manufacturing counties have higher population densities, with greater percentages of female-headed households, blacks, and persons who do not complete high school. As an industry, manufacturing employs more than twice as many rural people as farming does. Contrary to popular opinion, rural manufacturing is not primarily involved in the processing of food or the provision of farm outputs. In fact, only 3% of rural industries are closely tied to farming; the others (97%) produce textiles, munitions, and automotive and electronic components.

Changes are occurring in the manufacturing industry. Transportation and mechanized technology, for instance, are improving, thereby making it feasible to relocate manufacturing facilities almost anywhere in the world. Relaxed trade agreements, NAFTA in particular, have encouraged production outside U.S. borders. Consequently, along with textiles, many machinery, automobile, and computer components are produced abroad, then shipped back to the United States (outsourcing). Associated

with internationalization is global competition for low-skill and low-wage manufacturing jobs. Greater profit margins and higher-paying jobs are associated with manufacturing high-value products with short production runs and quick turnaround time—
for example, specialty medical equipment, electronic devices, and custom-made fur-
niture.

Remaining competitive requires that an enterprise have good, if not immediate, access to information, finance, and transportation systems. Such amenities tend to be more
accessible in urban than in rural counties, thereby giving the former an edge in a global
market economy. Rural manufacturers essentially are caught between two types of competition. On the one hand, they must contend with manufacturers hiring low-wage, low-
skill workers abroad. On the other hand, they must also contend with urban-based manufacturers hiring high-wage and highly skilled workers in this country. Still, the biggest
job growth rate in the manufacturing industry is occurring in some of the most rural
counties. Whether this trend will continue remains to be seen. Economists project that
competition from both foreign and metropolitan manufacturers will continue to be a significant factor in the future of rural manufacturing counties. Real earnings will suffer unless new ways are found to become more competitive through diversifying products,
modernizing production methods, enhancing management and finance practices, creating cooperative networks, and improving workers' skills. Ultimately, economic stability
or instability affects the health and well-being of individuals and families who live in rural manufacturing-dependent counties.

Services-Dependent Counties

Nationally, there has been a tremendous growth in the service sector, giving rise to
the term *service economy,* including jobs in transportation, public utilities, wholesale
and retail trade, finance, insurance, real estate, food, agriculture-related services, and education, health, and social services. This USDA county type derives 50% or more of its
income from service jobs. Unlike the farming and manufacturing sector, services-dependent counties are scattered across the nation and vary depending on a region's resources, location, and access to metro areas. For instance, in the Great Plains, jobs in the
services sector often are with regional or satellite offices of large urban-based trade, finance, communication, transportation, health care, and education enterprises. Communities located near natural amenities usually offer services that support the recreation,
tourism, and retirement industry. Given the dominant role that services-dependent counties ($N = 323$) play in the local economy, nearly half are listed as another county type:
specifically, retirement destination ($n = 70$) and federal lands ($n = 60$).

The economy of services-dependent counties is a mixed bag. Compared to other
non-SMSAs, services-dependent counties generally have lower unemployment rates, a
higher proportion of residents that have completed high school, higher median family incomes ($27,677), and higher per capita income ($14,384) but overall lower wages. The
fiscal discrepancy is somewhat startling! Partly it is explained by higher-salaried occupations usually associated with the recreation and retirement industries—specifically,

attorneys, health professionals, recreational outfitters, and engineers. In addition, migrating retirees tend to have higher incomes than do younger and longtime residents in services-dependent counties. Higher incomes in these counties can also be attributed to many residents' having more than one job. For example, an individual may work full time as a grocery store clerk and part time (moonlighting) as a tour guide at a local attraction, with both jobs paying very low wages. Some with higher incomes live in the small community because of its amenities but commute to work in high-salaried positions in a nearby metro area. Overall, the population in these county types has grown significantly and is projected to continue as the service industry expands. Nonetheless, the ability of this county type to thrive economically will depend on a region's unique features and its ability to capture a significant share of the services market.

Retirement Destination Counties

The presence or absence of natural amenities increasingly is important to the economic well-being of many rural counties. Mild climate, coastlines, lakes, mountains, and forested areas are attracting recreationists, tourists, retirees, businesses, and self-employed professionals who prefer a lifestyle offered by natural amenities. Concomitantly, these attractions are fast becoming important sources of employment and income for rural counties. Retirement destination counties ($N = 190$) tend to be found in the southern and western states. Hence, a large proportion of all who immigrate here are 60 years of age or older (15%). Many of these counties are located near military bases, reflecting retirees' preference to live near military-sponsored health care and shopping facilities. Other factors contributing to the expansion of retirement destinations include the overall improved health and life expectancy of our nation's people; earlier retirement with higher income levels; a preference for living in a smaller community; and improvements in rural transportation and communication systems that make remote regions more accessible to the public. Most longtime residents view the population influx favorably, but the situation raises concerns among others. More people increase the demand that is placed on aging community infrastructures (law enforcement, health care, roads, water, communication, sanitation, schools). Likewise, new residents can threaten historically steeped cultural values of longtime residents. Conversely, urban émigrés tend to have different expectations than longtime residents about access to specialized health care and social services. Different expectations often become a source of contention among the old-timers (insiders) and newcomers (outsiders).

Nearly all retirement counties have shown growth in jobs. However, these are low-skill, low-wage jobs that do not adequately provide for the needs of employees and their families. The influx of tourists and retirees who are at a higher socioeconomic level increases the demand, and hence the cost, of property, housing, and essential commodities. For example, in the intermountain area, several very small towns are becoming exclusive resorts for the world's wealthiest. Housing and food costs are superinflated, yet jobs in the local service industry (hotels, restaurants, casinos, recreation industry) pay very low or minimum wages to employees. Many service employees are foreign-born documented and undocumented workers. Likewise, long-established residents no longer can afford to live in their hometown, which an earlier family generation may have established.

Federal Lands Counties

Federal lands counties, predominantly found in western states, are defined by the USDA as counties in which at least 30% of the total land is owned by the government. In these county types ($N = 270$), property rights and conservation of natural resources are issues of great importance. People who live here are significantly affected by federal policies and regulations dealing with the use of the land, environmental protection, tourism, and recreation. As a result, county, state, and federal entities frequently are at odds over congressional proclamations, which can be tied up in the court system for decades. Essentially, political debates are couched in terms of economic development versus environmental protection. Also at issue is who has the right to use and benefit from federal lands versus who should pay for the benefits. A wide range of people and industries compete for that right, and all have a stake in the outcome—ranchers, miners, loggers, recreational users, tourists, conservationists, and environmentalists. Population changes, coupled with the increasing demand on natural resources, will escalate land-use debates, pitting recent urban émigrés against longtime residents and both against the state and federal governments.

In the last decade, the population in these counties increased significantly (9%), outpacing other non-SMSA counties (0.6%); this is attributable to their natural attraction for tourists and retirees. Here, the percentage of people age 65 and older has increased substantially (33%), but working-aged people also relocate to federal land counties. Nevertheless, the overall population density of this county type is relatively low (15.4 persons per square mile), though higher than in farming-dependent counties (11.8 persons per square mile). Federal lands counties often span a large area in which the population is unevenly dispersed. Only a few of these county types (14%) have cities with 20,000 to 50,000 people.

Federal lands counties for the most part are faring quite well when it comes to income and job situations. Compared to other non-SMSAs, the average poverty rate is lowest in federal lands counties. Families in these counties have a slightly higher family income ($27,923) than those in other non-SMSA counties ($25,848), though it is well below the urban average ($35,072). Job growth is strong, outpacing urban areas, but earnings per job declined more in federal lands counties than in other non-SMSA counties. These socioeconomic factors ultimately affect the health status of people in federal lands counties and the types of nursing services for clients who live there.

Persistent Poverty Counties

Poverty is a serious problem in rural areas. Persistent poverty counties are defined by the USDA as counties in which 20% or more of the population lived below the poverty level in each of the years 1960, 1970, 1980, and 1990 (Appendix F). Persistent poverty counties ($N = 535$) constitute nearly one fourth of all non-SMSA counties and contain nearly one third (32%) of the rural poor (2.7 million people). As dismal as this may appear, the number of counties with high concentrations of poverty has decreased dramatically (66%) over three decades, though some continue to be classified as persistent poverty. In 1990, poverty rates ranged from 20% to 63% in this county type, with an average significantly higher (29%) than for other non-SMSAs (18.3%).

Persistent poverty counties are heavily concentrated in the Southeast, Appalachia, and the Southwest and on Native American reservations. Here families have very low incomes and there is high unemployment. Although the number of jobs grew in poverty counties between 1960 and 1990, by 1990 it was still at about half that of other non-SMSAs. In persistent poverty counties, the per capita income was $2,500 lower ($11,056) and the median family income was $5,000 lower ($20,738) than in other rural counties. The unemployment rate for poverty counties in 1990 was significantly higher (8.5%) than in other non-SMSAs (6.6%). On reservations, in particular, unemployment is rampant, ranging from 75% to 95%. Unemployment, however, is only part of the problem and cannot be viewed in an isolated context in persistent poverty rural counties.

A high prevalence of low-skill, low-paying jobs in persistent poverty counties means that wages are not high enough to pull these families out of poverty. Of our nation's poor, more than 25% live in rural areas. Of those who are rural and poor, it is estimated that 30% to 40% work full time at year-round jobs; categorically, they are referred to as the near-poor and sometimes as the working poor. Compared to most other non-SMSAs, persistent poverty counties tend to have smaller and less urbanized populations. In fact, more than half of them are not adjacent to an urbanized area. Geographic isolation means that residents have less access to better paying jobs that may be located in an urban setting because of the lack of public transportation. Low income limits the possibility of private transportation too. Persistent poverty counties have disproportionate numbers of people with characteristics that make them vulnerable and prone to economic disadvantage, ultimately affecting their overall health status. Fewer people complete high school, which leaves them unprepared to participate in the economy. There also are high proportions of minorities and female-headed households. Historically, these groups have encountered problems in gaining access to economic and educational opportunities. Poverty is not strictly a racial issue, however. In all non-SMSAs and of those who are poor, significant numbers are Caucasian (80%), but overall there are fewer in poverty counties (56%). Compared to both the total U.S. and the urban population, non-SMSA counties have a disproportionate representation of people of color.

A major concern in persistent poverty counties is the high number of families who live on incomes below the federal poverty level. Closely aligned with family income is the lack of access to basic necessities, including adequate housing, nutrition, health care, education, public utilities, and social services. Most seriously affected by the inequities are children and the elderly. The availability of health care services correlates directly with economic development. The lack of either contributes to a spiraling cycle of impoverishment and vulnerability. A viable economic infrastructure is critical if residents are to be healthy, educated, and productive workers. Conversely, better paying jobs can help a family obtain basic services, which in turn enable them to become productive members

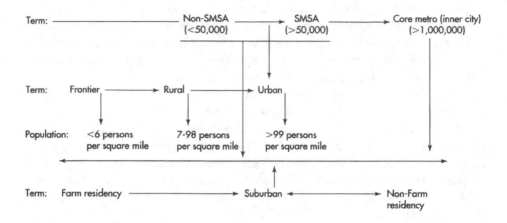

Figure 2.1. Rural-Urban Continuum

SOURCE: "Community Health Nursing in Rural Environments," by A. Bushy, in *Community Health Nursing*, edited by V. Stanhope and J. Lancaster, 1995, St. Louis, MO: C. V. Mosby, p. 317. Copyright 1995 by C. V. Mosby. Adapted with permission.

in their community. In both rural and urban areas, resolving intergenerational poverty requires that both economic and basic human needs be addressed (Chapter 6). Incidentally, persistent poverty counties often are the sites in which National Health Service Corps grant recipients—specifically, nurse practitioners, certified nurse midwives, and physicians—are placed upon graduation for educational loan payback assignments.

IMPLICATIONS

Having more than one definition for *rural* can lead to confusion among policy makers as well as health professionals. For nursing in particular, it creates challenges in developing a theory that fits the particular practice environment. For researchers, imprecise and conflicting definitions limit the reliability and generalizability of the findings to other rural populations (Baer, Johnson, & Gesler, 1997; Johnson-Webb, Baer, & Gesler, 1997). Still, the federal definitions can be used for

> ➤ Tracking population trends, numbers, and practice locations of health professionals
> ➤ Identifying health professional shortage areas (HPSAs) (Appendix E)
> ➤ Implementing appropriate services in a community
> ➤ Identifying special and at-risk populations
> ➤ Providing nursing care that fits the preferences of targeted populations

For example, even though 24% of the total population lives in regions identified as rural, about 12% of the nation's physicians practice there (Bureau of Primary Health Care,

1997). In other words, 20 million rural residents have restricted access to essential emergency and medical services. For nurses, federal definitions are useful to assess health risks of a target population, implement meaningful health promotion and primary health care, measure outcomes, and identify rural entrepreneurial opportunities.

RURAL-URBAN CONTINUUM

Historically, *rural* and *urban* have been viewed as unrelated dichotomies (Comartie & Swanson, 1995; Lee, 1991). There is, however, an inherent risk in this approach because wide variations can exist between, and within, rural as well as urban communities. A better approach might be to view residency on a continuum, ranging from very remote farm residency at one extreme to highly urbanized core metropolitan area residency at the opposing end (Figure 2.1). A continuum could enable researchers, demographers, and policy makers to address less discernible dimensions of rurality that are inherent in federal definitions. The Montana Rurality Index was developed to quantify access-related factors among a rural sample (Weinert & Boik, 1995). As for Urban Influence Codes (UICs), these expand the rural-urban continuum scale. The codes are based on a community's proximity to a metro area to determine its degree of urbanization (Baer et al., 1997; Comartie & Swanson, 1995). Readers having further interest in either of these measures can find additional readings in the references.

SUMMARY

This chapter examined commonly used definitions to differentiate rural from urban areas. There are a multitude of definitions of *rural* and *urban*. So many different definitions hinder analysis of clinical problems, implementation of essential nursing services for client systems in the rural environment, and the generalizability of research findings.

DISCUSSION QUESTIONS

> What do the terms *rural, urban, suburban,* and *frontier* mean to you? How are *rural* and *urban* defined in your state? What county types prevail, using USDA criteria? What are the socioeconomic and lifestyle characteristics of these communities, and how do they compare with the county types described in this chapter? Obtain and analyze morbidity and mortality rates associated with the predominant industries in a given region. Identify potential occupational and health risks for families and residents in these communities.

> Are there any health professional shortage areas (HPSAs) located in your state? Describe where these are located. Interview a nurse who lives and/or works in an HPSA, and ask about the resources, attributes, and challenges of delivering health care in that environment.

SUGGESTED RESEARCH ACTIVITIES

Complete a literature search on rural research in a specialty area of interest to you (e.g., oncology, critical care, community/public health, maternal-child, gerontology). Complete a meta-analysis of these articles as to how "rurality" is defined. Prepare a matrix to highlight characteristics of *rural/urban* definitions for these studies. What are areas of overlap? Inconsistencies? Common themes? How does this affect the reliability and generalizability of the findings? Prepare an integrated review, and submit the manuscript to a peer-reviewed nursing journal for publication.

REFERENCES

Baer, K., Johnson, M., & Gesler, W. (1997). What is rural? A focus on Urban Influence Codes. *Journal of Rural Health, 13,* 329-333.

Bureau of Primary Health Care. (1997). *Selected statistics of health professional shortage areas as of September 1996.* Washington, DC: Health Resources Services Administration.

Comartie, J., & Swanson, L. (1995). *Defining metropolitan areas and the rural-urban continuum: A comparison of statical areas based on county and sub-county geography* (Pub. No. AGES-9603). Washington, DC: U.S. Department of Agriculture.

Ellison, G. (1986). Frontier areas: Problems for delivery of health care services. *Journal of Rural Health, 8*(5), 1-3.

Hewitt, M. (1992). Defining rural areas. In W. Gesler & T. Ricketts (Eds.), *Health in rural North America* (pp. 25-54). New Brunswick, NJ: Rutgers University Press.

Johnson-Webb, K., Baer, L., & Gesler, W. (1997). What is rural? Issues and considerations. *Journal of Rural Health, 45,* 171-188.

Lee, H. (1991). Definitions of rural: A review of the literature. In A. Bushy (Ed.), *Rural nursing* (Vol. 1). Newbury Park, CA: Sage.

Office of Technology Assessment. (1992). *Rural health care: Defining "rural" areas: Impact on health care and policy research.* Washington, DC: Government Printing Office.

U.S. Department of Agriculture, Economic Research Service. (1995). *Understanding rural America* (Information Bull. No. 710). Washington, DC: Author.

U.S. Department of Agriculture, Office of Communications. (1997). *Agriculture fact book.* Washington, DC: Author.

Weinert, C., & Boik, R. (1995). MSU Rurality Index: Development and evaluation. *Research in Nursing and Health, 18,* 453-464.

CHAPTER 3

Theoretical Foundations for Nursing in Rural Environments

KEY TERMS

> Health belief model
> Hardiness
> Rural phenomenon
> Social support
> Networking theory
> Transculturalism
> Nursing theoretical concepts
> Long-timer/old-timer/insider, newcomer/outsider

OBJECTIVES

After reading this chapter, you will be able to

> Describe the rural phenomenon of interest to nursing and three dimensions that characterize it (occupational, ecological, sociocultural).
> Apply four concepts included in most nursing theories (health, person, environment, nursing) to the rural phenomenon.
> Identify theories from other disciplines that could be relevant to rural nursing.
> Discuss the need for developing a theory to guide rural nursing practice and research.

ESSENTIAL POINTS TO REMEMBER

> There is an ongoing debate as to whether rural nursing should be considered a specialty area or whether it is simply nursing that occurs in a rural setting. Development of a theory for rural nursing is in early stages of concept analysis. Relational statements are being refined among the concepts of health, person, nurse, and environment.

> ➤ Conceptual frameworks from other disciplines—specifically sociology, psychology, anthropology, and education—could be useful to guide nursing in the rural environment.
> ➤ A theory for rural nursing could be useful to guide practice and research with rural populations and is critical in making rural nursing a specialty area within the discipline.

OVERVIEW

Accurate and consistent descriptions of the nursing care needs of rural residents are affected by the way *rural* and *urban* are defined. Although there is agreement that a phenomenon and the population concerned must be clearly defined for theory development, when it comes to the phenomenon of ruralness there is no consensus on how this can be achieved. The cross-cutting issues identified in Chapter 1 must be reflected in a theory that focuses on rural nursing. This chapter summarizes the status of rural nursing theory development and presents an overview of frameworks from other disciplines that fit with the rural phenomenon.

THE PHENOMENON OF RURALNESS

Rural settings can be compared and contrasted with urban settings on three dominant dimensions: occupational, ecological, and sociocultural. Even though each is discussed separately, the three dimensions are interrelated and are a consideration for nursing practice, research, and theory development (Lee, 1991, 1998; Weinert & Long, 1987, 1991).

Occupational Dimension

The occupational dimension of ruralness has its origins in agriculture. This perspective is rapidly changing as economic diversity and the population increase in rural regions of the nation. Overall, the rural occupation base still can be described as labor of primary production. This labor requires direct and often daily interaction with the natural environment and can be classified as extractive: mining, forestry, fishing, agriculture. Other industries (Chapter 2) provide direct or indirect services for persons engaged in the extractive industries, such as supplying food, clothing, fuel, education, churches, health care, recreation, and entertainment. Regardless of the occupation for people who live there, employment in rural areas is characterized by a lack of clear separation between work and home life. Often, a sense of shared community prevails among residents in a one- or two-industry town. For example, the person who operates a service station may also be a volunteer fireman and an elected member of the city council. Nurses, too, assume a variety of roles, such as working in the local hospital, serving on the school board, and doing the bookkeeping for the family business. Social dynamics of this nature can be a double-edged sword. On the one hand, greater participation partly explains the increased sense of personal satisfaction expressed by residents—a feeling often shared by nurses who practice in a rural area. On the other hand, familiarity can pose threats to maintaining anonymity and confidentiality for the residents. Both of these social dynamics can create some unusual concerns for nurses and their rural clients.

Ecological Dimension

The ecological dimension of the rural phenomenon is the spatial apportionment of a population relative to other social structures (American Psychological Association, 1995; U.S. Department of Agriculture, 1995, 1997). Rural ecology is characterized by a low and widely distributed population within a larger geographical area. It is rare to find an area that is absolutely isolated, but so long as communication is not instantaneous and transportation involves cost, the potential exists for relative isolation in some rural regions. This dimension concerns geographical and spatial distance but does not take into consideration social connectedness versus social isolation. For example, even though families in a rural region may live many miles apart, they may still refer to each other as "neighbors." This may not be the case for urban residents. In fact, it is not unusual for families living in an apartment complex to be unacquainted with people who live next door or to feel alone and isolated.

Communities can vary widely as to their level of urban influence. Radio, television, and newspapers are available in most areas and play a role in characterizing rural ecological dimensions. However, urban residents usually have access to a range of cable channels, radio stations, and newspapers, whereas rural communities may have fewer choices, if cable service is even available. Or a rural community may not have access to a local Internet service provider (ISP) and may have to rely on a long-distance carrier. If there is a local ISP, rates can be more costly than in a more populated area. Likewise, access on foot to schools, libraries, shopping, fine arts events, or even a nurse practitioner at a neighborhood nursing center certainly connotes a different degree of availability than driving 30 or 40 miles to see a doctor, purchase groceries, and get repair parts for a piece of farm machinery. Rural residents living in states in the intermountain west and central plains tend to be the most remote from population centers. Aspects of the ecological dimension have implications for developing a theory that is appropriate to guide nursing practice and research in rural environments.

Sociocultural Dimension

The sociocultural dimension of the rural phenomenon tends to vary, reflecting the variety of cultures that characterize the United States as a whole. The following, however, are some sociologic features that are shared by many small communities. To reiterate, not all communities or all people who live in a small community perceive these features in the same manner. For example, because communities consist of a few people who often are related, day-to-day interactions in a small rural town occur in a variety of settings that tend to be less formal and more often face-to-face. Compared to residents of more highly populated areas, rural residents often have better access to extended family, who also may live in the area, partly explaining their preference for informal support systems. In some cases, this behavior may not be a matter of choice. Rather, it may be related to the reality that there are fewer formal social and health-related services in their small community. Also, formal health care agencies may be underused because the more conservative residents prefer to have local control and are more resistant to outside bureaucratic influence. Still, there are urban influences on rural consumers' attitudes, and generalizations about their lifestyle no longer are appropriate. Relocating urban residents are further diluting rural-urban sociocultural differences. In the process, these changes are creating unfamiliar and stress-inciting situations within traditionally stable communities. Ultimately, sociocultural along with occupational and ecological factors affect the health status and nursing care needs of people who live and work in small rural communities.

A THEORY FOR NURSING IN RURAL ENVIRONMENTS

Four concepts are common to nursing theories: person, environment, health, and nursing (Fawcett, 1984; Kalisch & Kalisch, 1986). When focusing on a particular phenomenon—in this case, nursing in rural environments—one must develop these concepts and their interrelationships (Table 3.1). Theory needed to guide rural nursing practice, education, and research is in its early developmental stage (Lee, 1998). Much of the preliminary work data is based on vignettes and anecdotes, using inductive approaches. Though useful and often quite revealing, these data are of rather limited value because they tend not to be systematically organized or analyzed. Furthermore, they are based on the experiences of only a few individuals in circumscribed areas of practice. Thus, the implications are extremely specific to location and situation. Deductive approaches, which take existing theoretical models and attempt to apply them to rural settings, also are fraught with problems in that the data may not fit with nursing practice in a particular environment. For instance, health care delivery models that succeeded in urban settings are not being accepted in rural communities, and nurses who focus extensively on high-technology and tertiary care models are finding it difficult to adapt to practice in rural settings where generalist skills are essential. Because nursing is a social phenomenon shaped by the society in which it is practiced, an understanding of rural persons along with their self-defined needs and preferences is essential to the development of a theory base for professional practice. Essentially, theory development requires the triangulation of quantitative and qualitative data, using inductive and deductive methods, to provide the total human perspective.

Person

It cannot be overstated that there are great differences between and among people in both urban and rural communities. But acknowledging that generalizations are difficult at best and risky at worst, we can nevertheless describe some frequently shared characteristics of rural people. Individuals can be affected by the environment in which they live as well as by genetics and lifestyle. Characteristically, people who live in remote ar-

TABLE 3.1 Core Nursing Concepts: Application to Rural Settings

Concept	General Themes	Rural Dimensions
Person	Genetic and biological variations Human relationships Values/views about humans at birth and death Who/which are valued most/least (individuals, related or nonrelated support systems) Human focus (doing, being, becoming) Spiritual relationship (control, subordination, harmony)	Diversity Multicultural population Familiarity among locals Preference for care by known person Newcomer (outsider)/old-timer (insider) dichotomy
Environment	Physical/social/cultural Values formation and orientation Time orientation (past, present, future) Belief systems and manifestations	Greater space between places Less dense population Diverse geographic terrain Orientation to the natural environment Occupations and recreation seasonal and cyclical
Health	Definitions of health and illness Major beliefs Worldview Healing practices Health and illness behaviors Taboos, rituals, rites of passage Health care systems, formal and informal	Ability to work Less emphasis on physical, more on spiritual Varies by culture Greater reliance on self-care and informal systems
Nursing	The professional nurse Nurse-client interactions Caring concepts and practices Provider culture	Lack of anonymity in the community Familiarity with clients Generalist nursing role that overlaps with roles of other health disciplines Multiple roles in the community

eas often develop independent and innovative coping strategies to compensate for the long distances from formal health care agencies (Bigbee, 1991; Lee, 1998; National Rural Health Association, 1997, 1998). When it comes to health care, self-reliance and independence have been demonstrated to be strong characteristics of rural dwellers, who often manage on their own or turn to family and friends for assistance rather than to formal agencies. A variety of reasons contribute to this behavior, including more access to families and less access to formal health care providers, lower incomes and resources to pay for services, and particular personality traits, such as hardiness. Hardiness as it relates to rural nursing is examined later in this chapter. Longtime residents (old-timers) in rural communities also are aware of, and sometimes reluctant to accept, outsiders (newcomers). This can contribute to dissension that sometimes occurs between the two groups, insiders (longtime residents) and outsiders (newcomers). It also raises questions regarding the health care-seeking behaviors and the expectations of the two groups. Questions also arise as to whether the changing demographic mix in rural areas (both inmigration and outmigration) is causing changes in these patterns of care seeking.

Environment

The concept of environment includes distance and isolation along with people's perceptions of the two. Both are relevant to rural residency. Moreover, the perception of their interrelationship is relative. For instance, rural dwellers who live long distances from a health care provider often do not perceive themselves as isolated or the service as inaccessible. And even though it may take longer to get somewhere in a rural area than in a city, it is not unusual for rural families to combine a number of activities into one day trip, such as going to town to see the doctor, pick up a prescription for another family member, obtain veterinarian supplies, attend a parent-teacher conference, purchase groceries, and enjoy a meal with an extended family member who lives there. Other dimensions of the country environment may be its health benefits or health risks. For example, a positive health effect may be less exposure to air and noise pollution and more opportunities for outdoor activities. Such factors also must be considered as dimensions of environment when refining a theory relevant to rural phenomena that can be used for implementing and evaluating nursing services.

Health

As a concept, health is defined and understood in a variety of ways and should be measured on more than a single dimension. In developing a rural nursing theory, one must understand health from the perspective of the rural consumer. Nursing faculty at Montana State University found the significance of "ability to work" in rural consumers' definition of health (Lee, 1998). This belief about health and healthiness has a role in their acceptance and use of providers and services. Rural people seemed to worry less about physical health and to be more likely to reject the sick role than urban dwellers. Variations in individuals' definition of health were found based on their age, gender, health status, and ethnicity. For instance, in defining health, older persons, both urban and rural, focused more on the absence of pain and fatigue and on their ability to function than did younger people. Rural women emphasized adaptation and coping in their definitions of health, whereas rural men focused on their ability to perform within a specific work role. Persons having chronic illness included emotional and spiritual well-being when defining health, whereas well respondents focused more on their physical health and ability to work. Definitions and perceptions of health among urban populations need further investigation to determine if these findings fit with rural populations who belong to different ethnic and cultural groups or who live in other regions of the nation.

Less than desirable outcomes, for example, often emerge when programs are planned and implemented without understanding how the targeted populations define health or how they seek and use health care services. One of the more serious errors is the application of programs from one community to another without recognizing the differences in a particular group's definition of health. One example of this error is the placement of urban-educated health professionals (viewed as outsiders) in the rural community. Another is the establishment, in a small community, of mental health or social services that residents do not use because of real or perceived threats of being stigmatized or stereotyped by others. Still another example is an urban-based health care institution's offering of outreach services at times when other activities take precedence: when field work, harvesting, or calving is going on in a community driven by agriculture; when fishers are out at sea in a fishing community; or when tourists are visiting a community that is dependent on that industry. Knowing how health is defined is of particular relevance for managed care organizations (MCOs) expanding into rural markets and has implications for advanced practice nurses pursuing an entrepreneurial venture such as a nursing center, solo practice, or a home care agency.

There are important ethnic (subgroup) variations in the definition of health among both urban and rural residents. Groups of particular concern to nurses in rural areas are Native Americans, Latino-Hispanics (particularly migrant workers), blacks (African Americans), Asians, Pacific Islanders, and other political and religion-based enclaves such as the Amish, Hutterites, or Mennonites. Cultural and linguistic competence is examined in Chapter 8.

Nursing

Dimensions of rural nursing are the lack of anonymity and the outsider/insider or old-timer/newcomer phenomenon. In particular, lack of anonymity is a common theme among rural nurses who report knowing many people in their care not only in the nurse-client relationship but in a variety of social roles, such as family member, friend, or neighbor. Thus, nurses must be able to provide professional care to people they know in a social and personal context. Acceptance into the community as a health professional also is linked to the outsider/insider or old-timer/newcomer phenomenon. For example, rural Vermont and Montana residents who had lived in the state for over 10 years but less than 20 years reported themselves as "newcomers" (Long & Weinert, 1989; Weinert & Long, 1991; Winstead-Fry, Tiffany, & Shippee-Rice, 1992). This example also has relevance for an MCO opening a rural outreach clinic staffed by nurse practitioners from an urban area.

Gaining the acceptance and trust of local people has been identified as a unique challenge that must be successfully negotiated by rural nurses before they can begin to function as effective health care providers. Rural nursing intersects with the practice domains of other health professionals' responsibilities, functions, roles, skills, and practice boundaries. Nurses in rural settings, for instance, may be expected to provide respiratory therapy, secure patients' medications from a stock supply, and even operate x-ray or other diagnostic equipment when other health professionals are not available. Rural nurses care for clients of all ages with a broad range of diagnoses and in a variety of settings that might be perceived as specialties by urban counterparts. The generalist role requires that rural nurses develop and maintain a broad range of competencies ranging from emergency care to maternal child care to gerontologic care. Obviously, these expectations pose challenges for the practicing nurse when educational opportunities are scarcer.

Proposed Relational Statements

Relational statements for the key nursing concepts of person, health, environment, and nursing have been proposed for the emerging theory for nursing in the rural environment. The following are examples of these statements (Lee, 1998; Long & Weinert, 1989, 1992; Weinert & Long, 1987, 1991):

➤ Rural dwellers tend to be independent and self-reliant in health-seeking behaviors. In the rural environment, help is usually sought by residents through informal rather than formal systems.

➤ Nurses in rural communities face much greater role diffusion than counterparts in urban settings. Nursing practice is significantly affected by a lack of anonymity within the community.

➤ Nurses in the rural practice environment frequently are under pressure to assume some of the functions that traditionally are in the realm of other disciplines. These can be as diverse as being expected to practice medicine when a physician is absent and being asked to shovel snow when the groundskeeper is unable to get to the hospital.

➤ Nurses in rural communities report a sense of always "being on duty." Because they lack the anonymity allowed urban counterparts, rural nurses are sought out by neighbors and friends as sources of health-related information in every conceivable context, including church, school, and community events.

The testing and validation of these relational statements are important in refinement of a theory for nursing in rural environments. Specific gender, age, ethnic, and socioeconomic groups must be studied to determine commonalities and differences among and within rural populations. A variety of research methodologies applied across various groups can assist nurse theorists in validating and refining the theory base for rural nursing practice.

BORROWED THEORIES RELEVANT TO RURAL NURSING

Theoretical models from the fields of anthropology, sociology, psychology, organizational sociology, and health education appear to be relevant to rural nursing. Areas of overlap among related theoretical perspectives warrant examination, as these can enhance nurses' understanding of the rural phenomenon and rural health issues. Examination of theories that are borrowed from other disciplines can facilitate developing and refining concepts that are unique to nursing with diverse rural populations. Relevant borrowed theories discussed in this chapter are the health belief model (HBM), social support (SS) theories, social network theory (SNT), partnership models, the concept of hardiness, and transcultural conceptual frameworks.

The Health Belief Model

The HBM emphasizes an individual's perceptions of the severity of a disease and his or her susceptibility to it as important in health-seeking behavior. The model also is useful for understanding preventive health and sick-role behaviors (Becker, 1974; Cobbs, 1976). Though not usually applied specifically to rural populations, the HBM can enhance understanding of rural health care issues and nursing in that practice setting. It highlights individual and environmental factors that must be examined to understand a person's or sometimes a group's health behaviors. These perceptions, for example, may be significantly affected by rural residents' emphasis on health as the ability to work. In this context, a nurse could speculate that rural persons' perception of severity of disease might be influenced by the degree to which an illness or condition interfered with their work: Thus, a rancher, coal miner, fisherman, or logger might view a fracture of the arm or leg as more serious than chronic hypertension because it would have an immediate effect on the ability to work at his regular job, whereas hypertension probably would not. Health, used as a core concept in a rural nursing theory, requires not only a definition but a careful analysis of all of its components. Perceived severity of disease, as well as a person's susceptibility to it, must be carefully examined within sociocultural and environmental contexts. That is, one must investigate when, and under what circumstances, rural residents perceive themselves as susceptible or resistant to a particular disease or health condition. The challenge for nurse scholars is to identify the unique features of the concept of health along with its interactions among persons and nurses within the rural context.

Social Support Theories

Theories describing social support systems also may be relevant in the development of a theory for rural nursing. One critical factor in achieving and sustaining a high level of function and life satisfaction in humans is the presence of supportive people. Social support is defined in terms of the exchange of information, material goods, services, emotional assistance, and problem solving. It is reciprocal and thus is returned by the person to those in the system who offered it. Social support has been described in such terms as *caring, friendship, community cohesion, neighborliness,* and *unconditional positive regard.* The quality of social support can affect a person's health outcomes such as recovering from hospitalization and illness, reducing pregnancy complications for women, protecting against psychological distress in adverse situations, and mediating the stress of maturational processes (Goeppingen, 1993; MacElveen, 1978). It seems that people having social support fare better than those who are without it. Mobilization of social support systems in times of stress is a widely recognized strategy and appears to be relevant for rural nursing practice (Tilden, 1985; Tilden & Gaylen, 1987).

However, there may be a darker side associated with it, and social interactions are not always benevolent or without cost. For example, domestic violence and substance abuse are serious public health problems. However, often these situations remain hidden by informal community systems. Tightly knit support systems may decrease the possibility that individuals or families will change their life circumstances, may promote a woman's remaining in an abusive relationship, or may enable people to continue any number of health-destructive behaviors. Persons with health conditions that are perceived to be associated with deviant behavior, such as HIV/AIDs (Chapter 10) and mental illness (Chapter 8), also can be detrimentally affected by informal social support systems. Consequently, the potentially negative as well positive dimensions of social support must be considered in the dimensions of environment, person, and health in the development and refinement of a theory to guide nursing in rural contexts.

Networks and Partnership Frameworks

Network frameworks, along with the health belief model and social support theories, may provide insights for developers of a theory for nursing in rural environments. Network theories emphasize informal structures, activities, and interactions within organizations (Goeppingen, 1993). Essentially, official structures and formal rules do not fully explain the activities and outcomes that occur within an organization. In other words, people are drawn together by personal characteristics, shared social roles, and common activities and interests. These serve as the impetus for human linkages and the eventual development of a network (partnership) that leads to actions and outcomes. Networks can develop across formal and informal organizations, including political, economic, occupational, and community groups. Such linkages play a role in health and social service agencies, providing a seamless continuum of care by blending informal support systems with formal services to meet the needs and fit the preferences of a rural community.

Theories that can guide nursing in the rural context should emphasize residents' preference for, and reliance on, informal support systems. Network theories, in turn, are a framework for examining partnering efforts between and among formal and informal support systems. In highly populated regions, networks tend to be larger, more diverse, and more complex. Urbanites tend to belong to and move among a sizable number of social networks. Rural dwellers in areas having a low population density tend to have fewer networks, but these have the potential of being more significant and powerful. Furthermore, personal interests and attributes, self-perceived roles, and shared interests are significant factors in determining group and individual actions within a small community. For instance, personal characteristics, such as the friendliness of a local physician or nurse practitioner, can be expected to have a greater impact on the successful development of a health care program in a sparsely populated area than in an urban center. Network frameworks are a sociological perspective for understanding how informal organizational processes influence the development and use of formal health care resources. A theory for rural nursing should emphasize nurses' ability to establish linkages (partnerships) and work within and among informal networks (Goeppingen, 1993; MacElveen, 1978).

Partnership is defined as a contract entered into by two or more people, in which each agrees to furnish a part of the capital and labor for a business enterprise. All share in the profits and losses. As a theoretical framework, partnership models have their origins in social support and social networking theories and community development processes

(Glick, Hale, Kulbok, & Shettig, 1996). Ultimately, the goal is for all partners to develop approaches that fit local health care preferences and needs.

Hardiness Theory

Another framework that could have relevance to rural nursing is hardiness (Allred & Smith, 1989; Antonovsky, 1979; Bigbee, 1991; Cabasset, Maddi, & Kahn, 1983; Kabosa, Maddi, & Kahn, 1982; Lambert & Lambert, 1987; Lee, 1983). Logically, it might explain aspects of the concept of person in a theory for rural nursing. In the dictionary, *hardiness* is defined as the state or quality of being hardy; a capacity for enduring or sustaining hardship and privation and the capability of surviving under unfavorable conditions; courage; boldness; and audacity. Horticultural science traditionally uses the term to classify annual crops as to the minimum temperature that can be withstood. Hardiness develops as a result of the "hardening" process, in which the plant increases its resistance to environmental stressors, especially cold and disease. Biologically, exposure to adverse environmental conditions, including temporary nutrient or water deprivation and cold temperatures, has been found to promote hardening.

The concept of hardiness has been applied to humans and animals to a lesser degree. Historically bold and daring adventurers were described as "hardy," as were sturdy breeds of animals. Consistently, themes of resistance and endurance under difficult situations appear in reference to hardy organisms. In humans, the concept of hardiness as a psychological resistance resource is consistent with the concept as it is generally used in plant and animal sciences. Essentially, it is an interaction of three personality characteristics: control, challenge, and commitment. Despite stress, the combined traits contribute to a personality that focuses not only on survival but on personal development and life enrichment. Hardy persons exhibit curiosity and find life experiences interesting and meaningful. They believe they are influential by what they say and do. This personality type views change as a normal part of growth and development. Accompanying an optimistic outlook, hardiness seems to help a person cope with stressful life and environmental events. Hardy individuals take decisive action to learn about changes, incorporate these into their lifestyle and belief system, and try to learn from the occurrences.

Relationships among the three elements of hardiness are a complex resistance resource in the stress-illness relationship. Essentially, faced with a stressful life event, the hardy person will attempt to change or modify that event (i.e., control) so that it is consistent with his or her life purpose (i.e., commitment), which will result in learning and personal growth (i.e., challenge). Subsequently, the life event can be cognitively reframed from that of a potentially illness-producing event to one that is health and growth promoting. Hardiness is a useful frame of reference for development of the core concepts of health and person in a theory that focuses on nursing in rural environments.

Transcultural Frameworks

In all settings, nurses must be able to work with multiple cultural and ethnic groups. Consequently, theoretical frameworks from anthropology can provide meaningful insights for rural nursing theory. In particular, Leininger's (1978, 1994, 1997) "sunrise model" includes concepts borrowed from anthropology, sociology, and biology and applies these to nursing. Transcultural nursing focuses on provision of care that is sensitive to the needs of diverse individuals, families, and communities. Interventions that are culturally appropriate decrease the possibility that the client will experience stress or conflict because of misunderstandings and misperceptions of rendered care. Cultural competence encourages the treatment of all people with respect, dignity, and responsibility, regardless of race, color, creed, religion, or handicap. However, before nurses can be sensitive to others who are of a different background, they must first reflect on personal beliefs, values, and traditions. Then they must make a dedicated effort to learn about cultures that are different. In this text, Chapter 7 presents strategies to provide culturally and linguistically appropriate nursing care for diverse rural populations. Nursing is particularly well suited to meet the needs of the growing diverse rural population. Nurses must have a broad theoretical knowledge base of the biological, psychological, and social sciences, combined with skill in family- and community-based services.

SUMMARY

This chapter focused on defining rural nursing's core concepts: health, person, nursing, and environment. Developing a comprehensive body of knowledge mandates collaboration among nurse researchers, theorists, educators, clinicians, and administrators in the discipline. Rural nursing theory is in an early stage of development, and the profession is challenged to refine and test concepts and relational statements. Attention must be given to areas that rural practice and theory have in common with nursing in general as well as to features that are unique. Moreover, scholars and practitioners must determine whether a single theory can address nursing in diverse rural settings with diverse populations. Finally, any theory designed to guide rural practice must integrate the cross-cutting issues described in Chapter 1. A theory should also include the three dimensions of the rural phenomenon: occupational, ecological, and sociocultural. The ultimate application of a rural theory is to serve as a guide for nursing education, practice, and research.

DISCUSSION QUESTIONS

➤ Select one of the borrowed theories described in this chapter. How can it enhance and refine the four concepts that are included in a theory for nursing? Explain your answer. How can a theory for rural nursing contribute to clinical practice, education, and research?

➤ Select a rural population and setting in your area. Discuss how nursing practice with that population, in that setting, fits with the concepts and relational statements put forth in the emerging rural nursing theory offered by Montana State University's nursing faculty.

SUGGESTED RESEARCH ACTIVITIES

➤ Locate research articles on the selected topic, specifically focusing on the variable "rural": for example, mental health issues in rural fishing communities, access issues to maternal child care in rural Appalachia, nursing interventions for rural women who abuse alcohol, or cancer in a particular rural group.

➤ Identify conceptual frameworks used by the researchers in the articles, and analyze how these models support or refute the core concepts of the emerging theory for rural nursing practice. Write an integrative review focusing on the core nursing concepts (health, person, nursing, environment), and disseminate your findings.

REFERENCES

Allred, K., & Smith, T. (1989). The hardy personality: Cognitive and physiologic responses to evaluation threat. *Journal of Personality and Social Psychology, 56,* 257-266.

American Psychological Association, Rural Health Task Force. (1995). *Caring for the rural community: An interdisciplinary curriculum.* Washington, DC: Author.

Antonovsky, A. (1979). *Health, stress and coping.* San Francisco: Jossey-Bass.

Becker, M. (1974). *The health belief model and personal health behavior.* Thorofare, NJ: Slack.

Bigbee, J. (1991). The concept of hardiness as applied to rural nursing. In A. Bushy (Ed.), *Rural nursing* (Vol. 1, pp. 39-58). Thousand Oaks, CA: Sage.

Cabasset, S., Maddi, S., & Kahn, S. (1983). Hardiness and health: A prospective study. *Journal of Personality and Social Psychology, 42,* 68-177.

Cobbs, K. (1976). Social support as a moderator of life stress. *Psychosomatic Medicine, 38,* 300-314.

Fawcett, J. (1984). *Analysis and evaluation of conceptual models for nursing.* Philadelphia: F. A. Davis.

Glick, D., Hale, P., Kulbok, P., & Shettig, P. (1996). Community development theory: Planning a community nursing center. *Journal of Nursing Administration, 35*(7/8), 44-50.

Goeppingen, J. (1993). Health promotion for rural populations: Partnership interventions. *Family and Community Health, 16*(1), 1-11.

Kabosa, S., Maddi, S., & Kahn, S. (1982). Hardiness and health: A prospective study. *Journal of Personality and Social Psychology, 42,* 168-177.

Kalisch, P., & Kalisch, B. (1986). *The advance of American nursing.* Boston: Little, Brown.

Lambert, C., & Lambert, V. (1987). Hardiness: Its development and relevance to nursing. *Image, 19,* 92-95.

Lee, H. (1983). Analysis of the concept of hardiness. *Oncology Nursing Forum, 10,* 32-35.

Lee, H. (1991). Definitions of rural: A review of the literature. In A. Bushy (Ed.), *Rural nursing* (Vol. 1, pp. 39-58). Thousand Oaks, CA: Sage.

Lee, H. (Ed.). (1998). *Conceptual basis for rural nursing.* New York: Springer.

Leininger, M. (1978). *Transcultural nursing: Concepts, theories, and practice.* New York: Wiley Medical Publishers.

Leininger, M. (1994). *Transcultural nursing education: A worldwide imperative.* New York: Wiley Medical Publishers.

Leininger, M. (1997). Transcultural nursing research to transform nursing education and practice. *Nursing and Health Care, 15,* 341-347.

Long, K. A., & Weinert, C. (1989). Rural nursing: Developing a theory base. *Scholarly Inquiry for Nursing Practice, 3,* 113-127.

Long, K., & Weinert, C. (1992). Rural nursing: Developing the theory base. In P. Winstead-Fry, J. Tiffany, & R. Shippee-Rice (Eds.), *Rural health nursing: Stories of creativity, commitment, and connectedness* (pp. 389-406). New York: National League for Nursing.

MacElveen, P. (1978). Social networks. In D. Longo & R. Williams (Eds.), *Clinical practice in psychosocial nursing: Assessment and intervention.* Norwalk, CT: Appleton-Century-Crofts.

National Rural Health Association. (1997). *HIV/AIDS in rural America: An issue paper, November 1997.* Kansas City, MO: Author.

National Rural Health Association. (1998). *Southeastern Conference on Rural HIV/AIDS: Issues in prevention and treatment.* Kansas City, MO: Author.

Tilden, V. (1985). Issues of conceptualization and measurement of social support in the construction of nursing theory. *Research in Nursing and Health Care, 8,* 199-206.

Tilden, V., & Gaylen, R. (1987). Cost and conflict: The darker side of social support. *Western Journal of Nursing Research, 9,* 9-18.

U.S. Department of Agriculture, Economic Research Service. (1995). *Understanding rural America* (Information Bull. No. 710). Washington, DC: Author.

U.S. Department of Agriculture, Office of Communications. (1997). *Agriculture fact book.* Washington, DC: Author.

Weinert, C., & Long, K. (1987). Understanding the health care needs of rural families. *Family Relations, 36,* 450-455.

Weinert, C., & Long, K. (1991). The theory and research base for rural nursing practice. In A. Bushy (Ed.), *Rural nursing* (Vol. 1). Newbury Park, CA: Sage.

Winstead-Fry, P., Tiffany, J., & Shippee-Rice, R. (1992). *Rural health nursing: Stories of creativity, commitment, and connectedness.* New York: National League for Nursing.

CHAPTER 4

The Community Health Assessment (CHA) Process

Building Partnerships

KEY TERMS

- ➢ Community-provider partnerships
- ➢ Community health assessment (CHA) process
- ➢ Team
- ➢ Facilitator
- ➢ Stakeholder
- ➢ Key informant
- ➢ Process (formative) evaluation
- ➢ Outcome (summative) evaluation
- ➢ Primary data sources
- ➢ Secondary data sources

OBJECTIVES

After reading this chapter, you will be able to

- ➢ Characterize provider-community partnership models.
- ➢ Analyze the role partnerships can play in providing appropriate health care services in rural and underserved communities.
- ➢ Compare and contrast the community health assessment (CHA) process with traditional community assessments.
- ➢ Examine the roles of the CHA process team and its facilitator in developing a competent community.

ESSENTIAL POINTS TO REMEMBER

- ➢ Partnering is an active process that is informed and flexible and that involves negotiated distribution (redistribution) of power among the partners. Negotiations occur throughout the partnering process and always are deliberate; they tend to be time consuming and are sometimes conflict ridden.

➤ The community health assessment (CHA) process includes systematic collection and utilization of data to identify, prioritize, and resolve a community's health-related concerns. The long-term goal of CHA process is to improve and promote the health of a community. Two characteristics of a successful CHA process are comprehensive scope and control by the community. Qualitative and quantitative data from primary and secondary sources are used to derive a comprehensive picture of the community's health status, resources, and needs.

OVERVIEW

Partnership is another recurrent theme in discussions about rural health and rural nursing. The previous chapter introduced the notion of networking and partnering within the context of social support and developing community competence. This chapter describes a tool that is useful to nurses for building and sustaining partnerships. The community health assessment (CHA) process is a systematic approach to identify, prioritize, and resolve a community's health-related concerns.

BACKGROUND AND RATIONALE

As reforms sweep across the nation, rural residents must be empowered to make informed decisions about the future of their local health care services. At stake is not only continued, and sometimes improved, access to care but the social and economic well-being of many rural communities. A popular approach to partner with and develop rural communities is the CHA process. The literature has numerous citations on community partnership arrangements that include nurses (Bureau of Primary Health Care, 1995; Frenn, Lundeen, Martin, Riesch, & Wilson, 1996; Glick, Hale, Kulbok, & Shettig, 1996; Glick & Thompson, 1999). For example, advanced practice registered nurses (APRNs) are collaborating with rural communities to offer outreach primary care and specialty services to uninsured and underinsured vulnerable populations, such as African American and Latino women and their children and the frail elderly. In other instances, APRNs partner with the school district and offer physical exams to student athletes and prenatal care to pregnant adolescents. In another state, nursing faculty partnered with an African American faith-based group to enhance health of children attending its annual Bible camp. The nurses, enrolled in a nurse practitioner educational program, served as role models, offered health classes that reinforce reading and math skills, and provided health assessments and immunizations to the campers.

On a broader scale, rural community partnerships study local health care needs, improve services, and build consumer support for the local health systems. The partnerships consist of civic leaders, public officials, local health care providers, and consumers who recognize the importance of health care in their community's economic development. Economic stability is a critical factor in the overall health and well-being of a community, particularly in persistent poverty counties and in those counties having agriculture as their predominant industry. Partnerships are an effective strategy for community economic development, addressing poverty and improving local residents' health status (Bogue & Hall, 1997; Bushy, 1995; Doecksen, Cordes, & Schaeffer, 1992).

On a national scale, the Bureau of Primary Health Care (BPHC), National Rural Health Association (NRHA), Centers for Disease Control (CDC), and Office of Minority and Womens' Health (OMWH) partnered to develop the *National Agenda for Rural Minority Health: A Strategic Planning Document* (NRHA, 1998). Nurses, physicians, national and state policy makers, and representatives from the predominant minority groups prepared this landmark policy-guiding document. The document includes strategies to empower communities to actively identify, prioritize, and resolve their health-related issues. Here, health is seen in the wider context, including educational, economic, political, and community infrastructures.

NURSES AS PARTNERS

Partnering strategies and familiarity with the CHA process are useful to nurses who work in a rural setting for making informed and community-appropriate decisions. Partnering activities, however, often take nurses into unfamiliar territory in that they require new types of skills and nontraditional roles. Different kinds of questions must be raised. The questions are not really new, for they have been asked for decades in public health: for example,

- ➢ What is the community of focus? How can the health of a community be measured?
- ➢ What factors directly and indirectly affect the health of community members and specific subpopulations?
- ➢ How can the community be engaged in assessing its health status and health risks and in prioritizing health problems?
- ➢ How can the community be motivated to accept responsibility for the health of its members?
- ➢ How can a community be empowered to drive change so that health care organizations will provide services that are appropriate and acceptable to local consumers?

Essentially, the CHA process is a useful tool to develop competence so that a rural community can arrive at solutions to its health-related needs.

THEORETICAL PERSPECTIVES

Theoretical underpinnings of partnerships were addressed in the previous chapter. This chapter highlights an approach that nurses may find useful in helping to build community partnership in a rural context. First, nurses must realize that health is not given by providers to a community. Rather, health is promoted through collaborative working relationships among health care providers, the community, and other private and public entities. A variety of terms are used to describe these arrangements, including *networks, alliances, coalitions, cooperatives, affiliations, joint ventures,* and *mergers.* Models vary from community to community, depending on the number of active participants, the organizational structures, and the scope of autonomy desired by each partner. Whatever the model, ideally all partners should have a similar goal: to develop an effective plan of action to solve a particular community health problem.

The term *collaboration* is derived from a Latin word meaning "to work together." Thus, partnerships comprise two or more organizations working together on a community issue or project that otherwise would have been undertaken by a single person or group. Partnering is an active process that is informed and flexible and that involves negotiated distribution (redistribution) of power among the partners. It is an informed process in that all partners must be knowledgeable of their own as well as others' perceptions, rights, and responsibilities. Each partner must learn to take the role of the other (self-other awareness) and to recognize similarities and differences, particularly those of culture, race, religion, political beliefs, disease conditions, socioeconomic status, and education. Partners must learn to effectively manage challenges that are posed by those differences and become knowledgeable about others' perspectives on issues of concern. Finally, the group makes decisions based on the actual problem, not only on the perceptions and positions held by people who are experiencing it. Partnerships must be flexible and build on the unique contributions that each partner brings to a given situation.

Because partnering is a dynamic process, the quality and quantity of contributions by partners will vary over time. For example, nurses in a provider-community partnership may be better able to contribute technical expertise and facilitate problem solving. Consumers, on the other hand, often have insights about the community as a whole, its particular health concerns, and its local resources. Community representatives, also referred to as *stakeholders,* along with the "average" person on the street, can reflect local cultural ways that an outsider—in this case, the nurse who is not indigenous to the community—may not easily grasp or fully understand. Anecdotal information often is more accurate than professionals' perceptions in determining whether a service is appropriate for the community.

Because every situation demands different contributions by each partner, the distribution of power in the partnership also is negotiated and renegotiated. Negotiations are deliberate, time consuming, and sometimes conflict ridden. Effective negotiating, like partnering, requires self-other awareness, flexibility, and sometimes mediation. Over time, partnerships evolve in their structure and effectiveness, but their mutual goal is to empower the community. The objective is to enable a community to assume responsibility for its health by understanding all of the impinging issues, thinking through possible solutions, and then making informed decisions that will positively affect the community as a whole.

THE CHA PROCESS

At first glance, the CHA process may seem similar to the community assessment that nursing students complete in traditional community health courses (Clark, 1998; Helvie, 1998; Smith & Maurer, 1999; Stanhope & Lancaster, 1999). There are some distinct differences, however, the most obvious being active participation on the part of the community and community control over the process. Another difference is that the CHA process extends beyond collecting community data. Rather, it begins with establishing rapport among partners. The process is ongoing, as the community assumes responsibility for planning, implementing, and evaluating programs that address local health concerns. Activities inherent in the CHA process are useful to arrive at answers and, ultimately, to implement quality services to fit the needs of a particular community. The community must, however, develop competence before its members take control of the process. Ultimately, all must work together to achieve mutually agreed-on outcomes for the community and the partners.

Even though the CHA process may seem similar to the traditional community assessment described in community health nursing textbooks, nurses should be aware that it is more complex. All of the activities in the CHA process require *active* community involvement to *systematically identify and resolve* the community's health-related concerns. Templates, or "canned CHA process models," are available to guide the multifaceted community-focused activities (Kansas Department of Health, 1995; Minnesota Center for Rural Health, 1996; University of North Dakota, 1992). Generic tools are designed to assist a novice through the process. A word of caution is in order, however. Each community must adapt the tools to fit its particular needs.

Even though there are eight distinct phases (see Table 4.1), CHA is not a linear process. Rather, the activities are interrelated, with an inherent feedback loop. First, there must be extensive and detailed planning. This is followed by a review of existing data, further data collection, and analysis and interpretation that guide the development and implementation of a community health plan. All the while, the process and outcomes are being monitored and evaluated. Modifications are subsequently made in the action plan, based on the outcomes of proceeding phases and community feedback. Partners then proceed to another phase, again planning, implementing, and evaluating the process and the outcome. To complete all of the essential activities, time frames must be delineated and adhered to; otherwise, little will ever be accomplished. Needless to say, the CHA process can require a significant amount of time, energy, commitment, and resources. Early on, organizers of the partnership must carefully project financial and staffing needs to effectively complete the CHA process in a particular community within a given period of time. The outcomes and how these are to be measured must be clearly stated.

Establish Partnership

Organizing partnerships is a new experience for many nurses. Where does one start? How does one proceed? How does one evaluate the process and its outcomes and make changes based on the collective data? Initiating partnering activities, exploring possibilities, sustaining a continuous effort, and adapting expanded solutions require a mind-set by all partners that departs from the status quo. Ideally, efforts to partner should be initiated by the community. In other words, the community should invite others to work with them to develop a plan of action to address issues that affect the health status of local resi-

TABLE 4.1 Overview: CHA Process

Phase	Objectives and Activities
Organize and establish community-provider partnership	Determine membership, organizational structure, purpose, goals, meeting times, and issues of concern related to initiating CHA process
	Identify community stakeholders and (potential) financial resources for CHA process activities
Involve and educate the community	Define the community
	Form and organize a CHA process team that represents the broad community membership
	Select a group facilitator
	Orient the CHA process team (plan/set up training/date)
	Establish consensus on CHA process mission, purpose, goals, outcomes
	Identify community resources (human, financial, technical assistance, supplies, work space)
	Develop a plan to keep community informed and involved throughout process
Review, analyze, and understand existing data	Obtain/review/compile/interpret
	➤ Community/county profile data
	➤ County map data
	➤ Health behaviors data
	➤ Local public funding data
	➤ Hospital discharge data
	➤ Environmental data
	➤ Occupational health/risk data
	Complete "at-a-glance" charts/publications on community's health status risks to identify real/potential problems
	As necessary, provide additional training for the CHA process team and the community
Collect additional community data	Assign data collection work to task forces
	Provide additional training to task forces, if necessary
	Conduct:
	➤ Community health opinion survey
	➤ Health resources inventory
	➤ Health and social services surveys
	➤ Health promotion/disease prevention surveys
	➤ Environmental health surveys
	➤ Health organization surveys
	Compile data from health:
	➤ Opinion surveys
	➤ Services surveys
	Complete "at-a-glance" charts/fact sheets on community perceptions

TABLE 4.1 Continued

Phase	Objectives and Activities

Analyze and interpret community data	Assign task force to analyze and interpret data
	Provide additional training as necessary
	Involve CHA process team in reviewing/discussing the analyzed:
	
	   ➚ Health status data
	
	   ➚ Health services data
	
	   ➚ Community perception data
	
	Identify major strengths, problems (5-10), availability of resources for each

Develop a community health plan	Determine the 3 to 6 most critical health problems
	
	Assign each problem to a work group that completes these activities (provide training as needed):
	
	   ➚ Identify contributing factors
	
	   ➚ Catalogue possible interventions
	
	   ➚ Identify community's health assets/resources
	
	   ➚ Identify potential barriers
	
	   ➚ Select interventions
	
	Formulate action plan for problem
	
	CHA process team:
	
	   ➚ Compiles and approves plan
	
	   ➚ Reports results to community

Implement community health plan	Acknowledge that assessment and evaluation are ongoing activities in the implementation plan Prepare community for any changes resulting from implementation of the plan Turn responsibility for implementing actions over to organizations identified in plan

Evaluate the implementation and outcome of the plan	Evaluate:
	
	   ➚ The process (formative evaluation)
	
	   ➚ The outcomes (summative evaluation)
	
	CHA process team discusses ongoing aspects of assessment

dents. Such discussions usually are grassroots efforts, initiated by concerned residents who subsequently consult with a university or state health planners.

Unfortunately, in many instances that is not how partnerships start. Rather, the process starts with providers, often using an institutionally generated questionnaire, to assess a community's level of satisfaction with existing services. Another way the process starts is nursing faculty who wish to expose students to a rural community or to pursue an independent research project focusing on some aspect of rural health care. These scenarios generally require that an "outsider" gain entrance into the small community to gather information that may be quite sensitive to some local residents. Often the community is never informed of or involved in the activities, even though residents will be affected by the findings. In other instances, a few respondents may reveal insights or share information that they believe the surveyor is seeking. This approach is not likely to elicit findings that are accurate, valid, or reliable in reflecting the community's perspective about a particular situation. In building a partnership, the organizational phase lays the foundation for all other activities that follow. It is crucial, therefore, that organizers gain active and passive support from local groups and community stakeholders. Nurses who live and work in rural communities often are in key positions to facilitate social networking, community development, and community competence. With encouragement, the informal discussions evolve into a structured community-provider partnership. Their mutual goal should be data-based decision making to improve the community's health status, and this can be facilitated with the systematic CHA process.

Select the Team and a Facilitator

Key stakeholders must be identified who are willing and able to assume a leadership role in motivating their community to become empowered and assume responsibility for the health status of all residents. The group may be a loosely organized or a highly structured health council or may be organized in some way between the two extremes. Hereafter, the term *team* will be used in reference to the core group that coordinates the CHA process. Membership on the team should reflect the community in terms of age, gender, income, race, geographic distribution, and political and religious preferences. All members should start on a level playing field. That is, there must be equal opportunity for team individuals to participate fully in discussions and have at least a basic level of knowledge of health care delivery and economics.

At the onset, each member of the team must be enlisted to accept responsibility for improving the community's health status and developing satisfactory solutions for its health concerns. Eventually, other community residents are called on to assist the team in implementing the various CHA process activities. The team is responsible for planning the overall activities and ensuring that these are completed as delineated in the organizational plan. Consistent with theories of change, there are enhancements (driving forces) that can support and barriers (restraining forces) that can inhibit creative initiatives put forth by the team. It cannot be overemphasized that the team should hire or appoint a facilitator who is adept at negotiation and conflict resolution and is familiar with the CHA process. This individual should have the skills to promote change (change agent), be sensitive to local cultural values, and be able to promote noncompetitive solutions that are appropriate for the community. In many instances, a nurse with advanced educational preparation in administration or community development who is living and working in the community fits these criteria (Lancaster, 1998).

The facilitator of the team has an important role in establishing trust and setting ground rules that are acceptable to all partners and community representatives. The facilitator should be aware that threats to an individual's sense of power must be minimized because the loss of even one person's perceived influence can be extremely debilitating to partnership efforts. Members of the team must learn to present ideas in a supportive manner that considers the self-esteem of other partners. Hidden agendas must be avoided, or trust and rapport among partners will quickly dissipate. The team should be encouraged by the facilitator to openly discuss actual as well as potential (perceived) consequences of each proposed solution. When examining anticipated outcomes, the facilitator should attempt to defuse emotional perceptions with quantitative assessments of the situation. Essentially, the goal of the team is to create win/win solutions for all partners. Obviously, an adept facilitator is critical in achieving this somewhat lofty outcome.

Define the Community

At the outset, the partners should agree on what is meant by *our community*. Subsequently, the team may wish to modify that preliminary definition to fit the parameters established by the community of interest. Generally, the concept of community is not limited to geographic location. In a rural setting, it could be the service delivery area enveloping the town, neighboring towns, a county, a district, or any combination of these. *Community* also may refer to a selected (sub)population within a broad geographical area, such as a racial, ethnic, or religious group. For a managed care organization (MCO) expanding into a rural region, boundaries of a community (catchment area) may cross county or state boundaries. In turn, community stakeholders and representatives must be involved in discussions with MCO administrators in defining local needs and preferences. Once boundaries are determined, coalition building occurs, with an exchange of ideas and shared solutions by the partners. This process may be part of developing a competent community. In early discussion stages, the community might consist of only two or three people who identify important issues with the current health care system. Members of the group share in the belief that others eventually will join and help resolve the problem. Informal community efforts can evolve into a more organized constituency (team). Nurses have an important role in getting the CHA process started, stemming from their professional ability to work between formal and informal networks and their role as information brokers in small communities.

Involve and Educate the Community

After a thorough orientation of the team to the CHA process, community building expands to integrate local residents. Their first order of business should be to inform the public of the partnership's existence and its role in addressing the community's health, economic, or social concerns. Public education can be done with the use of outside consultants, by the team, or both. As for the message, it can be disseminated in a variety of ways, including public service announcements on radio or television, feature articles in the local newspaper, or team members speaking to service, civic, and religious organizations about the mission and goals of the CHA process. Eventually, the team recruits volunteers from the community to assist in carrying out CHA activities. Volunteering is an effective strategy for the community to develop a sense of ownership and begin to accept responsibility for its overall health. It is prudent for the team to keep the public (community) informed about the partnership's vision and activities. The facilitator keeps the team focused and on schedule and anticipates barriers and driving forces in the CHA process.

Review and Collect Data

After the partners are oriented to the process and cohesiveness evolves, community data are collected and analyzed to glean insights on residents' health status. Such information can be obtained from existing federal and state data, using demographic, socioeconomic, and health indicators. Collection and review of data represent two of the more time-consuming activities of the CHA process but also create opportunities for greater community involvement. Furthermore, consumers in general and nurses in particular often are in positions to offer insights about the community that will facilitate and expedite the team's efforts. Data collection and review are not one-time actions because additional information often is needed as the CHA process evolves. Data are both qualitative and quantitative and are obtained from secondary and primary sources (Table 4.2).

Secondary data for the CHA process are compiled at regular intervals by federal, state, and local governments, as well as by health care and human service agencies. Secondary sources are categorized as health status risks, health services, and population data. Population databases can profile a community's demographic characteristics on such factors as age, gender, ethnicity, education, unemployment, and income levels. Depending on how the community is defined and the location of its boundaries, the team may need to compile a community-specific demographic profile from several secondary sources. These sources essentially provide a statistical profile of the community's residents and their health-related concerns and resources. However, secondary data often do not describe the human dimensions of a given situation. Consequently, the team may find that primary sources yield a more complete perspective of consumers' experiences with their health care system.

Primary data can be obtained from a variety of sources. The most common is the opinion survey, which seeks information about selected issues from a cross-section of community residents. Surveys can take the form of personal or telephone interviews, pencil-and-paper questionnaires, or combinations thereof and can serve a multitude of purposes.

For example, a survey can elicit perceptions about the most important issues experienced by local residents. Surveys provide an opportunity for residents to make valuable suggestions on how to effectively address the concerns. Careful planning accompanied by community input when developing a survey is an effective strategy to create awareness and motivate the public while at the same time obtaining relevant data. Survey data are useful in planning appropriate educational programs to inform the community about particular health risks, available resources to deal with these concerns, and specific prevention behaviors. Because of the many potential uses of the survey approach, the team may wish to seek outside consultation and technical assistance in developing a survey tool. To reiterate, community input is *essential* in the development of a survey to ensure that its norms, beliefs, values, preferences, and cultural nuances are reflected. Rural

TABLE 4.2 Data Sources for the CHA Process

Type	Secondary Sources	Primary Sources
Population and health status risks: describe profile and health status and risks of community or subgroups	Census reports State/local demographic data Crime reports Environmental risks Occupational injuries (OSHA/USDA) Behavioral health risk information (smoking/substance use/seat belt use, etc.) (CDC, NIH, USPHS, state health dept.) Hospital discharge data Emergency services reports	Reports/interviews with other health professionals (nurses, doctors, dentists, educators, veterinarians)
Health care system: describe local services and resources and their level of function in the community	Reports from ➤ Health institutions (organization/annual/ strategic planning) ➤ Local/county/state businesses ➤ Social service agencies ➤ Environmental services ➤ Transportation services ➤ Human resources agencies Public domain documents Financial resources Maps Telephone directories Lists of local resources	Formal interviews with health professionals, key informants Informal discussions with key informants and average citizens Delphi methods Nominal process methods
Community perceptions: describe local opinion on health issues, providers, and services	Reports from ➤ Bureau of tourism ➤ Economic/community development	Oral/written opinion surveys Focus groups Town meetings Public forums Informal (face-to-face discussions with stakeholders and average citizens) Media ➤ Feature articles ➤ Letters to the editor ➤ Call-in comments on local radio/television talk shows ➤ Internet user groups

nurses in particular often are able to make important contributions in refining the tool to fit local preferences. Telephone and face-to-face interviews are other ways to obtain in-depth information regarding residents' health concerns.

Key informants also are able to offer insights regarding specific community issues. For instance, residents with a particular illness can be interviewed about their experience in accessing certain types of services. Families who recently have had a family member involved in an occupational-related, machinery, or automobile accident usually can de-scribe in great detail how long it took for them to get emergency services. How far and how long did they drive to finally reach a doctor or nurse who could treat the emergency? Home care nurses might be asked about their experiences in locating senior African Americans in a southeastern persistent poverty county or the time it took them to find a Native American with chronic and poorly regulated diabetes who was living on a remote reservation in a midwestern state. What problems do they encounter when trying to pro-vide services to these highly vulnerable groups? Do their clients' homes have indoor plumbing, running water, electricity, or telephone services? How and from where do cli-ents obtain insulin and diabetic supplies? How do they take care of their nutritional needs? Local nurses often are able to offer anecdotal data to enhance statistical profiles from CDC, BPHC, Indian Health Services, or the state department of health.

Letters to the editor, feature newspaper articles, and call-in commentaries on radio or television programs are other sources of primary data. Thoughtfully selected small fo-cus groups are another strategy to elicit specific concerns of targeted consumers. Com-munity forums (town meetings) advertised and open to the public can elicit data from a cross section of community members. Their comments can be validated by designating interviewers to randomly ask an "average person on the street" for his or her views. Often such interviewees can substantiate, refute, expand, and enhance data that are obtained in more structured surveys, interviews, forums, and focus groups. Data collection methods for the CHA process must be decided with the following factors in mind:

> How can data collection methods be used to create awareness, educate, and implement change in the community?
> What resources (financial, salaried staff, volunteers, time) are available to collect, ana-lyze, and communicate the data?
> To what degree do primary and secondary data sources complement each other?
> How accessible are the data? What resources are available to analyze and interpret the data? How will the data be used and by whom?

Community perceptions are important and should always be considered. These per-spectives, however, should not be the sole basis for planning, especially if community views conflict with official health status data (e.g., data from the National Institute of Oc-cupational Safety and Health [NIOSH], CDC, or state or local departments of health). Sometimes the community must be educated about the problem because the residents are not aware that the problem exists or do not know the extent of its prevalence, as in the case of domestic violence, occupation-related injuries, teen pregnancies, or even poverty. Consequently, plan to carefully determine the resources and education that are required to collect data, and use them.

Analyze and Understand Data

Collecting data can be an arduous task, and sorting through the piles of information can be intimidating. Once data are collected, they must be compiled, analyzed, and interpreted for decision-making purposes. In the CHA process, this usually becomes an ongoing activity as the team and its facilitator integrate data from formative program evaluation. In brief, the procedures used for analysis of the data will depend on the collection methods and how the findings are to be used. Team members will have varying degrees of familiarity with analysis approaches. All members should have at least a basic understanding of the meaning of the data and how they are to be used. If outside consultants are used in developing the instruments, their services may include data analysis. The extent and costs for consultants' services should be made clear by the team or its facilitator when hiring negotiations take place.

Analysis means making sense out of reams of data. To begin, the team should review the community's perceptions from the opinion surveys. Ascertain whether public perceptions are congruent or incongruent with health status data. In addition to identifying problem areas, opinion data may indicate that the community must be better informed about services, educated about specific health-related issues, or encouraged to modify risky lifestyle behaviors. They also may need reminders about the purpose of the team and the short- and long-term goals of the CHA process. After analyzing the data, the team must synthesize the extensive information. Essentially, understanding the data is the bridge between the collection activities and development of a community-specific health plan. As with the other phases of the CHA process, volunteers from the community may be able to offer insights that will help to make sense of the data. Nurses often can provide relevant anecdotal information about vulnerable populations that do not have their views represented. They also may have ideas as to how the health plan can be tailored to fit the community's cultural and socioeconomic peculiarities.

Develop and Implement a
Community Health Plan

Once the data are analyzed and interpreted, the team reports the findings, and feedback should be encouraged to develop an appropriate community-focused action plan. Developing a plan of action probably is the most important aspect of the CHA process (Lancaster, 1998). During these activities, the multifaceted data are used by the team to identify areas of concern, prioritize these, and develop options for each according to local resources, assets, and deficits. For example, in one community, the CHA team members advocated building a new clinic to meet the needs of rural constituents in a persistent poverty county. However, in discussing these plans with residents in that region, it became evident that they did not need another clinic. Rather, the most cost-effective approach was improving the drivability of the county roads to make for easier access to the existing clinic. Even if the clinic was less than 5 miles away, most of the people could not get to the main roads due to impassible roads.

After consensus is achieved, the plan must drive community change. Also, the team must be able to implement change even with populations that prefer the status quo, as often is the case, especially in more geographically remote and persistent poverty counties.

If the community has been involved in the ongoing CHA process, implementation of the health plan should proceed smoothly. The best laid plans can go awry, however, especially when one is trying to modify entrenched culturally steeped behaviors. Flexibility as the situation requires is essential on the part of the team, the facilitator, and participants in the partnership. To evoke a sense of ownership as well as to inform the public, each problem in the health plan should be assigned to a working group of interested community volunteers. Through dialogue, they usually become aware of other community members who have an interest in this particular concern. Ultimately, each group is responsible for identifying contributing risk factors and possible interventions as well as driving and constraining community forces for each option. Volunteers often can determine the most effective ways to evaluate the change process and measure the outcomes of an intervention in relation to the community's health behaviors.

Evaluate the Process and Outcome

As the CHA process is carried out, the team should integrate opportunities for ongoing evaluation of the process (formative evaluation) and outcomes (summative evaluation). Again, community input is essential for developing appropriate goals and methodologies to ensure that data are valid and reliable and reflect the local perspective. Systematic and ongoing evaluation is critical for measuring short-term and long-term health-related outcomes. On the basis of feedback from all the partners, modifications are made in the plan to address the community's particular needs.

SUMMARY

Recent trends to downsize the federal government have led to the decentralization of power to the state and local levels. The CHA process is a systematic approach that promotes provider-community partnering to identify priorities and develop a plan of action to respond to those concerns. Nurses in rural communities are knowledge brokers and should learn the skills necessary to participate as a partner in the data-driven CHA processes.

DISCUSSION QUESTIONS

Contact your state department of health and determine if any community is implementing the CHA process. If so, review the team's final report and interview the team facilitator. Respond to these questions:

- ➢ Define the community.
- ➢ Describe the characteristics of the people who live there.
- ➢ Are there any community partnerships? If so, who are the community stakeholders?
- ➢ How are its activities financed?
- ➢ What data sources were/are used to complete the process?
- ➢ Identify potential education that the community requires to implement CHA process activities. By whom, where, and how could these programs be best delivered to the targeted population?
- ➢ What role did nurses have in the CHA process?
- ➢ Describe the evaluation methods.
- ➢ List projected community outcomes that emerged from the CHA process.

SUGGESTED RESEARCH ACTIVITIES

Survey a representative sample of a rural community to learn about their perception of the local health care delivery system.

- ➢ Compile, analyze, and interpret the data.
- ➢ Disseminate the findings to peers and other audiences in the community. For example, produce "at-a-glance" reports and fact sheets to present at a lunch meeting for local health professionals, a county commissioners' meeting, or a high school health education class.
- ➢ Write an article for the local newspaper based on your survey findings.

REFERENCES

Bogue, R., & Hall, C. (Eds.). (1997). *Health network innovations: How 20 communities are improving their systems through collaboration.* Chicago: American Hospital Association.

Bureau of Primary Health Care. (1995). *Models that work: 1994-1995.* Washington, DC: U.S. Department of Health and Human Services.

Bushy, A. (1995). Harnessing the chaos in health care reform with provider-community partnerships. *Journal of Nursing Quality Care, 9*(3), 10-19.

Clark, M. (1998). *Nursing in the community.* Norwalk, CT: Appleton & Lange.

Doecksen, K., Cordes, S., & Schaeffer, T. (1992). *Health care's contribution to rural economic development.* Rockville, MD: U.S. Department of Health and Human Services, Office of Rural Health Policy.

Frenn, M., Lundeen, S., Martin, K., Riesch, S., & Wilson, S. (1996). Symposium on nursing centers: Past, present and future. *Journal of Nursing Education, 35*(2), 56-62.

Glick, D., Hale, P., Kulbok, P., & Shettig, J. (1996). Community development theory: Planning a community nursing center. *Journal of Nursing Administration, 26*(7/8), 44-50.

Glick, D., & Thompson, K. (1999). Program and project management. In J. Lancaster (Ed.), *The nurse as a change agent.* St. Louis, MO: Mosby Year-Book.

Helvie, C. (1998). *Advanced practice nursing in the community.* Thousand Oaks, CA: Sage.

Kansas Department of Health and Environment. (1995). *Kansas community health assessment process: Overview.* Topeka, KS: Author.

Lancaster, J. (1998). *Nursing issues in leading and managing change.* St. Louis, MO: C. V. Mosby.

Minnesota Center for Rural Health. (1996). *Getting on the right road to rural health care: A community health development guide.* Duluth, MN: Author.

National Rural Health Association. (1998). *A national agenda for rural minority health.* Kansas City, MO: Author.

Smith, C., & Maurer, F. (1999). *Community health nursing: Theory and practice.* Philadelphia: W. B. Saunders.

Stanhope, L., & Lancaster, J. (Eds.). (1999). *Community health nursing.* St. Louis, MO: C. V. Mosby.

University of North Dakota School of Medicine, Center for Rural Health. (1992). *Networking and coalition building: Working together for rural action.* Grand Forks, ND: Author.

CHAPTER 5

Exemplar

A Framework for Rural Nursing Interventions

JERI W. DUNKIN

KEY TERMS

> ➤ Structural factors
> ➤ Sociocultural factors
> ➤ Health-seeking behaviors
> ➤ Financial factors
> ➤ Participation mediators
> ➤ Service utilization
> ➤ Outcome mediators
> ➤ Outcomes
> ➤ Adherence

OBJECTIVES

After reading this chapter, you will be able to

> ➤ Analyze sociocultural factors that can affect program planning and utilizing of health services by rural residents.
> ➤ Examine partnerships that are essential for successful nursing interventions with rural populations.
> ➤ Use effective strategies to facilitate nursing interventions in rural areas.
> ➤ Articulate potential health outcomes for rural residents in relation to health-mediating factors.

ESSENTIAL POINTS TO REMEMBER

➣ Sociocultural factors such as health beliefs, independence, level of trust, and belonging are critical for successful nursing intervention with rural clients.

➣ Structural factors such as availability and configuration of health care resources, transportation to them, and distance must be addressed when determining the best array of health services for rural clients.

➣ Participation mediators such as family roles, social support from informal systems, trust and acceptance, lack of anonymity, and isolation affect the utilization of health care services by rural clients; thus, they must be understood by nurses working with those clients.

➣ Multiple factors affect health services utilization. Understanding those factors can enhance nurses' abilities to assist rural clients.

OVERVIEW

This chapter highlights the interrelationship of multiple factors that can affect health-seeking behaviors and health outcomes among rural clients. The framework in this exemplar integrates content presented in the preceding chapters and serves as a reference point for subsequent chapters in this book. It integrates features of the rural phenomenon that nurses should consider when designing interventions for rural clients (Figure 5.1) (Dunkin, 1997; Dunkin, Stratton, & Holzwarth, 1992).

STRUCTURAL FACTORS

Structural factors refers to the accessibility of health care resources, both private and public, such as their availability and configuration, transportation to them, and distance, and the manner in which resources are accessed by targeted consumers. These factors are of particular importance in rural areas where there are high numbers of poor people.

With respect to *availability,* over the decades changes have occurred in the manner in which health care is delivered in the United States. For example, the post-World War II solution to health care access problems was expanding the supply of hospital beds. Later, in the 1960s, the focus was on increasing the supply of health care professionals. In the 1990s the federal government adopted a policy of capacity building at the local level, partly in recognition that Medicare and Medicaid entitlements would strain the health care delivery system by increasing the demand for medical care. Community health centers, the National Health Service Corps, and other programs were designed to increase the number of health care professionals in underserved areas. These mechanisms enabled local communities to take advantage of available public funds. Essentially, the legacy of this period was to measure access in terms of number of beds, facilities, and providers in relation to population (Institute of Medicine [IOM], 1993; National Center for Health Statistics, 1995).

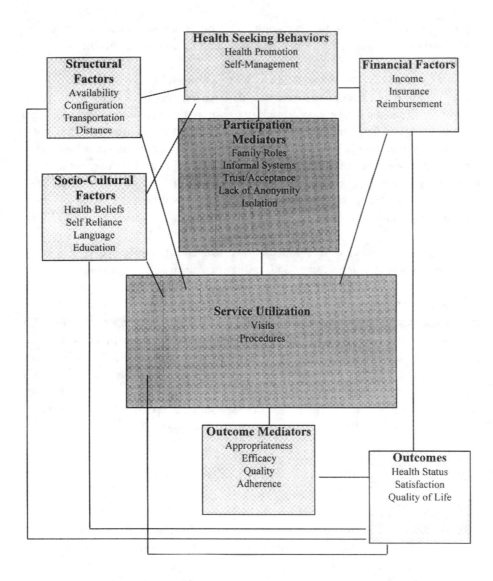

Figure 5.1. Factors Influencing Health Care Behaviors and Outcomes for Residents in Rural Environments

Configuration refers to how the health care services are grouped in a particular area. For example, are comprehensive and primary health care services accessible to local residents? Are specialty and tertiary services available in a more distant city? The manner in which health care resources were arrayed in the late 1990s may have been as important for improving access as was the production of hospital beds and health professions schools in previous decades. The current aim is to improve access by redistributing health resources in society and in the community. Outcomes are dependent on risk sharing among payers, patients, and providers and on a good balance between cost control and quality.

Transportation refers to the ability to get to and from health care services. Public transportation is not readily available outside large metropolitan areas in the United States. Therefore, the most common mode of transportation in this country is that of private automobiles. This can incur high costs, and people with low incomes may not be able to afford their own automobile. The lack of private transportation may be a significant structural barrier to health care because there are proportionately more residents living in poverty in the rural areas of America. Indeed, it is not unusual for clients in remote mining, lumbering, and fishing communities as well as Native American reservations, migrant camps, farms, and ranches to have limited access to personal or public transportation.

Distance to be traveled also is a factor in access to and utilization of care. It refers not only to miles but to terrain, weather, and familiarity with city driving. Consequently, distance along with transportation is always a consideration when seeking health care. Horner et al. (1994) described distance as a continuum category that ranges from going without through trying other options to travel the distance. It is not limited to miles to be traveled but rather reflects the depth or intensity of the health care resources sought. The concept of distance has great implications for nurses working in rural areas. For example, significant distances may separate rural clients from health care facilities and services. Therefore, assessing the influence of distance on clients' patterns of accessing care is important for nurses to help clients to use available resources more effectively to reduce the impact of distance (Henson, Sadler, & Walton, 1998).

SOCIOCULTURAL FACTORS

Sociocultural factors refers to such things as health beliefs, self-reliance, language, and education. Questions arise about equity of access when subgroups share characteristics such as education level or health-related attitudes, along with a systematic underuse of services that could make a difference in their health status. Rural dwellers are thought to be hardy, to possess a sense of connected independence, and to describe health in functional terms, such as the ability to do work (Chapter 3). These sociocultural characteristics provide a way to envision and describe rural residents in general (Running, 1998), but rural people and culture are as diverse as their landscapes. Therefore, health care practices must be considered in a sociocultural context.

Health beliefs are notions about health that an individual or group believes to be true. The beliefs may or may not be based on fact. However, they usually are based on sociocultural norms. Place of residence, too, may be a variable in the conceptualization of health within a group, in this case rural residents. *Self-reliance* and self-care have been identified as significant strategies used to cope with illness by rural persons. These are critical factors in their patterns of using health services and can affect health consequences. For example, rural dwellers often delay seeking health care until they are seriously ill or incapacitated. The time line for rural women may be as long as 14 days from the time of symptom recognition to professional contact but is shorter when a child is ill. This delay in seeking health care is consistent with rural dwellers' function-based definition of health (Chafey, Sullivan, & Shannon, 1998; Kirsch, Jungeblut, Jenkins, & Kolstad, 1993; Long & Weinert, 1989; Weinert & Burman, 1994; Weinert & Long, 1993; Winstead-Fry, Tiffany, & Shippee-Rice, 1992).

Language, too, can present problems for consumers—for instance, when non-English-speaking persons seek health care from a system that favors the English-speaking majority. Issues related to cultural and linguistic competence are extensively discussed in Chapter 7 of this text. *Education* refers to the years of formal schooling the individual has completed. Health care service utilization and health outcomes correlate with a person's educational level. For example, compared to urban residents, rural residents have fewer years of formal education, and a greater proportion do not have adequate literacy skills (Robertson & Minkler, 1994; Sissel & Hohn, 1996). Literacy is fundamental to delivering effective health care, but millions of Americans do not have the skills to read and comprehend health-related instructions that are provided by doctors and nurses. Therefore, nurses must consider such abilities, or the lack of them, when developing nursing interventions for targeted rural consumers.

FINANCIAL FACTORS

Financial factors include income, insurance, and reimbursement. *Income* refers to one's earnings in a given period of time and often is associated with health status. People in lower income brackets may not be able to afford health care insurance and so may delay seeking preventive health care. Poverty and its relation to health are examined in Chapter 6 of this text. Other financial factors that influence health care utilization and subsequent health outcomes are *insurability,* or the ability to obtain health insurance; *benefit coverage* (fully or partly subsidized by employers); and *reimbursement levels,* or the ability to have health care costs paid for in full. When insurance fails, it is the responsibility of publicly funded programs to act as a safety net by assuming the cost of that care. However, some rural factors may prevent residents from having that safety net. For instance, landholders may have little disposable income and hence may be among the *working poor.* In other words, they may be ineligible for public assistance programs. Being underinsured also can affect access. Insurance policies that do not cover preexisting medical conditions, require high copayments, or do not cover certain conditions such as mental health problems also can delay people from seeking necessary care.

HEALTH-SEEKING BEHAVIORS

Understanding a community's concept of health is critical to understanding clients' motivation for their health-seeking behaviors. *Health promotion* refers to the ability to have control over one's own behaviors to prevent illness or injury. *Self-management* is the ability to direct day-to-day activities that can enhance health. Generally, rural residents do not engage in health promotion activities to the same degree as urban counterparts. For example, they are less likely than their urban counterparts to use seat belts regularly, a difference that is reflected in the dramatically higher injury-related mortality rates in rural areas. Rural residents are less likely than their urban counterparts to exercise consistently, and they tend to be more obese. Fewer rural than urban residents smoke, but those who are smokers smoke more than urban dwellers (Bureau of the Census, 1995). In addition, rural residents use preventive screening services less often than urban residents. This difference may be related to decreased literacy skills, impaired access to these services, or beliefs about health and the ability to work (Michielutte, Dignan, Sharp, Boxley, & Wells, 1996). In other words, health promotion and disease prevention activities may not be seen as important as long as the person is able to work.

Rural dwellers often delay seeking health care until they are gravely ill or incapacitated. This delay may also be consistent with their function-based definition of health. Social support networks, often part of self-management strategies, can be motivating or detrimental to a person's care-seeking practices. For example, Crawford and Preston (1991) found that the family was an integral source of support for self-management for rural residents and women. Magilvy, Congdon, and Martinez (1994) described "circles of informal care" of both healthy and frail older rural adults. The circle included family, friends, and neighbors who provided assistance with meals, household tasks, shopping, personal care, health-related care, errands, transportation, and companionship. Formal resources were used only when self-management or lay resources failed to alleviate symptoms or when these intensified (Weinert & Burman, 1994). For nurses, planning a seamless continuum of care for rural clients implies the ability to link formal services with informal community networks.

PARTICIPATION MEDIATORS

In rural areas, numerous *participation mediators* (factors that influence participation in the formal health care system) are operative—among them, family roles, social support from informal systems, trust/acceptance of outsiders, lack of anonymity, and isolation. The mediator of family roles is exemplified in women's assumption of responsibility for the implementation and transmission of health care and knowledge (Dunkin et al., 1992). In rural areas, women often maintain links between the community and family by their active involvement in local groups. Women not only determine when outside help should be sought but select the provider, schedule appointments, and often arrange transportation. Their decisions may be influenced by the amount of time that will be lost to work and whether they have money to pay for the service (Carney, Dietrich, & Freeman, 1992).

That is not to say that rural families neglect their health. Rather, they may rely on *informal support,* which sometimes is described in such terms as *friendship, community cohesion, caring,* or *unconditional positive regard.* The rural environment is often considered to have strong informal support resources that enable individuals to manage health and illness. Historically, rural people identify neighbors and family as sources of support to sustain and promote health and well-being rather than using formal services or seeking care from professional caregivers. *Trust and acceptance* of outsiders have been core to the refinement of nursing concepts relative to rural clients. For example, rural dwellers may resist accepting help or services provided by "outsiders" or federal or state-sponsored agencies. If care is sought in the formal system, it will most likely be from a provider who is viewed as an "insider" and a perceived member of the community (Horner et al., 1994; Lee, 1998; Weinert & Burman, 1994). *Lack of anonymity* is another characteristic of small towns and sparsely populated areas, implying a lack of privacy in the lives of residents. Moreover, the lives of nurses and local residents are closely inter-woven, without a clear distinction between work and personal activities. Closely associated is *isolation* due to geographical remoteness. This too can compel rural residents to be more self-reliant, use more self-management interventions, and rely on informal systems for their health care needs. National and international perspectives on rural nursing are examined in more detail in Chapters 13 through 16.

SERVICE UTILIZATION

Service utilization refers to the participation in health care programming of some type where services are provided. Often it is measured as *visits* to a health care provider and use of *medical procedures* (IOM, 1993). However, availability and community support do not necessarily translate into use of the local hospital for health care. Some rural residents, particularly the more affluent and mobile, "outmigrate" or "out-shop." This connotes traveling to a larger town for health care, even though that same service is available locally. Consequently, rural residents who depend on local health care providers are disproportionately the indigent, aged, and less mobile (Rieber, Benzie, & McMahon, 1996; Shreffler, 1996).

OUTCOME MEDIATORS

Outcome mediators are those factors that affect the outcome of any health care service, such as appropriateness, efficacy, and quality of care and adherence to medical regimens. No matter how efficacious a particular health service may be, a good outcome cannot always be guaranteed, for a variety of reasons. For example, the treatment may be inappropriate for a patient, a certain percentage may not respond to the appropriate treatment, the skills of the provider may be below acceptable standards, or a client may not follow or adhere to the prescribed treatment regimen. Other mediators related to health outcome are explored in depth in Chapter 4.

OUTCOMES

Health outcomes are measured and defined in terms of health status, satisfaction, and quality of life. Outcome measures are complementary to measuring access, especially for complex chronic health problems. It can be difficult to track the services that are used by rural clients in order to measure the outcomes. Outcome assessments can provide insights about barriers that may impede access to services and nursing care. Careful thought must therefore be given to identify appropriate measures and methods to collect data that are valid and reliable relative to rural clients. To obtain the community's perspective, input must be sought from targeted consumers, and the tools must be culturally and linguistically sensitive (Brown, Renwick, & Nagler, 1996; Pan, Dunkin, Muus, Harris, & Geller, 1995; Stewart & Ware, 1992). Chapter 4 focuses on the community health assessment process. Chapter 18 examines research issues related to low sample size and isolated geographical areas.

SUMMARY

This exemplar presents a framework that incorporates features of the rural phenomenon that are pertinent to nursing in this context. It is an ever-evolving process that nurses can consider when designing interventions for rural clients. However, further investigation is needed to validate and refine the process so that it can be broadly applicable to nursing in a variety of rural situations and settings.

DISCUSSION QUESTIONS

➤ Discuss the relationship between health-seeking behaviors and outcomes for clients in rural environments. How might these differ across geographic locations? Identify strategies that nurses could employ to help ensure positive outcomes of a new prenatal program for poor young women in a given rural environment. What sociocultural factors might be considered critical to successful nursing interventions with clients in rural environments?

➤ How could the exemplar framework be used in developing a new primary health care clinic that you and several colleagues were planning to open in a rural area? How might this differ from developing a similar clinic in an urban area?

SUGGESTED RESEARCH ACTIVITIES

➤ Examine the health beliefs of rural residents across geographic areas in relation to their role performance. What is the relationship between geographic factors and participation mediators for these clients? Describe the similarities and differences in health-seeking behaviors among clients of various sociocultural groups who live in different geographic areas. What are the relationships among structural, sociocultural, and economic factors and rural families' patterns of utilization of health care services?

➤ Select three research articles that include a rural sample. Critique and analyze the framework in relation to the findings of each study. Develop a synthesis paper that compares and contrasts the consistencies and inconsistencies between, and among, the studies and the framework presented in this chapter.

REFERENCES

Brown, I., Renwick, R., & Nagler, M. (1996). The centrality of quality of life in health promotion and rehabilitation. In R. Renwick, I. Brown, & M. Nagler (Eds.), *Quality of life in health promotion and rehabilitation: Conceptual approaches, issues, and applications* (pp. 3-13). Thousand Oaks, CA: Sage.

Bureau of the Census. (1995). *Statistical abstract of the United States: 1995* (115th ed.). Washington, DC: Government Printing Office.

Carney, P., Dietrich, A. J., & Freeman, D. H. (1992). Improving future preventive care through educational efforts at a women's community screening program. *Journal of Community Health, 17,* 167-174.

Chafey, K., Sullivan, T., & Shannon, A. (1998). Self-reliance: Characterization of their own autonomy by elderly rural women. In H. Lee (Ed.), *Conceptual basis for rural nursing* (pp. 156-177). New York: Springer.

Crawford, C., & Preston, D. (1991). Differences in specific sources of social support for four healthy behaviors. In A. Bushy (Ed.), *Rural nursing* (Vol. 1, pp. 215-227). Newbury Park, CA: Sage.

Dunkin, J. W. (1997). Applying interventions in rural areas. In C. O. Helvie, *Advanced practice nursing in the community* (pp. 407-420). Thousand Oaks, CA: Sage.

Dunkin, J. W., Stratton, T. D., & Holzwarth, C. (1992). Assessment of family hardiness: A foundation for intervention. In S. B. Neister, J. M. Bell, S. L. Feetham, & C. L. Gilliss (Eds.), *Advances in the nursing of families* (pp. 247-255). Newbury Park, CA: Sage.

Henson, D., Sadler, T., & Walton, S. (1998). Distance. In H. Lee (Ed.), *Conceptual basis for rural nursing* (pp. 51-60). New York: Springer.

Horner, S. D., Ambrogne, J., Coleman, M. A., Hanson, C., Hodnicki, D., Lopez, S. A., & Talmadge, M. C. (1994). Traveling for care: Factors influencing health care access for rural dwellers. *Public Health Nursing, 11*(3), 145-149.

Institute of Medicine. (1993). *Access to health care in America.* Washington, DC: National Academy Press.

Kirsch, I. S., Jungeblut, A., Jenkins, L., & Kolstad, A. (1993). *Adult literacy in America: A first look at the results of the National Adult Literacy Survey (NALS).* Washington, DC: U.S. Department of Education, National Center for Education Statistics.

Lee, H. (Ed.). (1998). *Conceptual basis for rural nursing.* New York: Springer.

Long, K. A., & Weinert, C. (1989). Rural nursing: Developing a theory base. *Scholarly Inquiry Into Nursing Practice: An International Journal, 3*(2), 113-127.

Magilvy, J. K., Congdon, J. G., & Martinez, R. (1994). Circles of care: Home care and community support for rural older adults. *Advances in Nursing Science, 16*(3), 22-33.

Michielutte, R., Dignan, M. B., Sharp, P. C., Boxley, J., & Wells, H. B. (1996). Skin cancer prevention and early detection practices in a sample of rural women. *Preventive Medicine, 25,* 673-683.

National Center for Health Statistics. (1995). *Health, United States, 1994.* Washington, DC: Government Printing Office.

Pan, S., Dunkin, J., Muus, K. J., Harris, T. R., & Geller, J. M. (1995). A logit analysis of the likelihood of leaving rural settings for registered nurses. *Journal of Rural Health, 11,* 106-113.

Rieber, G. M., Benzie, D., & McMahon, S. (1996). Why patients bypass rural health care centers. *Minnesota Medicine, 79*(6), 46-50.

Robertson, A., & Minkler, M. (1994). New health promotion movement: A critical examination. *Health Education Quarterly, 21,* 295-312.

Running, A. (1998). Health perceptions of rural elders: "Landscapes and life." In H. Lee (Ed.), *Conceptual basis for rural nursing* (pp. 223-235). New York: Springer.

Shreffler, M. J. (1996). An ecological view of the rural environment: Levels of influence on access to health care. *Advances in Nursing Science, 18*(4), 48-59.

Sissel, P. A., & Hohn, M. D. (1996). Literacy and health communities: Potential partners in practice. *New Directions for Adult and Continuing Education, 70,* 59-71.

Stewart, A. L., & Ware, J. E., Jr. (Eds.). (1992). *Measuring functioning and well being: The Medical Outcomes Study approach.* Durham, NC: Duke University Press.

Weinert, C., & Burman, M. E. (1994). Rural health and health-seeking behaviors. *Annual Review of Nursing Research, 12,* 65-92.

Weinert, C., & Long, K. A. (1993). Support systems for spouses of the chronically ill. *Family and Community Health, 16,* 46-54.

Winstead-Fry, P., Tiffany, J. C., & Shippee-Rice, R. V. (1992). *Rural health nursing: Stories of creativity, commitment, and connectedness.* New York: National League for Nursing.

Part II
▬▬▬

Special Populations

Part II of this book builds on the information presented in Part I and focuses on special populations. Chapter 6 presents an overview of special and at-risk rural populations. Terms and definitions such as *persons with special needs, vulnerability, risk, disenfranchisement,* and *medical indigence* are discussed in relation to health and illness. Chapter 7 focuses on the continuum of cultural-linguistic competence. These skills are of critical importance for nurses if they are to provide acceptable and appropriate care to rural clients of other cultures. Concerns of the predominant rural minority groups are highlighted, specifically those of immigrants, migrant and seasonal farmworkers, African Americans, and Native Americans. Chapter 8 examines rural aspects of behavioral health care. It includes strategies to enhance the capability of rural providers and services by linking formal and informal resources, given that resources are often far and few between in rural communities. Another group with multiple health care needs is the homeless. Yet little has been written about homelessness in rural America. Chapter 9 describes the rural homeless and examines rural factors that contribute to their condition. The special needs of these rural families are discussed in this chapter.

Chapter 10 examines the health care needs and concerns of persons living with HIV/AIDS (PLWAs) in rural settings. Rural epidemiologic trends are described, along with the needs and concerns of persons living with HIV/AIDS in small and remote communities. Part II concludes with Chapter 11, which focuses on rural occupational health and safety. The information expands on the description, in Chapter 2, of U.S. Department of Agriculture rural county types based on their predominant industry. This chapter also discusses the National Institute of Occupational Safety and Health (NIOSH) rural initiative that targets farm-workers and their families. Part II, along with Part I, lays the groundwork for Part 3, which addresses international and futuristic perspectives on rural nursing.

CHAPTER 6

Special and At-Risk Rural Populations

KEY TERMS

- Risk
- At risk
- Disenfranchisement
- Distributive justice
- Hardiness
- Poverty threshold
- Poverty guidelines
- Medical indigence
- Vulnerability
- Intergenerational poverty
- Resiliency
- Poverty

OBJECTIVES

After reading this chapter, you will be able to

- Differentiate terms used to describe special populations.
- Characterize the health concerns of at-risk populations living in rural regions.
- Examine factors that contribute to health disparities among rural minorities.
- Identify individual and community resources that can counterbalance vulnerability.
- Implement nursing interventions for special populations using the advocate, activist, case manager, educator, counselor, collaborator, partner, and researcher roles.

ESSENTIAL POINTS TO REMEMBER

➤ The terms *vulnerable, at risk, special, disenfranchised,* and *medically indigent* often are interchanged in the literature, but the words have different connotations.

➤ Hardiness, resilience, and degree of access to formal resources and informal support networks can counterbalance risk factors that promote vulnerability.

➤ High-risk behaviors that some clients continue to engage in may be incomprehensible to others. Nurses must take utmost care to not judge another person before all the facts are understood, especially in cases where they have had limited experience with a health condition.

➤ Interventions to meet the needs of the vulnerable can draw on a variety of nursing roles, including advocate, activist, case manager, educator, counselor, partner, collaborator, and researcher.

OVERVIEW

This chapter presents common issues confronting special populations that are at risk and vulnerable for health problems. Commonly used terms are defined, and strategies to counterbalance these risk factors are described. Interventions to address these concerns are discussed in terms of nursing roles. This content integrates information from previous chapters and provides a basis for discussion in subsequent chapters focusing on rural minorities, health behaviors, HIV/AIDS, homelessness, and occupational health concerns.

TERMS AND DEFINITIONS

Even though the terms *vulnerable, at risk, special,* and *disenfranchised* are often used in health-related literature, they are difficult to understand. Moreover, they often are used interchangeably in health policy discussions and nursing literature. The way people define the terms is influenced by their societal values and attitudes about poverty along with their understanding of how socioeconomic status can be affected by genetic, environmental, and political factors (Sebastian, 1999; Sebastian & Bushy, 1999).

Persons With Special Needs

The notion of special needs is used in reference to individuals, groups, families, and communities who manifest social service and health care needs that are distinct, exceptional, and different from what is considered to be "ordinary" or "usual." Proportionally compared to urban, there are more persons with special needs in rural communities (National Center for Health Statistics, 1996). These individuals often are forgotten, discounted, or misunderstood, and they may or may not be at risk, vulnerable, or disenfranchised. In most cases, the community and families of persons with special needs have additional challenges in meeting their health care needs, whether emotional, economic, physical, or social (Aday, 1993, 1994; Conger & Elder, 1994; Dever, 1997; Garrison, 1998; Kotch, 1997).

Vulnerability

The vulnerable are members of society who are disadvantaged physically, psychologically, and socially. When used in health policy and nursing literature, the term *vulnerability* refers to persons or groups who are more likely to develop a problem and have a more serious outcome stemming from exposure to multiple risks. Vulnerable populations specifically identified in *Healthy People 2010* (U.S. Department of Health and Human Services [USDHHS], 1999) are high-risk mothers and infants, chronically ill and disabled persons, persons infected with acquired immunodeficiency syndrome (HIV/AIDS), the mentally ill and the disabled, alcohol and substance abusers, suicide- or homicide-prone individuals, the homeless, immigrants, refugees, and abusing families. In addition to being vulnerable, when living in a rural environment, these groups face even more challenges associated with access to care, scarce resources, and traditional cultural belief systems.

Risk

From the preceding discussion, it becomes evident that an element of risk underlies the concept of vulnerability. A population at risk includes persons for whom there is some probability that an illness event will occur within a given time period. Potentially, everyone is vulnerable to some degree. In other words, there always is some chance (risk) of developing some type of physical or mental illness or experiencing social isolation. Any of these events can drastically affect the course of a person's life. However, some groups and individuals are more at risk than others. Epidemiologically, the degree of risk for a specific condition in a particular person or population can range from very low to extremely high.

How can families and communities increase, or decrease, their risk and degree of vulnerability? There is no quick answer to this question. The downward spiral begins with a debilitating, chronic health or social problem that frequently leads to additional risks, with further degradation in health status in the vulnerable. Fractured family units place their members under tremendous economic, social, and emotional stress, and the interrelated effects amplify negative health outcomes. Compared to the norm, the vulnerable generally have fewer economic and social resources and are poorly educated and hence more likely to be unemployed, inadequately housed, and exposed to multiple health risks. These families have fewer resources to help them cope, and individual members are less able to respond effectively to the risks (Brownson, Baker, & Novick, 1998; Christoffel & Gallagher, 1999; Eggebeen & Lichter, 1993).

The vulnerable can be identified by their degree of risk of poor physical, psychological, and/or social health. For example, those at excessive physical risk include high-risk mothers and infants, the chronically ill and disabled, and persons with HIV/AIDS. Individuals with psychological risks include those with a mental illness or behavioral disorder. Families experiencing social risks include those with abuse, the homeless, immigrants, and refugees. These three risks, physical, psychological, and social, are not separate entities; their boundaries overlap and are diffuse and indistinct. In other words, poor health along one dimension (e.g., physical) is likely to be compounded by problems in other areas (e.g., psychological or social). Health care and nursing needs are greatest for persons having multifaceted problems, such as a homeless person who may also be diagnosed with a chronic mental illness or a person infected with HIV/AIDS who also is addicted to drugs. Essentially, the relative risk(s) for different groups will vary as a function of their material and nonmaterial resources. Risks to individuals and groups can be lessened, or counterbalanced, by cultural, demographic, economic, and social support. Likewise, schools, jobs, incomes, and housing that characterize a neighborhood affect the level of risk experienced by people who live in that community. Obviously, many factors interact to create and sustain vulnerability in rural families and how individual members respond.

Disenfranchisement

Disenfranchisement refers to the feeling, experienced by a person or group of people, of being separated from mainstream society. When this phenomenon occurs, a community or individual does not feel emotionally connected with society in general or to any group in particular. The notion of disenfranchisement suggests that a person or group does not have the essential resources to effectively manage a healthy lifestyle. In part, this may be attributable to not having well-established links with formal community organizations such as health care providers, social service agencies, churches, or schools. The disenfranchised usually also feel that they have fewer informal sources of support, such as family, friends, or neighbors. For example, the homeless often have few people they can call on for assistance. That is not to say, however, that all vulnerable populations are without social support resources. Many homeless families, especially in rural areas, report that they have reliable and consistent support from churches (faith-based communities), extended family, and neighbors, even though they may feel disenfranchised from society as a whole. In addition to perceived disenfranchisement, certain groups are hidden from society as a whole, perhaps even more so in remote areas.

Medical Indigence

Medical indigence refers to a serious inability to pay the costs associated with one's health care or the health care of one's family. Three rural groups are particularly vulnerable and affected by escalating health care costs and reductions in services: the elderly, children, and the medically indigent—of which there are ever-increasing numbers. The medically indigent do not have health insurance coverage, do not qualify for government assistance, and are unable to pay for their health care. It is estimated that more than 45 million people in the United States currently fall in the category of the medically indigent. The increasing numbers are attributable to the current economic situation. That is, although unemployment may be low, increasing numbers of people are working full time without health care benefits and in low-salaried jobs, such as jobs in the service industry or agriculture. Overall, their annual income is too high (above the federal poverty guidelines) to make them eligible for government assistance but is insufficient to purchase costly health insurance. Some have insurance but a plan that offers low reimbursement, requires high copayments, or does not cover certain conditions (Maurer, 1995; National Rural Health Association [NRHA], 1998a, 1998b, 1998c).

Although the elderly, children, and the uninsured have been spotlighted, many others are affected. Cost containment strategies, for example, are being implemented by employers to remain competitive. Consequently, employees are finding that their insurance benefits have been reduced or even eliminated. Some assume they are adequately covered until they experience a catastrophic illness or chronic disability or until they are confronted with unanticipated astronomical health care costs. Families experiencing these situations are referred to as the working poor or near-poor. For many, illnesses go untreated until acute symptoms manifest while preventive services are underused (Chapter 5). Such care-seeking behaviors are commonly encountered among families in rural areas where there is an even higher incidence of medical indigence. Long term, this pattern of health care utilization ends up being more costly for the families and society as a whole.

WEB OF CAUSATION, RISK, AND VULNERABILITY

The term *web of causation* is used extensively in public health and can be helpful to nurses for understanding the epidemiology of multiple risk factors that promote vulnerability and negative health outcomes in a given group. *Web of causation* suggests an interplay of multiple factors that directly and indirectly influence a specific health or social condition, whether in a rural or an urban setting. The epidemiologic approach also is evident in Dunkin's proposed framework for rural nursing and the health behaviors of rural clients (Chapter 5). Applying the concept of a web of causation to rural populations, poverty is closely associated with risk and vulnerability, and being poor affects the health of individuals, families, and entire communities. Often it is hidden; nonetheless, poverty exists in most communities and significantly contributes to other risk factors, thereby increasing certain individuals' degree of vulnerability. Of all persons in the United States who are poor, nearly half are younger than 18 years (about 40%), and about 11% are 65 years of age or older. Poverty is not limited to place of residence; rural and urban communities of all sizes and cultures have poor people living in their midst. Regardless of the setting, poor communities and neighborhoods have a higher proportion of minorities, single mothers, unemployment, and low wages (Friis & Sellers, 1999; Siegal & Doner, 1998).

Everyone has an idea about poverty, and usually it stems from personal experiences and cultural values. To gain an understanding of the real meaning of poverty and its impact on the daily life of rural clients and families, the nurse must first become aware of personal perspectives about the issues. Therefore, it is crucial to examine personal beliefs in relation to others' perspectives. A self-appraisal helps glean insights on what being poor really means, especially for the vulnerable. Learning about others' life situations can help one to be less judgmental and more accepting of others whose life and living situation may be different from that of the rural nurse.

Even though many people do not include financial resources in their notion of poverty, the federal government uses economic indicators to delineate what is adequate for a living wage, specifically *poverty threshold* and *poverty guidelines*. People who fall below the poverty threshold are considered to be poor. Federal poverty thresholds are updated each year by the Bureau of the Census and used primarily for statistical purposes: for instance, preparing estimates of the number of Americans in poverty each year. Nurses usually encounter government definitions of poverty when planning, coordinating, and evaluating services for clients who are vulnerable or at risk or who have special needs. Economic guidelines defining what is sometimes referred to as the *federal poverty level* are another way to define and measure poverty. The guidelines are revised annually by the U.S. Department of Health and Human Services and published in the *Federal Register* (USDHHS, 1998). This simple definition of *poverty* is used for administrative purposes such as determining eligibility for certain federal- and state-sponsored programs, such as Head Start, the Food Stamp Program, the National School Lunch Program, the Low-Income Home Energy Assistance Program, and Aid to Families With Dependent Children. Other agencies, however, do not use these eligibility guidelines, specifically agencies administering supplemental security income and tax credit programs.

The various disciplines describe poverty in still other ways. For instance, social scientists use the term *impoverished* to describe a variety of conditions related to home, environment, relationships, and material possessions (or the lack thereof), along with access to educational, occupational, and financial resources. Health care providers define poverty as not having sufficient financial resources to meet basic living expenses, such as food, clothing, shelter, transportation, and medical care. For almost half a century, economists and policy developers have used persistent poverty to categorize individuals, families, communities, and counties that are very poor (University of North Carolina, 1998; U.S. Department of Agriculture, 1995, 1997). For them, poverty is transmitted from one generation to another (*intergenerational poverty*). As for the best way to address the problem, the approaches are as varied as the definitions. It is an understatement to say that there is no quick fix for the pervasive poverty in our nation or worldwide.

ETHICAL AND LEGAL CONSIDERATIONS

There are innumerable ethical and legal issues related to poverty and the provision of care to vulnerable and at-risk populations. In fact, entire textbooks have been devoted to each of these topics, and space does not allow for discussion of the multiple, complex ethical and legal ramifications. Nurses in rural environments often find themselves in key positions to advocate for the vulnerable and help them become empowered to effectively solve their problems and be contributing members to society. However, a range of ethical and legal considerations must be understood. One of the more often encountered ethical issues centers on the allocation of scarce resources versus distributive justice. At the core of this value-laden issue are a number of questions: for example, who is most needy, worthy, or deserving to receive scarce resources? Who decides? Where does enabling behavior end? Or where does helping the needy to become more self-sufficient start? As resources become even more scarce, grappling with ethical issues will become paramount in our society, especially in underserved rural regions. Ethical issues related to nursing practice in rural environments are examined in more detail in Chapter 17.

There also is an array of corresponding legal issues associated with poverty. For instance, poor neighborhoods often experience more violence and crime. Consequently, legal situations may arise that center on maintaining confidentiality versus reporting criminal activity that nurses may encounter, such as domestic abuse, child neglect, gang and drug-related activities, and communicable diseases, especially HIV/AIDS. Space constraints do not allow for a comprehensive discussion of all of the associated legal issues in rural settings.

COUNTERBALANCING FORCES

Nurses should be aware that poverty includes a variety of conditions that can range from not having enough money to purchase essential life needs to not having enough money to buy material goods, services, and support systems that could enhance the quality of one's life. Understanding the particular characteristics of poverty is probably less important than the ability to accept, respect, and understand how a client's life situation influences his or her health status. Nurses should be sensitive to a client's risks as well as able to recognize the vulnerable person's resources that could address the problem at hand (Allred & Smith, 1989; Bigbee, 1991; Lambert & Lambert, 1987; O'Connor, 1994; Roos & Cohen, 1987). Successful nursing interventions build on resources that are available and acknowledged by the client. Health promotion research is focusing on factors that contribute to health and maintain long-term well-being. More specifically, negative risk factors must be balanced against health-enhancing factors such as resilience, hardiness, and support systems. These are not separate, self-sustaining entities but catalysts that enhance each other's effects.

Hardiness has been used to describe aspects of human resilience and has been discussed in some detail in Chapter 3 of this book (Allred & Smith, 1989; Antonovsky, 1979; Bigbee, 1991; Testa, 1998). Theoretically, hardiness is a combination of factors that keep some people from developing a problem even with exposure to a health risk. It is identified as a potential intervening factor in individuals and families (perhaps communities too) who seem to overcome the most adverse conditions and still lead meaningful lives. For example, hardiness may be a factor in why some persons with HIV infections survive for decades whereas others become very ill, or even die, within a short time after becoming infected. Dimensions of the concept of hardiness are control, commitment, and challenge. There may be additional aspects related to the dimension of control, or the lack of it, among at-risk and vulnerable groups, and these may be relevant to nurses in rural environments.

Support networks also can be counterbalancing and mediating forces to vulnerability. This topic is examined in Chapter 3 and is integrated in Dunkin's framework described in Chapter 5. To reiterate, support can be formal or informal. Furthermore, there is no prescription as to who should be included in a client's network or a family's circle of support (Magilvy, Congdon, & Martinez, 1994). Preference for and use of support vary by individuals, families, and communities and are culturally defined. For instance, some cultures have extensive social support networks, as in the case of many Native American, African American, and Latino families. The extent of these networks often becomes evident when a member of one of these groups visits the clinic or is hospitalized, accompanied by a contingent of relatives, frequently with several generations represented. Not everyone has such an extensive network, however. The nurse will find that some clients are unable to identify even one person in their support network. For example, one middle-aged homeless man, recently released from prison after being incarcerated for several decades, had lost all contact with his family. In another case, a 25-year-old man was diagnosed with HIV/AIDS in a large city in Florida. Upon visiting his parents in a very small southern town that was predominantly Baptist, he told them about his diagnosis and how the infection probably was acquired. They responded by asking him never to come back to their home or their little town because their religious beliefs could not condone homosexuality. Moreover, they probably would be ashamed if the community found out about his diagnosis or sexual orientation. Increasingly, faith-based communities in rural areas are assuming an active role in supporting congregation members as well as outsiders who have no such network.

NURSING ROLES AND INTERVENTIONS

Nurses have many roles in coordinating services and care for vulnerable clients and persons with special needs. When developing a plan of care for a client, it is important for the nurse not only to assess the multiple risk factors but also to identify mediating resources, such as individuals' resiliency and the quantity and quality of their support networks. (Chapter 3 addresses hardiness and self-reliance.) Assessment goes beyond helping the person identify formal and informal resources, however. It involves the use of a range of nursing roles, including those of advocate, activist, case manager, educator, counselor, partner, collaborator, and researcher. These roles are used to develop, implement, and evaluate interventions to fit vulnerable rural clients' particular needs and preferences. Aspects of these nursing roles are discussed in the remainder of this chapter (American Nurses Association, 1997; Hansen & Fisher, 1998; Sebastian & Bushy, 1999; Skelskey & Leshem, 1997; Stanhope & Lancaster, 1999).

Advocate and Activist

In the role of advocate, the nurse must first be sensitive to the health care needs of the vulnerable and have a broad knowledge of community resources and how to access these. A nurse also must possess the ability to communicate in a professional manner with, and for, a client to coordinate a continuum of services. A nurse needs persistence when acting on behalf of a client with special needs. Time and patience often are necessary to maintain contact with these clients and direct them to the appropriate resources. Political activism at the local, state, and national levels is another aspect of the advocacy role. Often nurses can make the greatest difference in the lives of those who are vulnerable and poor in the policy arena and with lawmakers.

Nurses who live and work in rural communities in particular are in positions to advocate with public and private entities to provide the necessary resources for new or more comprehensive services (Blendon, 1998). For example, it is not unusual for rural residents to personally know their elected officials. Often they live in the same neighborhood and attend the same church, or their children attend the same schools as the children of constituents. Consequently, opportunities often arise that allow other residents, in this case nurses, to formally and informally discuss health care issues with their elected congressional members. Generally, that is not the case in more populated communities, where residents may not even know the name of their lawmakers. During interactions with lawmakers, the nurse is first a professional role model with expert authority. Hence, the nurse is in a position to advocate for improving the economic and health status of rural populations with special needs.

Advocacy involves representing special consumer groups to regulatory organizations and even local health commissions. The nurse advocate publicly supports and sometimes opposes federal and state initiatives. This may entail grassroots lobbying for legislation that provides a financial safety net for people with catastrophic costs that are not covered by Medicare or health insurance. Sometimes it involves testifying against the views of an elected official who does not support a safe house for abused women, a residential home for the mentally challenged, or a halfway house for youth offenders. The overall goal of a nurse advocate is representing the vulnerable, helping these clients to solve problems, and developing appropriate strategies to address their concerns. To reiterate, advocacy and activism do not mean taking care of, enabling, or promoting long-term dependency. Rather, they mean helping people to learn how to help themselves by developing greater resilience and skills to more effectively deal with their concerns.

Case Manager

Another role for nurses who work with clients having special needs is that of case manager. Case management is a process in which services are organized and coordinated to meet a client's particular needs and to use scarce resources more effectively. In a rural area, case-managing a client can extend over a very long period, sometimes months or even years. Moreover, the nurse in the role of case manager will find that the need for formal and informal services often increases in intensity and complexity as a client is exposed to other health risks and stressful situations. The case manager, particularly one working with rural clients, must ensure that services are not overutilized or underutilized and that the care plan is modified to reflect life changes. Effective case management requires a broad base of knowledge concerning nursing roles, formal resources, and informal community support networks and an innate ability to integrate the three. Case managers are crucial in preventing and resolving confusion that can arise when a client has multiple members on his or her health care team. Confusion is especially problematic for rural residents who have been accustomed to having the same health care provider for decades but now must seek care in a large urban-based facility. Inherent in case management are the activist and advocacy roles described earlier, along with the educator and counselor roles.

Educator and Counselor

Two other important, often overlapping roles for nurses are those of teacher and counselor. Whether in rural or urban settings, and regardless of age, individuals may change risky lifestyle behaviors if they learn about the detrimental impact of these behaviors on their health. Education can be one of the most cost-effective and noninvasive interventions to inform consumers, regardless of their socioeconomic status, about pharmacotherapy protocols, health promotion, stress management, developmental changes, and symptom management of chronic health problems. Education, accompanied by counseling interventions, can be used by nurses in supporting clients with the grief process, helping them adjust to anticipated and unanticipated life events, and improving communication skills between family members as well as with health professionals. Education and counseling, in some instances, can be used to teach high-risk clients to ask appropriate questions of investigating agencies they encounter. The educator and counselor roles are important to enable clients to locate and access community resources.

However, an admonition is in order to rural nurses who must be expert generalists and resource brokers. Nurses cannot do it all! Client- and community-focused interventions must be developed to expand a nurse's range of effectiveness in using available resources. Nurses must partner with clients so that they can successfully negotiate health care and the health care-related systems.

Collaborator and Partner

Inherent in the collaborator and partner roles are those of educator, counselor, advocate, and activist. These roles can be used with clients as well as an entire community. On the one hand, case management usually involves the nurse's partnering with a client. On a wider scale, a nurse can partner and collaborate with providers from community-based agencies and citizen groups to address the particular concerns of populations with special needs to create a seamless continuum of care. Rural nurses must learn to partner with administrators and others from institutions outside of the health care arena, specifically education, housing, and employment bureaus. Collaboration can be useful to extend and enhance scarce resources, especially in medically underserved persistent poverty communities. Nurse should also learn to collaborate with private and nonprofit entities on community projects that focus on the needs of groups who are at risk for poor health outcomes. The challenge for rural nurses is to become as proficient in partnering-collaborating roles as with direct caregiving skills.

Researcher

The needs of special populations are growing, and there are no easy solutions to meet their needs, especially in rural areas with seemingly fewer resources. There is an urgent need for research on implementing and evaluating interventions that can be used with vulnerable and medically underserved segments of society. In many instances, rural populations with special needs must first be identified because they may be hidden or forgotten. Research is needed to develop a specific theory for rural nursing, for which there must first be adequate evidenced-based knowledge related to the rural phenomenon (see Chapter 3). In addition, outcome studies are needed to measure the health-related effects of existing community-based nursing interventions within a targeted population. Nurse scholars report that there are innumerable questions to be investigated regarding health concerns of rural clients, particularly at-risk groups that are highly vulnerable. Nursing research with rural clients is discussed more extensively in Chapter 18. At the end of this chapter, the reader will also find discussion questions and suggested nursing research topics that can serve as starting points for further study.

SUMMARY

This chapter highlighted health-related and nursing care issues of persons and communities with special needs. Relevant terms and definitions were examined, along with vulnerability-promoting risks that can affect the health of individuals, families, or an entire community. Using the advocate, activist, case manager, educator, counselor, and partner roles, nurses have a repertoire of skills to effect social change and meet the needs of vulnerable clients in the rural context.

DISCUSSION QUESTIONS

The following questions can be useful to complete a self-appraisal about what it means to be poor:

> ➤ How do you define poverty?
> ➤ Have you ever been poor? Describe what that was like.
> ➤ What words are used in your family when talking about poor or dependent families and individuals?
> ➤ Did your family make any particular efforts to help people who were poor?
> ➤ Describe a client whom you have cared for who was very poor.

➤ On what experiences or situations do you base your observations and ideas? Family? Friends? Classmates? Personal experience?

➤ What resources are available in your community to address the needs of the poor or vulnerable? Contact two publicly funded health-related or social service agencies. Discuss these agencies' criteria to determine who can or cannot receive certain entitlements. How do these agencies differentiate rural from urban?

SUGGESTED RESEARCH ACTIVITIES

➤ Describe the lifestyle and health risks of a vulnerable population in your community. For the conceptual framework, use the web-of-causation epidemiologic model or Dunkin's framework (Chapter 5). Develop, implement, and evaluate a community-focused nursing intervention that addresses an issue or issues identified in the previous study.

➤ Examine and compare rural and urban nurses' attitudes about poverty and caring for people who are poor.

REFERENCES

Aday, L. (1993). *At risk in America: The health and health care needs of vulnerable populations in the United States.* San Francisco: Jossey-Bass.

Aday, L. (1994). Health status of vulnerable populations in the United States. *Annual Review of Public Health, 15,* 457-509.

Allred, K., & Smith, T. (1989). The hardy personality: Cognitive and physiologic responses to evaluation threat. *Journal of Personality and Social Psychology, 56,* 257-266.

American Nurses Association. (1997). President embraces quality commission's consumer "bill of rights." *American Nurse, 29*(6), 18-19.

Antonovsky, A. (1979). *Health, stress and coping.* San Francisco: Jossey-Bass.

Bigbee, J. (1991). The concept of hardiness as applied to rural nursing. In A. Bushy (Ed.), *Rural nursing* (Vol. 1, pp. 39-58). Thousand Oaks, CA: Sage.

Blendon, R. (1998). Survey: Americans don't see poverty, health care as children's most pressing problems. *Nation's Health, 28*(1), 6.

Brownson, R., Baker, E., & Novick, L. (1998). *Community-based prevention: Programs that work.* Gaithersburg, MD: Aspen.

Christoffel, T., & Gallagher, S. (1999). *Injury prevention and public health: Practical knowledge, skills and strategies.* Gaithersburg, MD: Aspen.

Conger, R., & Elder, G. (1994). *Families in troubled times: Adapting to changes in rural America.* Hawthorne, New York: Aldine.

Dever, A. (1997). *Improving outcomes in pubic health practice.* Gaithersburg, MD: Aspen.

Eggebeen, D., & Lichter, D. (1993). Health and well-being among rural Americans: Variations across the course of life. *Journal of Rural Health, 9*(2), 86-98.

Friis, R., & Sellers, T. (1999). *Epidemiology for public health practice.* Gaithersburg, MD: Aspen.

Garrison, M. (1998). Determinants of the quality of life for rural families. *Journal of Rural Health, 14,* 146-153.

Hansen, M., & Fisher, J. (1998). Patient centered teaching: From theory to practice. *American Journal of Nursing, 98*(1), 56-60.

Kotch, J. (1997). *Maternal and child health: Programs, problems and policy in public health.* Gaithersburg, MD: Aspen.

Lambert, C., & Lambert, V. (1987). Hardiness: Its development and relevance to nursing. *Image, 19,* 92-95.

Magilvy, J., Congdon, J., & Martinez, R. (1994). Circles of care: Home care and community support for rural older adults. *Advances in Nursing Science, 16*(3), 22-33.

Maurer, F. (1995). Financing of health care for community health nursing. In C. Smith & F. Maurer (Eds.), *Community health nursing: Theory and practice* (pp. 110-138). Philadelphia: W. B. Saunders.

National Center for Health Statistics. (1996). *Health United States: 1996.* Washington, DC: Government Printing Office.

National Rural Health Association. (1998a). *Bringing resources to bear on the changing care system: Conference proceedings for the Second Annual Rural Minority Health Conference.* Kansas City, MO: Author.

National Rural Health Association. (1998b). *Healthy, wealthy and wise: Improving rural heath care and rural economies* [Videotape]. Whitesburg, KY: Appalshop Film & Video, 91 Madison Avenue, Whitesburg, KY 41858 (800-545-7467).

National Rural Health Association. (1998c). *A national agenda for rural minority health.* Kansas City, MO: Author.

O'Connor, F. (1994). A vulnerability-stress framework for evaluating interventions in schizophrenia. *Journal of Nursing Scholarship, 26,* 231-237.

Roos, P., & Cohen, L. (1987). Sex roles and social support as moderators of life stress adjustment. *Journal of Personality and Social Psychology, 52,* 576-585.

Sebastian, J. (1999). Vulnerability and vulnerable populations: An introduction. In M. Stanhope & J. Lancaster (Eds.), *Community health nursing: Promoting health of aggregates, families, and individuals* (3rd ed.). St. Louis, MO: Mosby-Yearbook.

Sebastian, J., & Bushy, A. (Eds.). (1999). *Health issues of special populations.* Gaithersburg, MD: Aspen.

Siegal, M., & Doner, L. (1998). *Marketing public health: Strategies to promote social change.* Gaithersburg, MD: Aspen.

Skelskey, C., & Leshem, O. (1997). Tuberculosis surveillance in long term care. *American Journal of Nursing, 97*(10), 16BBBB-16DDDD.

Stanhope, L., & Lancaster, J. (Eds.) (1999), *Community health nursing.* St. Louis, MO: C. V. Mosby.

Testa, K. (1998, January 18). Farmworkers' town: Hunger striking vegetable pickers seek pay raise. *Daytona News Journal,* p. 2A.

University of North Carolina, North Carolina Rural Health Research and Policy Analysis Center. (1998). *Mapping rural health.* Chapel Hill, NC: Author.

U.S. Department of Agriculture, Economic Research Service. (1995). *Understanding rural America* (Information Bull. No. 710). Washington, DC: Author.

U.S. Department of Agriculture, Office of Communications. (1997). *Agriculture fact book.* Washington, DC: Author.

U.S. Department of Health and Human Services. (1998, February 24). The 1998 HHS Poverty Guidelines. *Federal Register, 63,* 9235-9238.

U.S. Department of Health and Human Services. (1999). *Healthy people 2010: National health promotion and disease prevention objectives.* Washington, DC: Government Printing Office.

CHAPTER 7

Cultural-Linguistic Competence

Rural Considerations

KEY TERMS

- ➤ Culture
- ➤ Ethnicity
- ➤ Race
- ➤ Cultural-linguistic competence
- ➤ Seasonal and migrant farmworkers
- ➤ Documented/undocumented workers

OBJECTIVES

After reading this chapter, you will be able to

- ➤ Differentiate terms used to describe diversity (*race, ethnicity, culture*).
- ➤ Correlate national population trends and the potential impact of these on the rural health care delivery system.
- ➤ Characterize the cultural-linguistic competency continuum.
- ➤ Discuss cultural features of predominant rural minority groups.

ESSENTIAL POINTS TO REMEMBER

- ➤ Changing demographic trends are creating significant ethnocultural and racial diversity across the United States in rural as well as urban communities.
- ➤ To manage costs and ensure quality services, nursing care must be culturally and linguistically appropriate for rural consumers to be deemed as accessible and acceptable.
- ➤ Developing cultural competency is a nonlinear process, influenced by a nurse's life experiences and exposure to persons of other ethnocultural backgrounds.
- ➤ Ethnocultural factors should be included in planning, implementing, and evaluating a rural client's plan of care.

> ➤ Self-care and healing behaviors have an important place in the health care delivery system, and nearly everyone, including nurses, engages in some form of those practices.

OVERVIEW

Increasing diversity poses major challenges for the national health care delivery system in providing care to a multitude of minority groups. This chapter examines health issues of the predominant rural minorities, discusses cultural and linguistic competence, and applies common cultural features to rural minorities (National Rural Health Association, 1994, 1997, 1998a, 1998b).

BACKGROUND AND RATIONALE

White Anglo-Americans are projected to be in the minority sometime in this century, but it is impossible to predict precisely when this will happen. Demographically, there is a greater proportion of Caucasians in rural areas (about 82%) than in metropolitan areas (about 62%). As for the population mix of minorities, nonmetropolitan counties have nearly 4 million African Americans, almost 2 million Native Americans, about $\frac{3}{4}$ million Asians/Pacific Islanders, and 75 million of "other" races (Bureau of the Census, 1997). There are some regional variations, however. For example, some rural counties in the southeastern states are composed predominantly of blacks, several rural counties in the Central Plains states with an Indian reservation have high numbers of Native Americans, and Mexican American Hispanics predominate in a few rural counties located in southwestern states (University of North Carolina, 1998).

MINORITY HEALTH DISPARITIES

Despite the exponential development of biomedical innovations in the 20th century, epidemiologic reports reveal disparities in the health of minorities compared with that of the general population. Infant mortality among blacks and Native Americans, for example, is about twice that of whites in the first year of life. Hispanics and Native Americans are twice as likely as whites to have diabetes. This chronic condition leads to other more serious and costly medical problems, such as blindness, amputations, kidney disease, stroke, and heart attack. Other minority disparities include significantly higher incidences of cervical cancer, cardiovascular disease, HIV/AIDS, and incomplete immunizations. Dr. David Satcher in the U.S. Office of the Surgeon General has put forth a national goal to eliminate minority health disparities. Specific objectives focusing on those disparities are cited in *Healthy People 2010* (U.S. Department of Health and Human Services [USDHHS], 1999). The Minority Health Initiative is of particular importance for rural nurses because of the unstable economic climate of many rural communities and because of many residents', and especially minority residents', impaired access to health care services and providers.

PREDOMINANT RURAL MINORITY GROUPS

There are a great many minority groups across the nation, and space constraints limit discussing each in detail. This section highlights the health concerns of four predominant minority groups found in rural communities: immigrants, Latino farmworkers, blacks, and Native Americans. There is a very small rural Asian population, and little is documented on their particular health concerns. For that reason, that particular group is not discussed in this chapter.

Immigrants

Immigrants from all over the globe are entering the United States in record numbers. Until recently, most remained in metropolitan areas, but more of the new arrivals are settling in small-town America. This phenomenon is fostered by religious congregations' sponsoring the relocation of one or more refugee families into their little community. Such sponsorship generally is a positive experience for all involved, but that is not always the case. Anecdotal reports indicate that negative outcomes sometimes occur in small homogenous communities in their efforts to assimilate immigrants of other ethnic or racial origins, perceived as outsiders. Cultural conflicts, coupled with limited educational opportunities, inadequate social and health care services, and restricted job availability, can hinder immigrants' resettlement and acculturation in small towns. Most foreigners find American culture a complete contrast to their home country, and some U.S. citizens perceive immigrants' beliefs and worldviews to be as strange as the language they speak. Before arriving on America's shores, many immigrants endured traumatic life experiences associated with war, famine, loss of family and home, torture, and rape. Some lived for long periods in refugee camps under precarious hygienic and mental conditions. For some, those circumstances have contributed to problems in adjusting, and these immigrants' profound physical, emotional, and educational needs can further tax a rural community's precious resources (Ganey & DeBocanegra, 1996).

A slightly higher number of females than males enter this nation. They are younger than the national population as a whole, and more than two thirds are women of childbearing age. Even though many are poor, most immigrants are fairly healthy on arrival, but their lifestyle and health status deteriorate within a year. Deteriorating health probably is related to previous hardships coupled with social, economic, and cultural factors confronting them after they enter the United States. In addition to speaking another language, immigrants of different nationalities have unique epidemiological profiles, health beliefs, and expectations regarding health care. Their multifaceted needs and expectations have wide-ranging ramifications for rural health care systems in general and for nurses in particular. The reader having further interest in any of these minority groups is encouraged to seek out citations in the reference section of this chapter.

Migrant and Seasonal Farmworkers

Another rural minority group of concern to nurses is seasonal and migrant workers, many of whom speak Spanish and are of Latino origin. There is no accurate count, but a significant number are reported to be undocumented workers. In other words, they do not hold a federally issued "green card" permitting them to work in the United States. Documented or undocumented, most farmworkers come to the United States believing that they will have a better chance of improving their situation in life. Even though their lives are somewhat different, the health problems for migrant and seasonal farmworkers are similar in many ways (DeSantis, 1990; Galarneau, 1993; Huff & Kline, 1998; Miller, Clark, Albrecht, & Farmer, 1996; Mosocoso, 1998; Munet-Vilaro, 1998; Testa, 1998; Zabrana, 1996).

Seasonal farmworkers usually remain in one location and work with a particular crop, such as mushrooms in Pennsylvania, ferns and vegetables in Florida and California, or berries in the northeastern states, or they do meat processing in slaughter plants located in several midwestern (beef and pork) and southern (chicken) states. Some are able to rent housing that is provided by an employer, but most must find shelter elsewhere. Because they earn very low wages, it is not unusual for several families or a group of men to share housing costs. Often, to economize, they live in a makeshift shanty, trailer-camper, or small, substandard apartment or house. Migrant farmworkers usually travel in groups, following one of several migratory streams. They begin the route near the Gulf Coast, then migrate from worksite to worksite. The migrant stream moves northward, ending near the Canadian border. As fall and winter approach, migrants return to warmer climates to work with crop production in southern states.

The group usually consists of extended family members working for their "foreman," who negotiates jobs with crop producers. Extended family travel and work together, including grandmothers, grandfathers, aunts, uncles, and many children of all ages. Very young children work side by side with parents. It is not unusual to see breast-fed infants carried in slings by mothers as they work in fields. Sometimes a baby is placed at the end of the field along with other very young children who are unable to keep up with the adults. A few communities provide migrant schools and day care services for the children of farmworkers. Some regions have migrant health clinics to provide care to the workers, but in many instances these are some distance from the fields. Thus, the workers often are not able to get to the facility. Most will not take time away from the job to go to the clinic during daylight hours. Seasonal and migrant farmworkers live very difficult and arduous lives. They work from dawn to dusk for very low wages. Yet the goal for most adults is to provide better life opportunities for their children. Family is important for most Latino farmworkers, and many send a portion of their salary to elders who remain in their country of origin.

The agriculture industry has many inherent occupational risks, which vary with the crop being produced (Chapter 11). Essentially, the risks and injuries vary. For example, back injuries often result from stretching and lifting heavy produce. Farmworkers also can experience a wide range of symptoms associated with intense and prolonged exposure to highly toxic chemicals (herbicides, fungicides, pesticides, etc.) that are used in the agricultural industry. In addition, they have high incidences of skin disorders from extensive exposure to the elements. Urinary tract infections occur with greater frequency in women, due to the lack of potable drinking water and inadequate toilet facilities. Otitis media and dental caries are common childhood occurrences related to poor nutrition, irregular feeding patterns, and lack of preventive health care.

Other health risks are inherent in their migratory patterns. For instance, the group usually has one vehicle to transport its members. Hence, all of them crowd into an older-model vehicle, usually a pickup or van, which has no or not enough seat belts for all the passengers. Adults along with very young children are seen riding in the back end of a pickup truck as the vehicle travels along open highways. Consequently, vehicle accidents often involve multiple fatalities and injured passengers. These are some of the more prevalent health concerns, and space does not allow for a comprehensive discussion on the health issues of migrant and seasonal farmworkers (Morganthau, 1997).

African Americans

In the last 5 years, more information has become available on blacks in rural areas, and we are learning more about their health concerns (Barbee, 1993; Degazone, 1999; Krieger, 1996; Sebastian & Bushy, 1999; Strickland & Strickland, 1995; Williams, Lethbridge, & Chambers, 1997). Of all rural blacks, 95% live in the South. Of these, 97% are considered poor. Black women in the South are in the lowest-paying and least desirable jobs. They have poor perinatal outcomes and high rates of chronic problems related to obesity, hypertension, and diabetes, as well as a higher mortality rate from cancers, particularly breast cancer. Infection with HIV is an emerging problem in rural black women, but precise data are unavailable on its prevalence and incidence in this vulnerable group. There is great diversity among rural black communities, but compared to the U.S. population as a whole, most experience disparities in their health status. In fact, the largest number of health professional shortage areas (HPSAs) are found in this part of the United States (Appendix E). Many who live in these regions do not have access to even the most basic primary health care. The high school dropout rate is high in the African American community, as is the teen pregnancy rate. Recently the focus of federal and state initiatives has been on partnering with black faith communities to implement interventions that target socioeconomic and health issues. Perhaps the greatest strengths of African American families are their faith and the connectedness of family members to each other. In turn, these are resources on which nurses can build culturally appropriate interventions (Sebastian & Bushy, 1999; Strickland & Strickland, 1995; Williams et al., 1997).

Native Americans

Native Americans have the poorest overall health status of any racial minority on a number of health indicators—even with government and tribal interventions of many decades (Bell, 1994; Huff & Kline, 1998; Indian Health Service, 1995; Joe, 1995; Sebastian & Bushy, 1999). Overall, it is a young population, with the median age for women at 25.3 years and that for men at 21.1 years. Early mortality and high birthrates are factors that influence the demographic profile of Native Americans. In the years 1989 to 1991, the Indian birthrate was 68% higher than for all U.S. races, but Native Americans have the poorest perinatal outcomes and the highest neonatal mortality rate. As a group, Native American women have a lower life expectancy than other women but live longer than Native American men and men of other racial groups. More Indian women than men are divorced, separated, or widowed. About one fourth of all Native Americans list their residence on reservations, located predominantly in isolated rural areas of the United States. On most reservations, the travel time for residents to the nearest Indian Health Service (IHS) facility can range anywhere from 30 to 150 minutes. Of course, the time needed to get to a health care provider will vary depending on weather and road conditions and on whether the family has access to transportation. Unemployment is rampant on reservations, ranging from 45% to 95%. In addition to high incidences of abuse, accidents, violence, and suicide, Native Americans experience extreme poverty, illiteracy, cultural isolation, and discrimination. They have a very high prevalence of frostbite, tuberculosis, sexually transmitted disease, diabetes, cancer of the cervix, and cirrhosis of the liver. Many of these health conditions could be prevented though improved socioeconomic status, access to education, and lifestyle changes ("Indian Reservation," 1998).

THE CULTURAL-LINGUISTIC COMPETENCE CONTINUUM

Cultural-linguistic competence can be best described as existing on a continuum ranging from ethnocentrism to enculturation. Developing cultural-linguistic skills is a developmental process, and nurses progress at their own pace (Bushy, 1999; Sebastian & Bushy, 1999). Ethnocentrism, at one end of the continuum, is the prejudicial belief that one's own group determines the standards for behavior by which all other cultural groups are to be judged. At this level, the nurse devalues the behaviors and beliefs of other cultural groups or treats them with suspicion or hostility. The next level on the continuum is *cultural awareness,* an appreciation of and sensitivity to another's values, beliefs, practices, lifestyle, and problem-solving preferences. This is followed by *cultural knowledge,* at which level the nurse gleans insights about the society's organizational patterns. Next, the nurse will seek information on strategies to provide care that is acceptable by group members. Progressing along the skills continuum, a nurse eventually demonstrates cultural change and awareness of cultural relativity. *Cultural change* evolves with exposure to another group. Awareness of *cultural relativity* means that the nurse has an understanding of beliefs, values, and practices of a client from the context of another society's worldviews. *Cultural competence,* which is next on the continuum, is the most sophisticated level of skill. At this level, the nurse is aware of, sensitive to, and knowledgeable about another culture and develops a repertoire of skills to render care seen as appropriate by minority clients. Recently, the term *linguistic competence* has come into use. It encompasses complex interpersonal skills that integrate a society's linguistic preferences into nursing care, including the spoken and written word as well as nonverbal communication. *Enculturation,* at the far end of the continuum, refers to an outsider's complete internalization of a foreign culture. This level of assimilation, however, may hinder objectivity about the culture because the outsider has become an intimate member.

Developing cultural and linguistic nursing competence is a nonlinear process. Individuals progress at their own pace, which depends on life experiences, frequency of exposure to other societies, and receptivity to learning about differences. Like other skills, the ability to make culturally based interventions is learned and refined as a nurse progresses from novice to expert (Andrews & Boyle, 1997; Degazone, 1999; Grossman & Taylor, 1995; Stanhope & Knollmueller, 1997).

Race, Culture, and Ethnicity

In the literature, and in day-to-day discussions, the terms *race, culture,* and *ethnicity* often are used interchangeably, but they have different meanings. *Race* refers to skin color and biological markers that define membership in a Caucasian, Mongolian, Native American, or Negroid group. Biological markers include characteristics such as the color and thickness of the skin, hair texture, physical development patterns, and susceptibility to certain diseases. It is becoming more difficult for nurses to differentiate genetic variations because of increasing interracial and genetic mixing coupled with contextual variables such as socioeconomic status, nutrition, lifestyle, and climactic influences.

Ethnicity is the commonness of group members that stems from a shared history. Individuals within a racial group can differ in ethnic affiliation. Ethnicity, however, tends to be sustained by race, religion, and national origin and to be influenced by extenuating factors, including education, socioeconomic status, transportation, technology, and exposure to other cultures. Not all members of a society express the same degree of ethnicity. For example, the Bureau of the Census uses a group classification of "Hispanic," which is subdivided into "white" and "nonwhite" categories. However, the term *Hispanic* refers to a language that commonly is used in nations colonized by Spain in centuries past.

Culture refers to the values, ideals, and belief systems that emerge over time among a group of individuals. Often, but not always, the group shares a common ethnicity or race. Culturally based beliefs serve as a guide for an individual in defining his or her roles and responsibilities and how to deal with usual and unusual life events, such as birth, death, staying healthy, and coping with an illness. These behaviors are learned through routine day-to-day human interactions and by observing how other people respond to those events. Intergenerational transfer of a society's worldview begins early in life through caregivers. Ethnic and cultural variations can be obscured by skin color, and stereotyping is a consequence of not recognizing individual preferences.

DIMENSIONS OF CULTURE: RURAL CONSIDERATIONS

Dimensions of culture with particular relevance to rural minorities are highlighted in the next few paragraphs: social organization, assigned roles, naming, linguistic patterns, perceptions of space and distance, time orientation, control of the environment, and self-care behaviors. These also are elements of Dunkin's framework for rural nursing (Chapter 5).

Social Organization

The family is the basic unit of society, and cultural values influence how it is organized and the roles of each of the member. The concept of family is difficult to define. In some societies, for example, family consists of an extensive kinship network composed of many blood relatives along with those acquired through marriage. Other societies refer to all maternal aunts as "mother" and all paternal uncles as "father." Some Native Americans refer to all members in their clan as "cousins." A few tribes have an adoption ritual to incorporate someone in the family with whom they have a strong emotional bond. The adoptee subsequently is referred to as "brother," "sister," "son," or "daughter" by other family members. Along with highly structured nuclear and large extended networks, other family arrangements that the nurse may encounter are same-gender couples with or without children, grandparents raising grandchildren, blended families associated with remarriage, communal groups, and cohabiting elderly persons. Therefore, a culturally competent nurse will ask the rural client who constitutes his or her family and then include these individuals in planning, implementing, and evaluating nursing care.

Assigned Roles

Individuals' roles and associated behaviors are culturally prescribed, such as what is or is not expected of children. For example, in a persistent poverty community, education may take second place to supporting the family. Sometimes this is evidenced by school officials reporting student truancy, as in the case of some Mexican American farmworkers (Mosocoso, 1998). On closer examination, the nurse finds that one or more of the older children are kept out of school to care for younger siblings or to work with parents in the fields when the weather lends itself to planting or harvesting.

Gender role behaviors, too, are culturally defined and influence a family's health care-seeking behaviors. For instance, the decision maker regarding personal health problems among some African American families is a highly regarded elderly woman, whereas in Hutterite, Mennonite, Amish, and some Latino communities, such decisions are made by the dominant male in these patriarchal societies. Sometimes a person having more formal education, especially in a health-related field, is the designated family spokesperson. With immigrants, often the spokesperson is someone who understands English and is able to translate for them, even if he or she is familiar with only a few words. In many instances, children of immigrants become interpreters for adults because they learn English in school. Nurses should be aware, however, that in most cases cultural taboos govern who can discuss particular aspects of health, illness, and reproduction.

Role behaviors also dictate an individual's involvement in the treatment of sick family members. For example, in some societies only an older woman in the immediate family—specifically, a mother or a wife—can provide direct physical care. Other societies condone *machismo,* sometimes evidenced by a male's suspicions of other males who interact with his spouse and other females in the extended family, even possibly including male health professionals who provide care to "his woman" during pregnancy and childbirth. Consequently, this particular male-female interaction is cited by some Latino women as a barrier in obtaining timely prenatal and preventive health care. In turn, such barriers can reinforce the hiring of female nurse midwives and nurse practitioners for migrant health clinics and federally qualified health clinics serving Latinos with this cultural characteristic. In other instances, the entire extended family become active participants when one member is ill. This preference has important implications when a client arrives at the clinic or hospital accompanied by a very large extended family. Culturally steeped practices, if not acknowledged, can be a source of contention between the family and caregivers. Nurses who are not culturally and linguistically competent, however, may not even be aware of the cultural differences. Hence, the caregiver should not be surprised if a client chooses "the path of least resistance"—verbally agreeing with the nurse, doing what always is done in similar situations, and then expressing his or her dissatisfaction to others.

Naming

Cultural preferences influence naming and how a person is referred to. More specifically, some Latino societies use surnames from the mother, grandmother, and father, in a sequence that can vary from time to time and from person to person. In some Asian societies, the family surname comes before a birth name. Native Americans are named shortly after birth, but some select another title during a ceremonial rite of passage. Immigrants who have names that are difficult to pronounce or spell may shorten their names or select commonly used English ones to facilitate entry into mainstream society. Culturally based naming practices can lead to errors by health professionals stemming from differences between the information found in official records and that of a client's word-of-mouth report. Individual preferences with respect to name and title are determined and respected by the linguistically competent nurse. To ensure accuracy, the client's pronunciation and spelling should carefully be cross-referenced with the written information in the health records. Subsequently, nurses must ensure that the "right" treatment is administered to the "right" person.

Linguistic Patterns

Linguistic competence is the most sophisticated skill on the cultural competency continuum. A linguistically competent nurse has a basic understanding about societal communication patterns and is able to integrate that information when rendering care to minorities within the rural community. Communication is the use of language, vocabulary, grammar, voice qualities, intonation, rhythm, speed, pronunciation, physical gestures, and silence. Just as words in Spanish have several different pronunciations, regional nuances, and meanings across Hispanic populations, so do some words in English across English-speaking populations. Consequently, two people speaking in English may not completely understand or may even misunderstand each other. Needless to say, communication difficulties are intensified between people who speak different languages. They also can be extremely frustrating for a nurse when caring for a client who requires urgent attention.

The Spoken Word

Regardless of whether a setting is rural or urban, ideally, a nurse should know the languages spoken by all clients. This probably is not a realistic expectation for all nurses. But taking a foreign language course can be helpful when caring for clients of another background. Essentially, a formal course presents a classic form of language grammar and pronunciation that is not usually used in day-to-day communication, especially by persons with less formal education. Dialects are discouraged in such courses, and being able to read and write a foreign language does not ensure that a nurse will be able to communicate effectively with clients who speak in a dialect. Augmenting the spoken word with gestures and pictures can be a useful communication strategy. Sometimes translators are necessary to interpret what is being said by both parties, but locating one can be a challenge in a rural homogenous community. In some areas, a list of translators is compiled by social service agencies. Often forgotten are language teachers in local schools or nearby higher education institutions. When several clients in a community speak the same language, it is prudent to have English-translation dictionaries readily available for staff reference in a clinic or hospital. If knowledge is limited about anatomy, physiology, and the disease process, or if medical jargon and acronyms are used by the speaker, the translator may not be able to understand what is being said. Translators should be objective and able to deliver an accurate interpretation of what was stated by both parties. The nurse, in turn, must use language that both client and translator can understand.

The linguistically competent nurse is aware that communication is based on cultural rules that dictate who can or cannot discuss certain personal health matters. Often the parameters are set by age, gender, family position, and the problem of concern. In some societies, for instance, children and males are not allowed to talk about reproductive matters. In other cultures, male health professionals should not speak to a woman unless she is appropriately attired—for example, by having the face, legs, or feet covered by particular garments. Linguistic competence also involves being sensitive to others' unwritten social courtesies. For example, an elderly Latino farmworker who speaks very little English arrives at a rural health clinic to see the doctor for his chronic lower abdominal pain. A young female nurse enters the treatment room with the intent of completing a "routine" intake assessment. Upon hastily greeting the gentleman, she asks about his presenting symptom, using an efficient and direct-questioning approach. The client is startled by the seemingly intrusive queries of a complete stranger. For him, personal questions of this nature are perceived as disrespectful, especially because this nurse is younger and of the opposite gender.

Among some rural Appalachians, a typical response to direct questions about symptoms of an illness is telling a story that metaphorically describes the problem and its multiple effects on the individual. The person often talks extensively about circumstantial themes related to the event, expecting the nurse to extract the essence of the health problem. Others enumerate the preceding day's or week's events, interspersing accounts of symptom development up to the present moment.

Obviously, it takes time to interpret clients' linguistic patterns, and there is no single approach to initiating conversation. Therefore, to demonstrate linguistic competence, the nurse must establish mutual rapport, be sensitive to linguistic preferences, and allocate adequate time to meet a client's expectations in the discussion.

Nonverbal Communication

Obviously, nonverbal communication patterns also are culturally steeped. For example, speaking very softly, with a slightly bowed head and downcast eyes, may be indicative of respect and deference among some Native Americans. To some nurses, those behaviors could demonstrate shyness, slyness, or dishonesty. Conversely, direct and prolonged eye contact by an adult male could be interpreted as self-confidence, especially by some white middle-class American nurses. Or that same behavior could be construed as overt aggressiveness, disrespect, contempt, or even a sexually oriented gesture. Head nodding by elderly Asian immigrants during a conversation is another frequently misinterpreted behavior by nurses. The nodding gesture does not necessarily mean that the client understands what is being said. Rather, it probably indicates respect for the speaker, even if the client does not understand a word of what is being said. One situation that nurses in rural practice may encounter with some Anglo-American families is having another spokesperson who responds to questions even when these are directed to the client. For example, a wife or adult daughter responds to questions directed to her spouse or father. These are but a few of the many culturally steeped linguistic patterns the nurses can expect to encounter when caring for persons of another cultural background. Linguistically competent nurses are sensitive to cultural nuances (Sebastian & Bushy, 1999).

The Written Word

A useful strategy for nurses is to write out specific verbal directions for a client describing the treatment plan. However, inadequate literacy skills pose serious challenges for many clients that the nurse encounters. Surprisingly, among all nations in the world, the U.S. literacy rate dropped from 1st place in the 1960s to 49th place in 1997. Functional literacy means an ability to read and write at least at a fifth-grade level (Morganthau, 1997; USDHHS, 1999). Of all adults in the United States, about 90 million (48%) have inadequate literacy skills. Of these, about half are functionally illiterate or have marginal literacy skills. In pragmatic terms, someone who is functionally illiterate is not able to read a newspaper, use a bus schedule, write a check, identify an expiration date on a driver's license, read street signs, or read a clinic appointment card, much less understand the written material on a prescription or in a discharge plan. Most are not able to function in a job that requires even the most basic reading and writing skills. Nurses should be aware that limited literacy affects health behaviors. For example, the person is less likely to obtain preventive health care, adhere to recommended treatment regimens, and keep appointments and is more likely to delay seeking professional care until he or she is quite ill. There is stigma associated with illiteracy, and many people hide the problem because they are ashamed or embarrassed. Of the illiterate, the majority never tell their spouse (67%) or children (53%). Over time, most learn to recognize symbols or key words, rely on a child or a spouse who is able to read, and offer very little information in day-to-day social interactions. Although precise numbers are not available, anecdotal reports suggest that compared to those in urban areas, rural residents, especially racial minorities and immigrants, have a higher rate of functional illiteracy. It also is easier in a small community for a person to hide his or her inability to read because day-to-day activities tend to become routine in a more controlled environment.

Essentially, a nurse should not assume that a client can read even the most simply written document or follow complex instructions. Furthermore, people may not be fully literate even if they say they completed high school. Increasing numbers of elderly and families cannot afford eye care and glasses. Linguistically competent nurses are aware that print size in written materials is very important when preparing and disseminating educational materials. Likewise, the health care environment (clinic, institution) should be assessed to determine potential and real cultural and linguistic barriers. For instance, do posters and pictures reflect the clientele being served, such as Mexican American Latinos, Native Americans, blacks, or Asians, and are reading materials written in their language? Are consent forms and instructional materials written at a level that can be understood, perhaps even in another language? Linguistically friendly materials are less likely to frustrate clients, especially those having inadequate literacy skills.

Perception of Space and Distance

The ways space and body boundaries are perceived are culturally based and are an important dimension of linguistic competence. Spatial preferences are exhibited as "comfort zones" for different kinds of human interactions, such as day-to-day business transactions, intimate situations, and nursing care. Generally, compared to males, females do not have as many restrictions placed on them regarding space and touch, but there are cultural variations. For instance, compared to Anglo-Americans, in day-to-day social interactions, some Latinos prefer less distance and often touch the person with whom they are interacting. In other societies, a common practice among males as well as females upon meeting a new acquaintance of the same gender is lightly embracing him or her. This gesture is highly uncomfortable to some Anglo-Americans, especially men, who prefer more space and are unaccustomed to being touched even by family, much less a complete stranger. A firm handshake is the accepted greeting among some European cultures. This gesture, too, surprises many mainstream Americans. Culturally competent nurses are aware that invasion of a client's personal space may be evidenced as discomfort: for instance, during a physical examination or an intervention that involves body touching.

Time Orientation

Time and how it is perceived relative to daily life vary from one group to another and among group members. More specifically, societies tend to be past, present, or future oriented. It is with *utmost caution and at the risk of risk of stereotyping* that general statements can be made regarding time orientation. To illustrate dimensions of linguistic competency, several examples are provided about time orientation. But these examples should not be construed by the reader as the norm for a particular racial group.

For example, some middle-class Anglo-Americans are future oriented; therefore, they may be willing to work hard and delay gratification for some anticipated goal. Their time perspective can influence lifestyle choices too. One example of a future-oriented client making a lifestyle choice would be the person who adheres to a rigorous physical fitness program in order to eventually appear more attractive or increase the years of life. Another would be the pregnant woman who is highly committed to delivering her child using "natural processes." She attends Lamaze classes, exercises, and does everything that is deemed to be "right." Yet another might be the new mother who has decided to breast-feed her baby until it is a year old. For any of these three future-oriented clients, not achieving the desired outcome, whether gaining weight, undergoing an emergency cesarean section, or experiencing an unanticipated circumstance that requires bottle-feeding the child, can result in high levels of stress and depression.

Present-time orientation may be exemplified in an African American with a chronic health problem. For example, an individual may be aware of how debilitating symptoms of the health condition, such as hypertension or diabetes, can be when they are out of control. Still, at a family gathering such as a reunion or holiday, he or she will eat particular "ethnic" foods traditionally served at the event. Even though the foods are acknowledged to be high in salt, animal fat, or sugar that contributes to uncontrolled symptomatology, there are emotions associated with it: In other words, those foods are "in the spirit of the happening." Despite the possible consequences of erratic blood sugar levels, increased blood pressure, and congestive heart failure, the person will opt to eat the food.

As for cultures with a past orientation, these include some Native American tribes, Alaskans, and Asians/Pacific Islanders having a worldview of life as a circular phenomenon. Deceased relatives are considered active participants of the extended family; hence, they are given great deference by the living. Family members in the nonearthly spiritual realm are believed to provide guidance to living relatives. Hence, it is not unusual for a client with a past-oriented perspective to incorporate healing practices on the advice of a deceased relative. This preference can lead to great bewilderment of a future-oriented nurse, especially if the client has an emotional or behavioral health problem.

The linguistically competent nurse is aware that time orientation can lead to misunderstandings when rendering care to clients of a minority background, such as performing a prescribed intervention. The long-standing adage "A watched kettle never boils" also refers to time perception. Essentially, when people are waiting for something to happen, they perceive time as passing very slowly—as in the case of patients who report that their call light was on for hours before staff finally responded. Patients may expect to receive a medication at the *exact* moment it was scheduled, whereas the nurse adheres to the hospital policy for medication administration, namely that most medications can be administered within a window of time from one half-hour before to one half-hour after they are scheduled. The adage is further illustrated by the statements of overextended nurses with multiple role responsibilities that "the more work I have to do, the faster my day seems to pass." For them, free time is very limited; relaxation time is perceived to be a luxury, occurring rarely and passing all too quickly.

Some societies expect that an individual will fulfill personal responsibilities within a given range of time. Conflicts emerge when a client prioritizes responsibilities differently than the nurse would: for instance, when the client does not adhere to scheduled appointments or follow through with recommended immunizations for children. Linguistic competence means acknowledging clients' time orientation and integrating it into the nursing plan of care.

Perceived Control of the Environment

Understanding the degree of control that people of a particular society perceive themselves to have over their environment and nature is another aspect of cultural-linguistic competence. More specifically, some cultures perceive humans as having mastery over nature, others believe they are dominated by it, and some have a worldview of living harmoniously with nature.

For example, individuals who perceive that humans have mastery over nature are likely to believe they can overcome most natural forces. This can be exemplified by the client's strong belief in the ultimate success of medicine and biotechnology such that he or she expects a malignancy to be cured with a surgical intervention. Those believing they are subject to nature might be viewed by the nurse as fatalistic or helpless. This frame of reference is sometimes evident in the attitudes of minorities living in persistent poverty counties or women not leaving an abusive relationship. Over time, both groups may believe they have little control over what happens to them. This perspective also provides insights about a client who does not adhere to prescribed treatments or preventive care such as getting a mammogram, a pap smear, prenatal care, or immunizations or wearing a seat belt or a cycle helmet. Time orientation may be one contributing factor to some minority health disparities, such as the finding that rural black women are diagnosed later with breast cancer and have higher mortality rates from it than their Caucasian counterparts.

Societies having a worldview of living in harmony with nature believe that illness is the result of the two not being in balance. Those holding this perspective believe that Western medicine primarily relieves symptoms but does little to address the source of the problem. Disease, in this instance, is a manifestation of not living in balance with the environment. When harmony and balance are restored within the client, good health may be an outcome. In such instances, cultural-linguistic competence involves integrating contemporary medicine with traditional healing in the care plan—for example, by including an indigenous or spiritual healer.

Self-Care and Healing Behaviors

An important dimension of cultural-linguistic competence is acknowledging the use of ethnocultural self-care behaviors in society. Resources and rituals used for healing vary among groups and are influenced by environmental and economic factors. Even mainstream Americans use a wide range of alternative healers and healing practices. Some of the more popular are herbal, chiropractic, magnetic, and massage therapies, hydro- and aromatherapies, spiritual and psychic healing, rolfing, osteopathy, meditation, visualization, and use of veterinarian products such as lotions and ointments for muscles and joints, pain, and skin conditions, antibiotics, and oral analgesics. Self-care and complementary healing practices reportedly are used more often by rural people than by urban counterparts. Partly, the finding could be associated with the high cost of health care and limited access to services. The culturally competent nurse therefore assumes that most people, including health professionals, engage in self-care, especially when they are feeling sick.

BECOMING COMPETENT

In light of the growing diversity nationally and in rural areas, the nurse must learn how to effectively work with people who have different beliefs and preferences (Leininger, 1978, 1991, 1994, 1997; Lester 1998).

Developing Self-Other Awareness

Before accommodating to another's belief system, nurses must understand something about their own cultural and ethnic background. Self-other awareness helps to deflect cultural conflicts in day-to-day life as well as during highly unusual events. Information on other cultures can be obtained from recreational and professional literature. An open and nonjudgmental attitude is a critical step in learning about other cultures. Talking with people who have more knowledge about and exposure to other cultures is another strategy to learn about their worldviews. Ask questions! Most people enjoy telling others about their culture if the inquiry is made with an intent to learn. If possible, seek explanations of how and why specific rituals are used in certain situations.

The most effective strategy is to actually interact with people of a particular background *on their turf* (natural environment) at social events as well as in their homes. Even by becoming highly involved in a community's social and political activities, it is not likely that an outsider will learn all of the important facts about a different culture before making at least a few blunders. Rather, he or she will learn gradually by working within a community over a period of time. Eventually, with a desire to learn, less obvious values and expectations become more obvious. For example, through formal and informal communication exchanges, the nurse becomes aware of and sensitive to rural clients' manner of interacting with various kinds of health professionals, their self-care practices, and their use of alternative healers.

To overcome cultural barriers to health care, nurses must acquire ethnocultural knowledge that can explain why clients engage in certain practices to promote health or treat an illness. It can be difficult to learn about persons who are not part of a community's mainstream unless the nurse actively seeks out those (sub)groups (Miseer, Sowell, Phillips, & Harris, 1997). The importance of assessing rural catchment areas cannot be overstated to establish the existence and needs of underrepresented cultural groups within the larger community. Some minorities are easy to identify because they are isolated by a geographical boundary, biologic or racial features, lifestyle, attire, religion, political views, language, leisure activity, or occupation. For example, generally it is not too difficult to identify an Amish or Mennonite group in the Midwest, or the Puerto Rican Latino and Asian community within a large city. But other groups, such as Laotians, Vietnamese, Italians, Poles, Irish, Jehovah Witnesses, Orthodox Jews, Latter-day Saints, Seventh-Day Adventists, and smaller Native American tribes, are not as obviously found in a given region and do not appear to have such a distinct lifestyle. Essentially, cultural and linguistic competence involves a dedicated effort on the part of a nurse to learn about rural minorities by interacting with them in their natural settings—where they live, learn, work, play, and pray. Real-world experiences should be augmented with theoretical information about a minority's worldview.

Recruiting Minorities to the Health Professions

Much cultural insensitivity in the health care system is attributable to low percentages of minorities entering the health professions, specifically as advanced practice nurses who eventually will practice in a rural community. Historically, schools of nursing reflected a homogeneous student body, with a predominance of Anglo/Euro-American students. Currently, schools of nursing recruit and retain minority students with varying degrees of success. The nursing profession, by virtue of its dominant culture representation, reflects the attitudes of the greater majority, that being white, middle-class women. Current and projected demographic and social changes challenge nurse educators to produce culturally and linguistically competent administrators, clinicians, theorists, and researchers, especially to work with rural underserved communities. Who can better present the ethnocultural perspective of a minority than persons who are of that background? Minorities must therefore be encouraged to enter the health professions. Nurses of minority backgrounds, especially in leadership roles, are in ideal positions to serve as role models to others in their community. Nursing education programs with their own tradition-based culture must encourage diversity among faculty and within the student body while preparing nursing students to practice with cultural sensitivity.

In addition to planning and delivering care, the cultural perspective must be taken into consideration when measuring satisfaction and the appropriateness of nursing services rendered to targeted consumers, particularly in rural catchments. Acceptability means that a particular service is offered in a manner that is congruent with the ethnocultural values of a target population and perceived as desirable and familiar to persons receiving it. Cultural factors that evoke consumer satisfaction go beyond clients' dietary and pastoral care preferences or manner of requesting analgesics to include their definitions of health, illness, self-care, and effective and ineffective professional care. Ethnocultural factors influence the appropriate time of seeking health care and the manner in which one interacts with a professional provider. Consumer satisfaction surveys often use rating scales of "satisfactory"/"unsatisfactory" or "acceptable"/"unacceptable," with little attention devoted to why a group perceives care as such. Furthermore, developers of the tool may not even consider respondents' reading abilities or understanding of the rating scheme. Suffice it to say, traditional evaluation approaches often are not culturally or linguistically sensitive, so the data probably are not valid or reliable with rural subgroups. The community must validate the appropriateness of outcomes and their measurement (Chapters 4 and 18).

SUMMARY

This chapter examined issues surrounding diversity in the United States. Cultural-linguistic competence means effectively responding to the needs and preferences of minorities, especially those having special health care needs. The process begins with self-other awareness and evolves to implementing nursing interventions that mesh with rural clients' health beliefs and expectations, even when these are different from those of the nurse.

DISCUSSION QUESTIONS

➤ Describe population changes that are projected for your catchment area. How might these affect rural nursing practice in the next 10 years, 20 years, and 50 years?

➤ Identify a minority subgroup in your practice setting. Describe particular ethnocultural practices that you have encountered associated with their health beliefs, health care-seeking behaviors, and expectations. What physical assessment skills are needed for differential diagnosis purposes? Compare and contrast the overall health of the minority group that you have chosen to that of the community and nation as a whole. If there are differences, speculate on potential reasons for them.

➤ Discuss biological markers that may differentiate one racial group from another and that may be evident in a physical assessment.

➤ Develop an action plan to increase your level of cultural and linguistic competence. Where do you fall on this continuum? What changes will you need to make to progress to a more sophisticated competency level in your professional development?

SUGGESTED RESEARCH ACTIVITIES

➤ Identify the most prevalent health conditions in your catchment area that could be attributed to racial or ethnic genetic predisposition. Develop strategies to integrate ethnocultural preferences into your nursing care plans. Design formative and summative methods to evaluate these interventions.

➤ Explore the self-care practices of a particular minority population in your catchment area. Disseminate your findings in a professional nursing journal.

REFERENCES

Andrews, M., & Boyle, J. (1997).Competence in transcultural nursing care. *American Journal of Nursing, 97*(8), 16AAA-16DDD.

Barbee, E. (1993). Racism in U.S. nursing. *Medical Anthropology Quarterly, 7,* 346-362.

Bell, R. (1994). Prominence of women in Navajo healing beliefs and values. *Nursing and Health Care, 15,* 232-240.

Bureau of the Census. (1997). *Population profile of the United States: Annual report.* Washington, DC: Government Printing Office.

Bushy, A. (1999). Cultural and ethnic diversity: Cultural competence. In J. Hickey, R. Ouimette, & C. Venegoni (Eds.), *Advanced practice nursing: Changing roles and clinical application (pp. 91-106).* Philadelphia: J. B. Lippincott.

Degazone, C. (1999). Cultural diversity in community health nursing practice. In M. Stanhope & J. Lancaster (Eds.), *Community health nursing: Promoting health of aggregates, families and individuals* (pp. 117-134). St. Louis, MO: C. V. Mosby.

DeSantis, L. (1990). Fieldwork with undocumented aliens and other populations at risk. *Western Journal of Nursing Research, 12,* 359-372.

Galarneau, C. (1993). *Under the weather: Farmworker health.* Rockville, MD: National Advisory Council on Migrant Health.

Ganey, F., & DeBocanegra, H. (1996). Overcoming barriers to improving the health of immigrant women. *Journal of American Medical Women's Association, 51*(4), 155-160.

Grossman, D., & Taylor, R. (1995). Cultural diversity on the unit. *American Journal of Nursing, 95*(2), 64-67.

Huff, R., & Kline, M. (1998). *Promoting health in multicultural populations: A handbook for practitioners.* Thousand Oaks, CA: Sage.

Indian Health Service. (1995). *Regional differences in Indian health.* Rockville, MD: U.S. Department of Health and Human Services.

Indian reservation tackles epidemic of teen suicide. (1998, February 8). *Daytona News Journal,* p. 5A.

Joe, J. (1995). The health of American Indian and Alaska Native women. *Journal of the American Medical Women's Association, 51*(4), 41-45.

Krieger, N. (1996). Inequality, diversity and health: Thoughts on "race/ethnicity" and "gender." *Journal of the American Medical Women's Association, 51*(4), 133-136.

Leininger, M. (1978). *Transcultural nursing: Concepts, theories and practice.* New York: Wiley Medical Publishers.

Leininger, M. (1991). *Cultural diversity and universality: A theory of nursing.* New York: National League for Nursing.

Leininger, M. (1994). Transcultural nursing education: A worldwide imperative. *Nursing and Health Care, 15,* 254-261.

Leininger, M. (1997). Transcultural nursing research to transform nursing education and practice: 40 years. *Image: Journal of Nursing Scholarship, 29,* 341-347.

Lester, N. (1998). Cultural competence: A nursing dialogue. *American Journal of Nursing, 98*(8), 26-35.

Miller, M., Clark, L., Albrecht, S., & Farmer, F. (1996). The interactive effects of race and ethnicity and mother's residence on the adequacy of prenatal care. *Journal of Rural Health, 12*(1), 6-18.

Miseer, T., Sowell, R., Phillips, K., & Harris, C. (1997). Sexual orientation: A cultural diversity issue for nursing. *Nursing Outlook, 45,* 178-181.

Morganthau, T. (1997, January 27). America 2000: The face of the future. *Newsweek,* pp. 58-61.

Mosocoso, C. (1998). The Mexican way. *Daytona News Journal, 73*(305), pp. 1C, 6C.

Munet-Vilaro, F. (1998). Grieving and death rituals of Latinos. *Oncology Nursing Forum, 25,* 1761-1763.

National Rural Health Association. (1994). *A shared vision: Building bridges for rural health access: Conference proceedings.* Kansas City, MO: Author.

National Rural Health Association. (1997). *A national agenda for rural minority health: A strategic planning document.* Kansas City, MO: Author.

National Rural Health Association. (1998a). *Bringing resources to bear on the changing care system: Conference proceedings for the Second Annual Rural Minority Health Conference.* Kansas City, MO: Author.

National Rural Health Association. (1998b). New presidential initiatives on health disparities highlighted at NACHC meeting. *Rural Health FYI, 20*(3), 28-29.

Sebastian, J., & Bushy, A. (Eds.). (1999). *Health issues of special populations.* Gaithersburg, MD: Aspen.

Stanhope, M., & Knollmueller, R. (1997). *Public health and community health nurse's consultant: A health promotion guide.* St. Louis, MO: C. V. Mosby.

Strickland, W., & Strickland, D. (1995). Coping with the cost of care: An exploratory study of lower income minorities in the rural south. *Family and Community Health, 18*(2), 37-51.

Testa, K. (1998, January 18). Farmworkers' town: Hunger striking vegetable pickers seek pay raise. *Daytona News Journal,* p. 2A.

University of North Carolina, North Carolina Rural Health Research and Policy Analysis Center. (1998). *Mapping rural health.* Chapel Hill, NC: Author.

U.S. Department of Health and Human Services. (1995). *Health United States.* Washington, DC: Government Printing Office.

U.S. Department of Health and Human Services. (1999). *Healthy people 2010: National health promotion and disease prevention objectives.* Washington, DC: Government Printing Office.

Williams, R., Lethbridge, D., & Chambers, W. (1997). Development of a rural health promotion inventory for poor rural women. *Family and Community Health, 20*(2), 13-23.

Zabrana, R. (1996). The under-representation of Hispanic women in the health professions. *Journal of the American Medical Women's Association, 51*(4), 147-153.

CHAPTER 8

Behavioral Health Care

Rural Issues and Strategies

KEY TERMS

➤ Behavioral health
➤ Mental hygiene
➤ Farm stress
➤ Code of reciprocity
➤ Reciprocal behavior
➤ Contingency planning
➤ Self-reliance
➤ Neighborliness
➤ Managed care organization

OBJECTIVES

After reading this chapter, you will be able to

➤ Discuss the prevalence of behavioral health disorders in rural communities.
➤ Describe the etiology and symptoms of farm stress.
➤ Characterize social structures and how these can affect rural clients who need behavioral health care.
➤ Develop strategies to protect confidentiality and anonymity for rural providers and clients using behavioral health services.

ESSENTIAL POINTS TO REMEMBER

➤ Experts estimate that of all people diagnosed with a medical problem, from 5% to 20% have some type of behavioral health disorder.
➤ Rural residents experience high incidences of depression, alcohol abuse, domestic violence, incest, and child neglect, exacerbated by stress-producing rural occupational and economic situations.

➢ The term *farm stress* refers to emotional and physical responses among some in the agriculture industry.

➢ Nurses have an important role in educating the community about mental health and recognizing the symptoms associated with emotional disorders and mental illnesses.

OVERVIEW

This chapter presents rural issues surrounding behavioral health, which encompasses mental hygiene, emotional problems, mental illness, psychiatric disorders, substance abuse, and dependency-control issues. Recurrent themes cited in Chapter 1 reemerge in the provision of behavioral health services, namely conflicting data on the mental health of rural residents, delivering care to a few in a large geographical area, and recruiting, retaining, and educating health professionals. Upon closer examination, nurses often are surprised by the array of social and behavioral health resources that actually exist in small communities that they may not have been aware of before. This chapter concludes with strategies that nurses can use to reduce fragmentation of services and enhance the care continuum for rural clients needing behavioral health care.

BACKGROUND

The term *behavioral health* has only recently come into use and therefore may be unfamiliar to some readers. Historically, mental health and substance abuse have been treated separately and often unequally. Funding priorities have changed from one year to the next, depending on congressional members' personal experiences with mental illness. Early in the 1990s, funding priorities shifted to more effectively reduce national health care costs. Consequently, providers of mental health and substance abuse services partnered to deal with shrinking budgets and shifting power structures. Ultimately, the goal was inclusion of mental health and substance abuse in primary health care as opposed to treatment of the mind and body as separate entities; thus, the concept of behavioral health emerged. Unfortunately, along with other cost-managing initiatives, behavioral health again has been relegated to a back seat and has sometimes been completely neglected among the working poor. Yet many rural residents have behavioral health problems.

Experts estimate that of all people diagnosed with a medical problem, from 5% to 20% have some type of behavioral health disorder. Further, these individuals visit a medical provider twice as often as counterparts without such symptoms. Incidences of psychiatric illness, emotional disorders, and substance abuse usually are reflected as "treated prevalence." In other words, there is a "head count" of clients who actually use the mental health system in a given region. But this approach raises questions about the reported rural prevalence because services may not exist or may not be physically accessible to those residents (Flax, Wagenfeld, Ivens, & Weiss, 1997; Goldberg, 1996; May, 1998; Murray & Keller, 1991; National Institute of Mental Health, 1993; U.S. Department of Health and Human Services [USDHHS], 1994, 1996a, 1996b, 1996c, 1997; Wagenfeld & Wagenfeld, 1990).

Morbidity and mortality reports suggest that rural residents experience high incidences of depression, alcohol abuse, domestic violence, incest, and child neglect. These symptoms are exacerbated by stress-producing rural occupational and financial situations, especially among residents in economically fragile areas, such as counties dependent on one industry (e.g., manufacturing, agricultural, fishing, mining). Education on mental hygiene and symptom recognition of behavioral health disorders may not be available to these residents either.

The term *farm stress,* which came into use during the 1980s, refers to socioeconomic factors in the agricultural industry that cause a range of emotional and physical responses in people who are directly or indirectly involved with that occupation. However, the symptoms are not unique to that particular industry (Elkind, Carlson, & Schnable, 1998; Elliott, Heaney, Wilkins, Mitchell, & Bean, 1995; Gunderson et al., 1993). Families involved in other occupations experiencing an economic crisis, particularly the lumber, fishing, and mining industries, report similar responses.

Successive years of poor crops and low prices have increased stress for farmers and their families. Behavioral health specialists in those communities report that farmers and their families are reluctant to seek professional care. Although they are highly vulnerable to depression and stress-related illnesses, farmers are socialized to bear their burdens alone. They tend not to talk about their difficulties because of pride and/or shame, even though the economic difficulties are not their fault. Farmers must be encouraged to talk about the stress-producing economic situation and their family members' responses to it. Along with education, 24-hour hotlines have been established to enable farmers and their families experiencing high levels of stress to have access to professional counselors.

Symptoms of farm stress include depression, emotional distress, illness, marital conflicts, increased violence, substance abuse, accidents, and suicidal ideation, especially among adolescent and young adult males. An exemplary fact sheet on farm stress that includes signs, symptoms, and management interventions is shown in Table 8.1. Isolation always has been a problem for farm families, and the situation is compounded when there is no money for recreation and entertainment. Further, some families believe that extra money should not be spent on recreation and entertainment. Figures for the prevalence of behavioral disorders in rural communities are for the most part estimates, based primarily on anecdotal reports of professionals who provide outreach services in rural areas (Bartlett, 1993; Graham, 1998; Human & Wasum, 1991).

AVAILABILITY OF PROVIDERS AND SERVICES

In economic terms, sparse population often limits the array of providers along with the social and behavioral health services in a catchment area. More specifically, the cost per client visit tends to be higher in sparsely populated areas than in more populated settings having a greater client (volume) base. The financial instability of rural hospitals contrib-

TABLE 8.1 Fact Sheet on Farm Stress

Each person responds differently to stress. The most effective intervention will vary from one person to another, depending on the situation. Remember to reinforce positive steps that can be taken when a situation seems hopeless to the person/family experiencing excessive farm-related stressors.

Signs and Symptoms	Interventions
Inability to relax	Exercise.
Difficulty sleeping	Eat a balanced diet.
Irritability, restlessness	Take time off to relax.
Anger out of proportion to the situation	Avoid alcohol and drugs.
Inability to eat or overeating	Avoid isolating yourself.
Alcohol and drug (substance) abuse	If physical problems persist, consult a health professional.
Abusive behaviors (verbal/physical)	
Sexual problems	Obtain a physical exam.
Blaming self or others	Seek professional counseling (mental health, financial).
Wanting to be left alone (isolating, withdrawing)	Separate things that can be controlled from those beyond control.
Failing to attend family, community, or church functions	Deal with problems; avoidance only complicates matters.
Seeming more "accident prone" or involved in an accident that caused or could have resulted in serious injury or death	Base decisions on accurate information.
	Set priorities; proceed step by step.
Unexplained headaches	Don't try to solve everything at once.
Upset stomach	Talk to friends, family, or pastor to obtain another perspective that can lead to practical solutions or alternative options.
Chest pains	
Chronic back or neck pain	
Cold hands and feet	Get involved. Becoming active on issues, especially injustices, can promote self-healing.
Muscle tension	
Skin disorders	
Other unusual physical symptoms	

utes to the scarcity of behavioral health services as well. Of all rural behavioral health professionals, nearly half (40%) are hospital based compared to less than one fifth (18%) for the nation as a whole. Consequently, the array and quality of rural services are dependent on the stability of small hospitals, many of which are on the verge of closing because of tenuous financial situations. Particularly lacking are personnel with advanced education, especially advanced practice psychiatric nurses and clinical specialists in other behavioral health specialties areas (USDHHS, 1997).

To reduce fragmentation of services while responding to the provider shortages, rural professionals often must function in a variety of roles. For example, a psychiatric nurse practitioner employed by a multicounty mental health center wears many hats: advocate, case manager, grant writer, crisis worker, administrator, marketing expert, counselor, therapist, consultant, and educator. Several times a month, the nurse provides outreach services to schools and senior centers within the multicounty district. One nurse may report that the role diversity allows her to use a range of professional skills with many opportunities to learn new things. However, another nurse not having this personality bent may find that the multiple roles are a deterrent to developing a professional specialty, and this may lessen her job satisfaction.

Because of the geographic, cultural, social, and economic factors described in the preceding chapters, rural communities have disproportionate numbers of vulnerable people who require help to conduct their everyday lives. Yet many who need social and behavioral health services are less able to advocate on their own behalf because they are limited by a disability or have special needs. Social structures, third-party reimbursement practices, and a person's ability to procure entitlement funds are other deterrents to seeking care.

Sometimes a much needed community-based resource is not available because rural health professionals do not have "grantsmanship skills." Writing is a critical element in procuring external funding from public and private agencies to implement community-based behavioral health activities. Such skills evolve with practice along with dedicated time by a writer to produce a fundable proposal. Developing successful grant-writing skills may not be a realistic expectation for professionals who already are overextended by excessively large client caseloads and multiple responsibilities. Nurses, in particular, may not have access to continuing education offerings on writing techniques and exposure to the current "buzzwords" that are essential in preparing a competitive grant. But telecommunication technology is making information more equitably accessible so that many nurses in rural areas are finding Web-based government resources very useful in identifying funding sources and preparing a competitive grant proposal.

Community political structures, too, may resist outside help. Interestingly, the formal and informal power structure in homogenous rural communities often is vested in an elite portion of the local population. These individuals may remain unaware of the particular needs of the underprivileged who live among them. Resistance frequently is evidenced by community leaders' not supporting a grant proposal to fund a new program that will meet the needs of a vulnerable population. Thus, powerless rural minorities may experience human service needs to which the more affluent and powerful majority may not be sensitive or sympathetic. In many instances, rural social structures advocate a solid work ethic and stigmatize those who seek public assistance ("going on welfare"). Consequently, residents who need professional care may not even seek, or accept, services that are available and locally accessible.

Acceptability also can be influenced by the urban orientation of behavioral health professionals. A negative or elitist attitude on the part of a provider can perpetuate difficulties in relating to the rural environment and the people living there. Insensitivity, for instance, can exacerbate clients' mistrust of an outreach worker who already is perceived as a community "outsider." Conversely, a cool reception by the community will perpetuate feelings of isolation and nonacceptance among health professionals who work among these residents.

LINKING FORMAL AND INFORMAL RESOURCES

Nurses who work with rural clients having behavioral health care needs must develop the skills to link formal and informal support systems to coordinate a seamless array of services. From a theoretical perspective, social support can be characterized as a three-tiered system. The first tier, sometimes referred to as "neighborliness," includes support behaviors that are volunteered by family and friends. The second tier consists of support from organized community groups, such as faith congregations, women's clubs, civic organizations, or volunteer fire and emergency medical services (EMS). Services in both tiers usually are volunteered without financial remuneration. There is, however, an unwritten code of reciprocity among participants, sometimes seen as an "insurance policy" should a similar event occur in their lives. Examples of reciprocal helping actions include volunteering time, transportation, food, material goods, and sometimes money to help defray a family's medical costs, funeral expenses, or expenses associated with destruction by natural catastrophes. The third tier includes formal services, specifically those sponsored by governmental agencies and sometimes a philanthropic donor. Financial remuneration is expected for services rendered by these providers, though often on a sliding scale based on income.

Shifts in the rural population mix are creating some unusual behavioral health care needs for these communities. For example, counties classified as persistent poverty and those having agriculture as the predominant industry frequently have limited employment and educational opportunities for residents. This situation is forcing productive adults to move elsewhere to find a job or attend school. Left behind are single mothers, the elderly, and dependent individuals with physical or emotional disabilities. Conversely, an influx of newcomers ("outsiders") is creating social upheavals in other small communities, but they lack the resources to deal with the issues. Both of these changes can disrupt long-established informal helping systems and create a need for new kinds of health care and social services by the community. Especially lacking are mental health services for the elderly and children, including services to diagnose and treat emotional and behavior problems.

SELF-RELIANCE VERSUS DEPENDENCY

Historically, neighborliness and self-care helped people to survive in austere, isolated, and rugged environments, as reflected in the statement "We take care of our own." This comment implies a preference for receiving care from familiar people. Rural residents have had a preference for primary relationships and reciprocal support (kith and kin) as opposed to use of formal (bureaucratic) services (Lee, 1998; Rogers & Burdge, 1985; Stein, 1989). In some ways, this preference affirms a sense of self-reliance. But with natural helping networks being disrupted, rural residents are forced to rely on services that originate in the third tier of support. Friends and family can be beneficial in eliciting health promotion and compliance behaviors. For instance, a close-knit family can be highly supportive to someone with a behavioral disorder by motivating him or her to take prescribed medications or keep a follow-up appointment. Other times, an overly solicitous family can discourage a sick individual from getting better, perhaps enabling the sick role. Over time, the family may become immune to deviant (dysfunctional) behaviors exhibited by one of its members. The family is no longer able to be objective about the loved one's idiosyncratic behaviors as he or she progresses to pathology. The family may not even be aware that the person poses a danger to him- or herself or others. A similar situation can occur in a community that is homogeneous and close-knit, often the case in a one- or two-industry-dependent town. The community as a whole can develop a tolerance for risky lifestyle activities, such as excessive consumption of alcohol, indiscriminate use of firearms, unsafe sexual practices, or corporal punishment.

Mental illness, too, may be viewed by the community as the weakness of a particular family ("skeleton in their closet"). Stigmatizing reinforces a need to "hide" the problem and promotes the unspoken admonishment "What happens in the family stays in the family." This attitude is of particular significance in small rural towns where most families have a shared history—living, working, and struggling together for generations. To maintain integrity, it is important not to let everybody in town know about a family problem, particularly substance abuse, domestic violence, incest, mental illness, or alternative sexual practices. Even with extensive public education, much remains to be done to eradicate the stigma of behavioral disorders and mental illness in our nation. Consider the case of Billy Joe, a client who lives in a remote Appalachian town with fewer than 800 residents. Recently the psychiatrist from the regional mental health center diagnosed his condition as bipolar depression. While responding to questions about his family's history, Billy Joe tells the outreach advanced practice psychiatric nurse his story:

> I hear from old-timers around town that, every now and then, Uncle Tom, great-grandpa, and another cousin made and sold moonshine, drank a lot, were big spenders, and tore up the town. They all spent time in the state hospital too. The family never talks about them. When someone brings up the topic of mental illness, they change the subject. Neighbors tell me that my mental problem is our family's weakness.

Billy Joe's story demonstrates one of the ramifications of familiarity among the residents of a close-knit community. This example also shows how social structures might hinder individuals from accessing services that are offered in the community, even if these are needed.

ADVOCATING A WORK ETHIC

How a group defines health and illness is culturally based, and this too affects individuals' care seeking for behavioral problems. For example, some rural people define health as the ability to work and do what needs to be done. One can infer that, for them, illness probably means not being able to do one's usual work. The association between work and health reinforces the rural work ethic and probably dictates attitudes regarding leisure activities, such as viewing relaxation as frivolous when there is work to be done and putting family needs before individual health and well-being (Lee, 1998; Stein, 1989).

With respect to mental illness, a family may continue to deny the problems of one of its members as long as that person is able to complete his or her work. Over time, expectations of the person are modified by family members to accommodate their loved one's degenerating abilities. Consider the case of a 31-year-old man, Jackie, who lives in a small town located in a southern state. Townsfolk say, "Jackie is strange. . . . He sees and hears things that aren't there." His mother, however, disagrees with local residents, as evidenced by this comment that she made to the psychiatric nurse at the county mental health office:

> How can people around here talk about him that way? Jackie always helps dad with the farm work. Oh, he drinks a little when he gets to a bar. But he goes into town only once in a while. . . . He never has had much interest in girls. Jackie always has been so different from our other five children . . . more sensitive . . . religious. He is so dependable about helping with the work. Most of the time dad thinks Jackie does really good work!

Obviously, a strong work ethic has distorted these parents' perception regarding the healthiness of their son. More than likely, Jackie's ability to complete assigned tasks influences whether mom and dad encourage him to obtain professional treatment too. The following are examples of other activities sometimes relegated to a secondary position to work. (The comments are from my own personal correspondence with residents from various rural communities.)

➢ Obtaining education, evidenced by comments such as "I'm keeping the kids home from school to help out at home."
➢ Participating in hobbies and leisure-time activities, described by some as "a waste of time and money."
➢ Seeking professional care for nonemergency services, exemplified by the remark, "I'll go to the doctor on the next rainy day, when we can't get into the fields."
➢ Keeping follow-up health care appointments, evidenced by the following remark: "I'm feeling fine—so why should I drive 100 miles to have a social worker tell me that I'm doing alright?"
➢ Obtaining prescribed medications and complying with recommended dosages, exemplified by the following comment: "Annie says she isn't hearing voices. We can wait until the harvesting is done to get her prescription filled. Then we'll have more money too."

IMPLEMENTING AND EVALUATING NURSING SERVICES

Nurses involved in implementing and evaluating behavioral health programs must be sensitive to the cultural values of groups within a rural community. A comprehensive community assessment is critical in identifying consumers' real and perceived needs and obtaining their insights about the most effective ways to meet these. Some communities, for instance, abide by religious doctrines that dictate behaviors for Sunday or reproductive practices. Problems arise when an individual's lifestyle conflicts with these mandates, leading to guilt, stress, depression, and other emotional disorders. Other results of doctrinal beliefs that nurses may encounter are regulations mandating that stores remain closed on Sundays ("blue laws"), terrorist-type actions against family planning clinics, and electing of officials who oppose entitlement services ("welfare programs"). These dynamics influence the manner in which a service is used (utilization patterns) and should be addressed when implementing and evaluating behavioral health services and programs (Baradell, 1995; Center for Mental Health Services, 1993).

Because behavioral health services tend to be limited in less populated areas, those that are available should be congruent with the values of a target population. This principle reinforces the need for measuring and documenting outcomes of behavioral health interventions and consumers' satisfaction with the program and the providers. As for managed care organizations (MCOs), they are asking for data in terms of treatment outcomes about the product their dollars are buying. In an era of cost management, government funding agencies are demanding similar accountability from health care providers. The information deficit on the health status of rural people coupled with the subjective nature of behavioral disorders reinforces the importance of evaluating the usefulness and appropriateness of services. Nurses, in particular, are challenged by consumers and administrators to demonstrate outcomes for nursing interventions. The mandate is even greater for those in rural practice because the cost per visit/service may be higher due to low client volume. Incomplete or nonexistent outcome data further deter MCOs from enrolling rural consumers and offering mental/behavioral health benefits in their plans (Chapter 12).

ENSURING ANONYMITY AND CONFIDENTIALITY

News travels quickly through a small community because there are fewer people, most of whom are acquainted. Most small towns have an active "local grapevine" that passes along information about the community's sick members, especially those with behavioral health disorders. Informal networks can pose challenges in ensuring confidentiality and anonymity for professionals and their clients. For instance, it is not unusual for confidentiality issues to arise because of the location of the mental health clinic. When it is publicly visible, passersby and vigilant neighborhood observers may take note of whose car is parked by the clinic and even how often clients visit and how long they remain inside. Similar problems can occur with family planning clinics. It is not unusual for residents to recognize others in the community by the kind of car(s) they drive. Careful consideration must be given by planners as to the best location for behavioral health services to ensure confidentiality and anonymity for clients. It may, for example, be prudent to establish a mental health clinic within a building that houses other health and social service agencies or in a general office building with a lot of activity.

Confidentiality issues also can arise from the high visibility of health professionals among local residents. For instance, when an advanced practice nurse in a behavioral health specialty has gained entrance and has become well accepted by the community, confidentiality and anonymity concerns can arise when the client openly acknowledges problems to the nurse in a public place. It is not unusual for a client or someone in his or her family to stop and "chat," for instance. Where interactions are spontaneous and informal, a resident may not think it unusual to telephone the nurse's home or even broach health concerns while in a grocery store, at a service station, or at a church or school function. To prevent such situations from occurring, nurses must educate clients as to what constitutes a "real" crisis and the process to be followed if an untoward event occurs. Likewise, a nurse should learn to tactfully evade these sensitive conversations. For example, the nurse could display an interested attitude while tactfully bringing up a subject of mutual interest such as children's activities, current events, or even the weather.

CLIENT SATISFACTION AND PROFESSIONAL BURNOUT

Nurses who have gained acceptance from the community usually find that this contributes to having satisfied clients. Client satisfaction coupled with health professional shortages can, however, lead to high caseloads for the advanced practice psychiatric nurse. Occasionally, a nurse reports that she or he has been on call for weeks, months, or sometimes even years. However, "on call" does not necessarily mean the nurse will actually see a client; rather, it means being available should someone need care. Cellular phones and digital paging have done much to free health professionals from the tether of being on call and make them still available to clients with urgent needs. Obviously, a nurse can become "burned out" by unremitting professional demands if practice limitations are not delineated. Therefore, when considering practice in a professionally underserved area, the advanced practice nurse should identify someone who can and is willing to provide backup coverage. Collaborative arrangements can prevent burnout, allow a practitioner to have a personal life, and demonstrate to clients the need to set personal boundaries.

RECOMMENDATIONS

The following commonsense approaches have been found to be useful by nurses in coordinating an array of mental health and psychiatric services for rural clients living in underserved regions.

Avoid Duplication of Services

Interdisciplinary collaboration is critical to reduce turf disputes between the various providers and agencies within a geographical region (Chapter 4). Further, nurses working in a behavioral health setting must be flexible with expert generalist skills. These nurses usually work with clients of all ages having a myriad of problems, emotional as well as physical. They are specialists in their knowledge about community resources, whether formal agencies or informal circles of support, and how to access these (Human & Wasum, 1991; May, 1998).

Develop Meaningful Discharge Plans

Urban-based nurses often are not familiar with social networks and behavioral health programs that exist or are offered as outreach in rural catchment areas. For that matter, neither are most nurses who live and work in rural communities knowledgeable about services that are locally available. Advanced practice nurses in behavioral health specialties must assume an active role in disseminating to peers information on regional resources. That kind of information can assist other nurses in making appropriate referrals and developing meaningful discharge plans for rural patients. Recently, small communities have started compiling a database listing of regional and local resources such as social services and other health-related programs, addresses, telephone numbers, and, when available, Internet sites. Comprehensive directories include a list of services provided by each agency, its providers, their credentials, and, when possible, e-mail addresses. Some rural communities with an Internet home page include hypertext links to resources listed in the database. User-friendly Web-based information enables clients to access relevant health information. Technology is especially useful in more remote regions for clients to maintain contact with a health care provider as well as peers in their support network. Once developed, continuing education programs should be offered to nurses on the database along with strategies to prepare clients to access Web-based information (Association of Telemedicine Service Providers, 1999).

Consider Case Management and Contingency Planning

Case management is well suited for rural clients needing behavioral health services and has been successfully used by public health nurses for decades. This model of care delivery can help to decrease duplication of services, promote interdisciplinary collaboration, and integrate formal services with informal support for a client. Case management also is appropriate for clients who live in a region having limited resources, provider shortages, and restricted access to services—all characteristics of many rural communities. Furthermore, this approach meshes nicely with rural people's preference for having someone they know minister to them. Case management is a partnership model. To be effective, clients must actively participate with a nurse, in the role of case manager, to develop their discharge plan and anticipate potential adverse events. Crisis situations can arise when rural clients lack available or accessible services to manage their mental health problem. For example, in many frontier regions there is no pharmacy in the area from which to purchase prescription medications. Neither is there a dietitian or an occupational or physical therapist with whom to consult regarding medication side effects. Psychiatrists and social workers may have an office that is located several hours away. Thus, in an emergency, they may not be available to a client. Remoteness is exacerbated when clients have restricted transportation capabilities, as may be the case for some of the elderly, those taking psychotropic medications, or those with seizure disorders.

It is prudent for a nurse, in the role of case manager, to negotiate a contingency plan (contract) that clearly states what the client will agree to follow should events go awry or a crisis occur. Increasingly, regional mental health centers are providing 24-hour toll-free crisis (telephone) services much like the farm stress "hotlines" described earlier in this chapter. This strategy can be especially useful to deal with many unanticipated events, but not every event that may arise. Other situations to consider in the contingency plan are that the client may not have telephone services in the home and so may be unable to access the crisis line. Professional outreach services may be available only at designated intervals in the community: for example, every 2 weeks or once a month. Essentially, a case manager-client contingency plan should be explicitly written in culturally and linguistically appropriate language; explained by the nurse to the client and reinterpreted by the client in his or her own words; and then "tested" by role-playing each option with the client and all those who agree to participate in the plan. Finally, the contract should be signed by the client, the case manager, and everyone else in the contingency plan.

Anyone placed on medication always should have explicit education regarding his or her pharmacotherapy regimen and its potential side effects. Rural clients may require additional considerations because they have restricted access to pharmacy services. For instance, seriously depressed persons having a potential for self-harm usually are dispensed a limited supply of medication to reduce the risk of overdosing. Logistical barriers such as not having access to transportation to a pharmacy or laboratory may result in a client's needing a greater number of doses dispensed directly to them. For risk management purposes, a responsible individual should be identified in the contingency plan who will be in contact with the client on a regular basis. This person should be educated so that he or she can monitor the client's behavior patterns and medication practices and, if necessary, secure extra supplies of medication in a safe place. At designated intervals, the person can give additional medication doses to the client as directed by the case manager or pharmacist. Obviously, this individual must be highly committed, motivated, and well informed about the responsibilities and must agree to be involved in the client's plan of care. An alternate may be needed if the first individual is not always available. Examples of people who usually can be reached in a small community are the sheriff, a clergy member, a public health nurse, a dependable neighbor, or a family member.

When negotiating the contingency plan, the case manager should discuss medication noncompliance with the client. For example, it is not unusual for a client to feel "good" after taking psychotropic medications for a period of time. If family members are not educated about these behaviors, they may believe the client is "back to normal" and thus no longer needs to take medication. This phenomenon seems to occur with greater frequency when clients do not have the financial means to purchase prescribed medications. In the contingency plan, the nurse can list situations taking precedence over a client's reluctance to take medications or to adhere to prescribed dosages. If necessary, the nurse can specify negotiated interventions to alleviate medication side effects such as ataxia, akathisia, nausea, or tardive dyskinesia. For some clients, it is helpful to outline behaviors that can occur when they are not taking the prescribed medications, such as hearing voices, frightening certain family members, and wanting to hurt themselves or someone else. It is not unusual for nurses in the role of case manager to work with some rural clients for years. Interestingly, nurses often report this extended professional relationship to be one of their most rewarding experiences.

Coordinate Follow-Up Appointments

When scheduling follow-up care, consider a client's occupation, lifestyle, and home situation, especially if he or she lives a great distance from behavioral health professionals. In the contingency plan, a nurse case manager should delineate procedures in the event that the client does not keep an appointment, such as calling a mutually agreed-on neighbor, minister, or sheriff or even going to the home. Sometimes writing down the consequences may be effective to remind the client what can happen if he or she does not adhere to the treatment plan.

Educate the Community

Nationally, knowledge about mental hygiene, symptoms of behavioral disorders, and treatment options for these conditions is lacking, and this is even more the case among professionally underserved populations. Advanced practice nurses in the behavioral health specialties must make a sustained effort to educate the public on these important health concerns. Strategies to reach targeted vulnerable groups center on collaborating with their informal support networks and well-established formal health care organizations in the community. Nurses must learn to present health promotion and disease prevention content so that it is congruent with a community's cultural beliefs. Sometimes this involves having highly sensitive content validated by a well-respected community member, such as a pastor in the faith community or an esteemed elder in the extended family. When implementing a program (in the third tier of social support), it may be prudent to interface the new services with established informal structures (first and second tiers of social support) (Bartlett, 1993; Campbell, 1998; Jones, Luchok, & McKnight, 1998; Levin, Blanch, & Jennings, 1998).

For example, a nurse could collaborate with a farm women's organization to implement a communitywide educational initiative on recognizing depression, responding to farm stress, and preventing suicide. Or several rural nurses could partner with the local chapter of the Women's Junior League to establish a safe house in the community for victims wanting to leave a violent relationship. Partnerships of this type can facilitate a community's acceptance and use of a new bureaucratic program. Partnerships also enhance the likelihood of obtaining a grant to implement a rural community-based or community-focused program. Health information is better accepted by rural families when obtained by a woman, especially when it is first sanctioned by the faith community or local women's group, such as a homemakers' club or church circle. Those organizations remain important sources of information on health promotion and symptom recognition of behavioral problems. Women, mothers, daughters, and wives tend to be motivated to learn about emotional health and occupational injuries that can be devastating to a loved one. Likewise, business owners usually are amenable to participating in initiatives that benefit members of their community. For example, bartenders, beauticians, and barbers can learn to recognize depression and make referrals to a mental health professional. Most respond favorably to a nurse they know who is spearheading a local health initiative (Sidani & Braden, 1997).

Provide Continuing Education for Health Professionals

Continuing education (CE) on behavioral health topics may not be available or readily accessible to professionals in rural practice. Further, CE programs that are offered may not be relevant to rural practice. Local health departments, social service agencies, and mental health clinics usually are an integral component of state and federal organizations. Hence, that affiliation can facilitate bringing an outside speaker to offer CE on a variety of mental and behavioral health topics to nurses working in more remote areas. Consultants from the state department of mental health, for instance, are knowledgeable about regional services along with state-of-the-art pharmacotherapeutic interventions related to mental hygiene and behavioral health conditions. They may also have insights on potential funding sources and techniques for writing a competitive grant to develop and sustain these kinds of services. An often forgotten resource for CE is community health nurses. They tend to be aware of prevalent behavioral health concerns in the region and may be willing (even eager) to talk to peers about those disorders.

Further, to expose students, nurse administrators of behavioral health agencies should invite nursing faculty into their institutions. Perhaps one or two faculty members will be willing to provide CE programs to nurses in clinical practice. Collaboration is essential in exposing undergraduate students to rural environments and developing preceptorship arrangements for nurses pursuing an advanced practice degree, especially a behavioral health specialty. Particularly lacking is representation from minority communities. Their input is essential to effectively assess, diagnose, and treat behavioral health disorders in individuals who have a different cultural belief system, particularly African Americans, Native Americans, Asians, and Hispanics of diverse ethnic backgrounds. Ultimately, early exposure should result in a greater number of graduates choosing rural practice. Educator-administrator-clinician partnerships may also lead to nursing research opportunities that focus on the rural phenomenon. This could lead to writing a competitive grant proposal that benefits the community and the proposal writers in institutions and agencies (Baer & Bowers, 1998; Campbell, 1998; Sallis & Owen, 1998; Schornstein, 1997; Solari-Twadell & McDermott, 1998).

Conduct Research

As with many other health-related concerns and nursing interventions, there is a critical need for research to obtain the rural perspective. To complicate matters, there are no reliable data on the actual incidence and prevalence of behavioral health disorders in rural communities. In recent years, the problem of "farm stress" has been brought to the forefront, and national efforts are underway to educate rural communities and health professionals in rural settings about the signs and symptoms associated with stress-induced conditions. An entire text could be devoted to nursing research needs in the areas of behavioral and mental health in rural communities. There are several suggestions at the end of this chapter, and Chapters 17 and 18 may provide other insights on evidence-based interventions that focus on behavioral health promotion, mental illness prevention and symptom management, and the human responses to family members who are mentally and emotionally challenged.

SUMMARY

This chapter examined issues surrounding behavioral health care in rural environments. Well-informed, articulate nurses can provide relevant anecdotal information on specific problems of concern to the community. The most urgent need at this time is the development of health policies that will integrate behavioral health with primary care. For nurses, this means actively engaging in the advocate and educator roles to inform policy makers as well as voters about the rural perspective on behavioral health issues and interventions.

DISCUSSION QUESTIONS

➤ Interview a nurse administrator in a rural mental health clinic to obtain his or her perspective on the most prevalent disorders that present in the facility. What are the most effective and most frequently used resources? Who funds these services (federal, state, local government, philanthropic donors)? What criteria are used to evaluate the program, services, and client outcomes?

➤ Review two health insurance policies/plans, and determine if behavioral health services are covered. Identify the benefits/limitations in the plan, such as indemnities, deductible, number of paid visits allowed per year/per enrolled member, hospitalization, medications, exclusion of certain diagnoses, and other therapies. What are the similarities, differences, and costs among the plans?

SUGGESTED RESEARCH ACTIVITIES

➤ Identify a rural client with a family member who has a chronic mental illness. Learn about his or her lived experience with the health care delivery system as the disease progressed. How did the family cope? What adaptations were made to accommodate the needs of the ill person? How did extended family respond? The community? What has been the person's greatest source of support? Disappointment? What advice does he or she have for others in similar predicaments? Disseminate your findings.

> ➤ Select a rural community and make a list of its behavioral health resources
> that will be useful to providers and consumers. Link these to the community's
> Internet home page. Prepare a hard copy for those who do not have Internet
> access.

REFERENCES

Association of Telemedicine Service Providers. (1999). *1998 report on U.S. telemedicine activity.* Portland, OR: Author.

Baer, M., & Bowers, C. (1998). Using a nursing framework to measure client satisfaction at a nurse-managed clinic. *Public Health Nursing, 15*(1), 50-59.

Baradell, J. (1995). Clinical outcomes and satisfaction of patients of clinical nurse specialists in psychiatric/mental health nursing. *Archives of Psychiatric Nursing, 9,* 240-280.

Bartlett, P. (1993). *American dreams, rural realities: The family farm in crisis.* Chapel Hill: University of North Carolina Press.

Campbell, J. L. (1998). *Empowering survivors of abuse.* Thousand Oaks, CA: Sage.

Center for Mental Health Services. (1993). *The journey of native American people with serious mental illness: Executive summary of the First National Conference at Albuquerque, April 1993* (Pub. No. 3878a). Boulder, CO: Western Interstate Commission for Higher Education.

Elkind, P., Carlson, J., & Schnable, B. (1998). Agricultural hazards reduction through stress management. *Journal of Agromedicine, 5*(2), 23-32.

Elliott, M., Heaney, C., Wilkins, J., Mitchell, G., & Bean, T. (1995). Depression and perceived stress among cash grain farmers in Ohio. *Journal of Agriculture Safety and Health, 1,* 177-184.

Flax, J., Wagenfeld, M., Ivens, R., & Weiss, R. (1997). *Mental health and rural America: An overview and annotated bibliography.* Washington, DC: National Institute of Mental Health.

Goldberg, R. (1996). *Integrating behavioral health services with general medicine.* Alexandria, VA: Manisses Communication Group.

Graham, L. (1998, December 13). Where have all the small towns gone? *Parade Magazine,* pp. 6-9.

Gunderson, P., Donner, D., Nashold, R., Salkowicz, L., Sperry, S., & Whitman, B. (1993). The epidemiology of suicide among farm residents or workers in five north-central states, 1980-1988. *American Journal of Preventive Medicine. 9*(Suppl. 1), 26-33.

Human, J., & Wasum, K. (1991). Rural mental health in America. *American Psychologist, 46,* 232-239.

Jones, M., Luchok, K., & McKnight, R. (1998). Empowering farm women to reduce hazards to family health and safety on the farm. *Journal of Agromedicine, 5*(2), 91-99.

Lee, H. (Ed.). (1998). *Conceptual basis for rural nursing.* New York: Springer.

Levin, B., Blanch, A., & Jennings, A. (Eds.). (1998). *Women's mental health services: A public health perspective.* Thousand Oaks, CA: Sage.

May, J. (1998). Clinically significant occupational stressors in New York farmers and farm families. *Journal of Agricultural Safety and Health, 4*(1), 9-14.

Murray, J., & Keller, P. (1991). Psychology in rural America: Current status and future directions. *American Psychologist, 46,* 220-231.

National Institute of Mental Health. (1993, June). *Creating community: Integrating elderly and severely mentally ill persons in public housing* (DHHS Pub. No. ADM-86-1466). Washington, DC: Government Printing Office.

Rogers, E., & Burdge, R. (1985). *Social changes in rural societies.* Englewood Cliffs, NJ: Prentice Hall.

Sallis, J., & Owen, N. (1998). *Physical activity and behavioral medicine.* Thousand Oaks, CA: Sage.

Schornstein, J. (1997). *Domestic violence and health care.* Thousand Oaks, CA: Sage.

Sidani, S., & Braden, C. (1997). *Evaluating nursing interventions.* Thousand Oaks, CA: Sage.

Solari-Twadell, P., & McDermott, M. (1998). *Parish nursing.* Thousand Oaks, CA: Sage.

Stein, H. (1989). The annual cycle and the cultural nexus of health care behavior among Oklahoma wheat farming families. *Culture, Medicine and Psychology, 6,* 81-89.

U.S. Department of Health and Human Services. (1994). *Rural issues in alcohol and other drug abuse treatment* (Technical Assistance Pub. No. 10, DHHS Pub. No. SMA 90-2063). Washington, DC: National Mental Health Service Knowledge Exchange Network.

U.S. Department of Health and Human Services. (1996a). *Innovative community based services for older persons with mental illness* (DHHS Pub. No. SMA 94-5003). Washington, DC: National Mental Health Service Knowledge Exchange Network.

U.S. Department of Health and Human Services. (1996b). *Responding to the needs of people with serious and persistent mental illness in times of major disasters* (DHHS Pub. No. SMA 96-3077). Washington, DC: National Mental Health Service Knowledge Exchange Network.

U.S. Department of Health and Human Services. (1996c). *Training manual for human service workers in major disasters* (DHHS Pub. No. SMA 90-538). Washington, DC: National Mental Health Service Knowledge Exchange Network.

U.S. Department of Health and Human Services. (1997). *Bringing excellence to substance abuse prevention in rural and frontier America.* (1996 Awards for Excellence Papers, PHS Pub. No. SAMHSA 270-93-0004). Rockville, MD: Government Printing Office.

Wagenfeld, M., & Wagenfeld, J. (1990). Mental health and rural America: A decade review. *Journal of Rural Health, 7,* 707-22.

CHAPTER 9

America's Lost Population

The Rural Homeless

KEY TERMS

> Homelessness
> Homeless persons
> Chronic mental illness

OBJECTIVES

After reading this chapter, you will be able to

> Characterize homelessness and homeless persons.
> Differentiate features of the homeless population in rural and urban communities.
> Describe outcomes of homelessness on the health of individuals, families, and rural communities.
> Identify community resources in rural areas to help meet the needs of the homeless.

ESSENTIAL POINTS TO REMEMBER

> It is difficult to count the homeless population, but it is estimated to be anywhere from 350,000 to 2.5 million people in the nation. Estimates of the proportion of the homeless who are rural range from 7% to 14% of the total homeless population. As in urban areas, the homeless in rural areas include families with children, runaways, women with and without children, single adult men, the elderly, the mentally ill, and veterans.

> Informal structures that exist in many small communities often support relatives, neighbors, and friends without a home, but their life situation usually is uncertain. This phenomenon contributes to rural homeless persons' being forgotten or hidden.

➢ Partnerships among public and private entities at local, state, national, and international levels may be one strategy to develop and enhance support services for the rural homeless.

OVERVIEW

The Rural Homeless: America's Lost Population (National Rural Health Association [NRHA], 1996) described the complex interplay of policy decisions and economic circumstances that contribute to this desperate human phenomenon in rural areas. This chapter discusses homelessness in general, highlights issues of the rural homeless, presents nursing implications, and suggests resources that exist in most small communities (Acquaviva & Lancaster, 1999; American Public Health Association, 1997; Ratnesar, 1999; Rosenheck et al., 1998).

BACKGROUND AND DEFINITIONS

Homeless persons have been labeled as vagrants, tramps, deviants, and victims. The names have changed with society's interpretations of its moral and social responsibility for the poor and homeless. There are no precise figures on the number of homeless in the United States, and even less is known about those in rural areas. Furthermore, the operational definition that is used determines both the size and the characteristics of the homeless population. Even though health and policy planners do not have reliable statistical data, the popular media offer extensive anecdotal evidence of the daily hardships that must be endured by the homeless. Human interest stories abound in newspapers about individuals and families who live in their vehicles, in abandoned buildings, and on the street, not to mention the associated problems of petty crime, prostitution, abuse, panhandling, and begging. For the most part, publicity centers on the plight of urban homelessness. Even more interesting is that some who live on the street and in subterranean areas of cities do not refer to themselves as homeless. Rather, they refer to themselves as people without houses and report having a home, though in a rather nontraditional sense.

Given the vague nature of homelessness, how is it officially defined? In 1987, the Stewart B. McKinney Homeless Assistance Act (Public Law No. 100-77) described homelessness as a lack of shelter and a homeless person as someone who lacks a fixed, regular, and adequate nighttime residence (National Coalition for the Homeless [NCH], 1987, 1989; National Institute of Mental Health [NIMH], 1992). Using the preceding criteria, in 1987 the Bureau of the Census (1994) estimated that there were between 500,000 and 600,000 homeless. Of these, the rural homeless constitute 7%. To glean some insights into why this is a hidden population in rural communities, homelessness should be defined in broader terms than simply not having a fixed place of residence. For example, the definition should also include individuals temporarily staying in shelter-affiliated housing, with friends or relatives, in informal church-sponsored arrangements, in vehicles, in improvised shelters (e.g., storage sheds, garages), or in vacated farm buildings. Other overlooked rural homeless are those who stay in a tent or camper in an isolated area and families who are facing farm foreclosure and imminent eviction from their home. It is important to stress that these estimates exclude more than 2 million rural people who live in substandard housing (First, Toomey, & Rife, 1990).

The definition of homelessness is blurred by the growing numbers of transient homeless people who view their situation as temporary. They travel the highways seeking steady employment, while barely eking out a subsistence with part-time or casual labor. Transient people are not categorized among the homeless, nor are they migrant or seasonal workers (Chapter 7). Hence, they do not fit into any precise statistical category. Largely, the transient homeless often are featured in stories in small-town newspapers. These distressing reports often focus on the plight of a family living in their vehicle and going from town to town as they seek to improve their life situation. Even though they are not categorized as homeless according to federal definition, they remain poorly and insecurely housed. The above examples reinforce some demographers' views that the rural homeless probably are significantly undercounted.

DESCRIBING THE RURAL HOMELESS

The homeless often are portrayed in stereotypes, such as the substance abuser sleeping on an open grate; the panhandler soliciting money in a business district; the disheveled middle-aged man wearing army fatigues standing in the midst of an intersection with a placard stating, "Vietnam veteran—willing to work for food"; the deinstitutionalized bag lady; and the runaway teenager hitching a ride to an undetermined destination. These are well-recognized images that, for the most part, are associated with the urban homeless. The rural homeless in America include families with children, children who have been abandoned and runaways, single women and female heads of households, migrant and seasonal farmworkers, elderly and mentally ill people with no one to care for them, and veterans. Images of the rural homeless are either absent or poorly defined (Foster, 1993; Gladden, 1991; Preston & Child, 1997; Sobel, 1998).

Compared to the urban homeless, the rural homeless include a larger proportion of the working (near) poor, whites, and women with children. The percentage of intact two-parent families is greater. Adult men among them are more likely to have been recently employed but less likely to have served time in the military or a correctional institution. They are less visible, often living out of a vehicle in a public parking lot, in a "borrowed" camper parked in the yard of a friend or relative, or in a tent located in an isolated setting. "Family" is a recurrent theme among these hidden homeless, yet its role and impact in a rural context are not fully understood. Compared to metropolitan areas, rural counties report that persons are homeless for a shorter time. Family dissolution and marital conflicts are the most often cited reasons for their current housing situation. The incidence of chronic drug and alcohol abuse also seems to be lower among the rural homeless than among their urban counterparts.

It is important to emphasize that there are regional variations in the incidence and demographic features of the homeless. Because of recent urban-to-rural population changes, existing data probably are outdated. In rural communities located in warmer climates, one is more likely to see homeless people in public places such as national parks, hitchhiking along the highway, or going through the dumpster of a restaurant. This may not be the case in northern states, especially during the colder season. Some leave their community to find work, all the while living in their one possession, a vehicle. These living arrangements make it difficult if not impossible to count or track rural persons who are without homes. Shelters virtually are nonexistent in rural areas, and homeless persons are less likely to congregate at predictable sites. Moreover, the curious subculture of the homeless with its primitive informal support system does not have a similar counterpart in agriculture-dependent counties.

Rural communities tend to be tight-knit, with many of the residents sharing an intergenerational history and a tradition of mutual aid and cooperation. Consequently, a dislocated family may temporarily take up residency with extended family, friends, or coworkers. Sometimes the homeless family spends a few days, weeks, or even months at one place, then moves on to another in order to disperse the burden. Anecdotal reports indicate that in small towns the faith community (congregation) often becomes the first resort for its needy families. This may involve several families informally agreeing to care for members in the congregation who need assistance. Or local residents may be aware of abandoned farmsteads or seasonal vacation homes for temporary refuge. Sometimes these are inhabited with the proprietor's knowledge but often without prior approval. Of families facing farm foreclosure, some continue living in their house until the property is sold and wait for an eviction notice. Others take to the road in search of a job, living in their car but regarding their homeless situation as temporary. Precariously, the family may survive on wages from low-paying odd jobs or seasonal work provided by one of the adults in combination with charity offered to them by private and public entities. A significant percentage of the rural homeless use camping facilities as temporary living sites. In particular, at one campground located in a national park, more than half of those who were at the site during one particular time indicated that they were homeless and in search of a job (NRHA, 1996; Patton, 1988). It is highly unlikely that these campers are counted by the Bureau of the Census in the category of "homeless."

Health issues affecting the homeless are numerous, and their nursing care needs will vary from one shelter to another and from community to community. Individually and as a group, health problems and nursing care needs of homeless persons are influenced by genetic, demographic, behavioral, and environmental factors, such as season, climate, geographic location, and terrain. Common health problems and nursing needs that are cited in the literature on homeless populations are summarized in Table 9.1. This is not to say that every homeless person experiences all of these conditions, and there are regional variations. For example, strep throat may be more prevalent in children living in the intermountain area, scabies on an Indian reservation, and hypertension in the black elderly. Compared to the general population, the nurse can expect to encounter a higher prevalence of substance abuse, tuberculosis, HIV/AIDS, hepatitis, and chronic mental illness among the homeless, whether they are rural or urban.

CONTRIBUTING FACTORS

Homelessness is not the result of one or even a few factors. Rather, it is a human outcome of multiple factors that interact in complex ways, creating additional risks and perpetuat-

TABLE 9.1 Common Health and Nursing Concerns of the Rural Homeless

Vision-related problems	Lost, broken glasses
	Old prescriptions
	Not having the money to see the eye doctor
	Eye infections
Dental-related problems	Caries
	Abscesses
	Periodontal disease
	Broken missing teeth/dentures

Nutrition-related concerns

➢ Malnutrition
➢ Anemia
➢ Obesity
➢ Iron deficiency anemia
➢ Hunger

Psychological-emotional disorders

Diagnosed mental illness

➢ Schizophrenia
➢ Personality disorders
➢ Bipolar depression
➢ Eating disorders
➢ Anxiety disorders

Undiagnosed mental health problems/illness

➢ Depression
➢ Insomnia
➢ Anxiety
➢ Attention deficit disorders
➢ Learning disorders

Substance use/abuse/dependency

➢ Mind-altering street drugs
➢ Over-the-counter medications
➢ Alcohol
➢ Prescription medications

Chronic health concerns

Hypertension

➢ Undiagnosed
➢ Uncontrolled: essential and secondary

Diabetes mellitus

➢ Types I and II

Gastric disorders

➢ Duodenal ulcers
➢ Cirrhosis/pancreatitis (alcohol related)

Cardiovascular problems

➢ Arrhythmias
➢ Coronary artery disease
➢ Congestive heart failure

Respiratory disorders

➢ Asthma
➢ Bronchitis

Neurologic problems

➢ Seizure disorders
➢ Noncompliance/side effects of psychotropic medications
➢ Parkinson's disease
➢ Alzheimer's disease

(Continued)

TABLE 9.1 Continued

Infections	Sexually transmitted
	➢ Chlamydia
	➢ Herpes
	➢ Gonorrhea/Syphilis
	➢ Pediculosis pubis
	➢ HIV/AIDS
	➢ Hepatitis
	Upper respiratory
	➢ Colds
	➢ Influenza
	➢ Tuberculosis
	Eyes (conjunctivitis)
	Ears (otitis)
	Skin/bone infections (chronic)
	Genitourinary
Musculoskeletal and integumentary system disorders	Dermatologic
	➢ Idiopathic rashes/infections
	➢ Allergies
	➢ Diaper rashes
	➢ Impetigo
	➢ Herpes
	Burns
	➢ First and second degree
	Frostbite
	➢ Feet, fingers, toes
	Trauma (often alcohol related due to falls or domestic violence)
	➢ Blunt trauma
	➢ Fractures
	➢ Lacerations
	Miscellaneous
	➢ Scabies
	➢ Pediculosis
	➢ Athlete's foot
	➢ Ringworm
	➢ Thrush
	➢ Hepatitis
	➢ Typhoid
Social and developmental concerns	Behavior disorders
	➢ School-related problems
	➢ Erratic attendance
	➢ Failure to thrive
	➢ Failure in school
	➢ Attention deficit disorders
	➢ Depression/anxiety
	➢ Enuresis
	➢ Sexual abuse

TABLE 9.1 Continued

Education-counseling needs	Health promotion—age and situation dependent
	Anticipatory guidance—age and situation dependent
	Illness prevention—age and situation dependent
	Modification of lifestyle behaviors
	➤ Incomplete immunizations
	➤ Growth and development
	➤ Parenting skills
	➤ Minor health problems/emergencies
	➤ Nutrition
	➤ Birth control
	AIDS/HIV
	➤ Hepatitis
	Medications
	➤ Monitoring
	➤ Procuring
	➤ Effects/side effects
Legal issues	Financial counseling
	Legal assistance
Pregnancy-related issues	Undiagnosed pregnancy
	Genitourinary problems
	➤ Infections
	➤ Trauma
	Diabetes
	➤ Undiagnosed
	➤ Uncontrolled
	Substance use/abuse/dependency
	➤ Alcohol
	➤ Smoking
	➤ Mind-altering drugs
	➤ Caffeine
	➤ Over-the-counter medications
	Family planning
	Domestic violence
	➤ Issues/intervention
	Nutrition
	➤ Inadequate
	➤ Malnutrition
	➤ Education needs

ing vulnerability (Chapter 6). Again, the web-of-causation framework is helpful to identify factors that contribute to homelessness. Likewise, Dunkin's framework described in Chapter 5 of this book is useful for developing interventions that are appropriate for rural populations.

Fragile Economies

Poverty, associated with shifting economic infrastructures, is a recurrent theme among homeless persons. The continuing decline of the family farm coupled with low prices for agricultural products affects most people in a small town and is often reported as the precipitating cause of homelessness. (Refer to Chapter 8 for additional information on the signs and symptoms associated with farm stress.) Even though less than 2% of Americans live on farms, fragile economic infrastructures often are negatively or positively affected by that industry. In small towns, "main street businesses" are indirectly and often directly affected by the region's predominant industries, whether timber, agriculture, fishing, mining, manufacturing, or tourism. Persistently lower-than-average median family income and stagnating economies contribute to rural people's becoming homeless. Family dissolution, drug and alcohol abuse, deinstitutionalization of the mentally ill, and earlier release from correctional facilities are other causes. The homeless situation is further intensified by inadequate support networks and financial resources in sparsely populated rural states. Along with enhancing social and health care services, creating new jobs with living wages is critical for dealing with rural homelessness (NRHA, 1996).

Housing Situations

In rural communities, the available housing situation contributes to the homeless phenomenon. Shelter facilities, usually associated with urban homelessness, are virtually nonexistent in rural communities because building and maintaining these on a per capita basis are not cost-effective. Elected officials of small towns, already in economic straits, may be reluctant to offer generous benefits for fear of becoming magnets for the homeless. Affordable housing, especially rental properties, is especially difficult for the poorest of the poor to obtain. Nationally, the vacancy rates in nonmetro areas are twice (16%) those of metro areas (8%). Careful analysis reveals that rural vacancies are not really "vacant"; rather, these holdings are for seasonal, recreational, or occasional use by tourists, vacationers, or migrant workers. Essentially, in metro areas, housing vacancies are more likely than in nonmetro areas to be rental units (39% vs. 15%) (NIMH, 1992; Ohio Department of Health, 1985). The Agency of Housing and Urban Development (HUD) reports that nearly half of all rural minorities (about 1.4 million) live in substandard housing and that many of them pay more than one third of their annual income for it (NIMH, 1992).

Veterans' Issues

Veterans, in particular those of the Vietnam era, are another segment of the homeless population who often must deal with some additional challenges in remote rural areas (Loy, 1997; Mooneyhan, 1997; NCH, 1987, 1989; NIMH, 1992). It is not unusual for this group of homeless men to have a dual diagnosis, that is a posttraumatic stress disorder along with substance dependency. They often have problems in accessing Department of Veterans Affairs (VA) services due to the distance. Veterans' needs may include food, shelter, clothing, transportation, safety, and security. Furthermore, their basic sub-sistence needs cannot always be met by personnel in VA-sponsored clinics. To better ad-dress the needs of rural veterans, increasingly the VA is contracting with providers in the private and public sector within rural catchment areas to provide essential services to veterans. Likewise, VA Vietnam Veterans Outreach Centers (Vet Centers) provide read-justment counseling to veterans and, in some cases, their families.

Chronic Mental Illness

A significant segment of the homeless are mentally ill. Therefore, health profession-als and policy makers alike must address the special needs of this group (Chapter 8). Of the more than 600,000 adults who are homeless on any given night, about one third are suffering from severe mental illness. Of the homeless mentally ill, between 10% and 15% are schizophrenic, and at least as many have manic depressive disorders. Untreated, mental disorders can cloud thoughts, sap motivation, and turn a person's emotions into engines of terror, rage, and despair. Severe mental illness often means a lifelong waxing and waning of symptoms for afflicted persons and their families. Chronic mental illness affects virtually every aspect of a person's life. Significant numbers of these individuals have problems with self-care, money management, education, work, family relation-ships, and social interactions, and those with children face a multitude of parenting chal-lenges. Most of the debilitating symptoms could be managed with ongoing treatment and rehabilitation, but many chronic mentally ill persons resist pharmaco-medical inter-ventions.

The mentally ill suffer from additional burdens that exacerbate the symptoms that sustain homelessness. Foremost are the lack of an adequate income, diminished social support, and the frequent presence of alcohol and/or other drug-related problems. Con-tributing factors are lack of affordable and appropriate housing, continuous medical treatment, fragmentation of services, stigma, community resistance, discrimination, and limited resources. Outreach treatment for homeless mentally ill persons who are of a ra-cial or ethnic minority is further hampered by cultural and language barriers (Chapter 7). Once housed, many lack adequate support systems to sustain community living and pre-vent another lapse into homelessness. Helping the chronic and severely mentally ill to es-cape the plight of homelessness entails multidisciplinary efforts to improve nearly every dimension of life (Lemal, 1998; NIMH, 1992; Wagner, Menke, & Cicone, 1994).

Availability of Resources

A continuum of services for homeless persons is needed, including emergency shel-ters, rehabilitation services, and permanent housing. In other words, once immediate shelter is provided, attention must focus on finding a job and addressing work/life skill deficits that sustain chronic dependency. Table 9.2 lists potential resources for the needy and homeless that are available in many, if not most, rural communities. Lack of support services contributes to extended homelessness. In particular, the rural poor may encoun-ter culturally based obstacles when seeking assistance, such as the stigma associated with accepting charity and publicly funded resources. Associated with this view is the

TABLE 9.2 Potential Resources for the Homeless in Rural Environments

Needs	Resources and Strategies to Help Address Needs
Eyeglasses	Lions Club and some church groups recycle glasses Some optical retail outlets/franchises donate glasses Local ophthalmologist and optometrists may volunteer services for indigent eye care Health department may provide screening for children Department of Veterans Affairs
Child care	Local church, women's group may provide occasional services Human service departments may arrange temporary foster care in case of emergencies Become familiar with state policies regarding under what circumstances children can be reunited with parents after their situation is stabilized
Transportation	Become familiar with local transportation services for the needy and disabled (e.g., local health care facilities, outreach services to/from agencies) Some area transit systems offer discounted monthly passes for the homeless; in these cases, promote a bus ticket donation drive in community Church groups and/or veterans' service organizations may provide transportation service (e.g., Baptist church provides transportation for parish members, AMVETS, Legion Club, VFW, health care system van to satellite facilities, cab companies may have reduced fares for social service/health agencies)
Clothing	Identify local organizations that provide clothing (e.g., St. Vincent DePaul for families; Junior Women's League provides career clothing for women seeking employment; Christian women's groups provide newborn and infant layette) Other sources (e.g., a retail store donates school clothes to needy children; local dry cleaner collects winter coats from the community and cleans them, then donates garments to needy Veteran or fraternal organizations provide clothing for men
Advertising, marketing, employment opportunities	Use public site or bulletin board at sites where homeless may be (e.g., campgrounds, church vestibules, neighborhood grocery stores, quick-stop gas stations, fast food restaurants) to disseminate information Print notice in another language if necessary (e.g., Spanish, Laotian, Russian, Slavic) State and local employment service public service announcements on the radio/television Identify sites where homeless clients, or those without these services, can make/receive telephone calls for job contacts/interviews Remember the potential effectiveness of the informal grapevine to disseminate information to targeted homeless group Partner with local library for clients to use Internet for job searches, etc. Help clients complete job applications and resumes and identify an address to receive mail Identify/refer clients to career development programs at local schools, community colleges, and businesses (e.g., displaced homemakers' program, farmers' reeducation program, PELL grants, scholarships) When planning for community services, survey to determine local needs and priorities and the most effective way to reach targeted group
Legal	Contact local bar association to assist in identifying lawyers who may be willing to perform free legal services in emergency cases Most counties have legal aid societies/services that will provide a legal representative to low-income individuals

---

TABLE 9.2 Continued

Needs	*Resources and Strategies to Help Address Needs*
	Be familiar with state court-ordered commitment process for institutionalizing persons posing a danger to themselves or others
Housing	HUD provides funding for homeless with Supportive Housing Shelter Plans Care (Contact regional HUD representative for details) Coordinate with local churches, private citizens, hotels, and civic/service organizations for sheltering/housing the homeless Provide safety education on carbon monoxide poisoning, heat exhaustion, or frostbite for persons who live in their vehicles, tents, or campers
Food	Senior centers may prepare meals (elderly) School lunch programs (children) Local restaurants may donate a hot meal in an emergency to clients referred by a charitable organization Be familiar with the WIC and food stamp program eligibility and application process Help community organize a Second Harvest site where food can be collected, safely stored, and disseminated in an efficient manner Identify churches, service groups, and community action agencies that distribute food or food vouchers or operate food pantry
Social service referrals	Network with other social service, health care providers, and community leaders to identify a continuum of services to which the homeless can be referred Prepare a "street sheet" for select homeless groups (e.g., families, veterans) that lists community services, locations, and how to get to these Develop a database of local resources, the services each offers, to whom, location, and contact persons; disseminate to local agencies and providers who work with the homeless
Health care	Identify physicians, nurse practitioners, dentists, optometrists, social workers, and other types of health care providers who are willing to donate services to care for the indigent at a designated site (e.g., homeless clinic, nursing center) Negotiate with pharmacy to get a discounted rate for medications that are needed by the indigent Invite faculty in a nearby school of nursing, school of medicine, or other health discipline to partner with the community to provide services Establish a school of nursing–sponsored nursing center to provide services in areas where homeless come (e.g., church basement, school)

rural work ethic, with its expectation that people be self-sufficient. Inherent in this cultural value is the unwritten admonishment that an adult should be able to deal with his or her own problems. For those unable to do so, there is the fear of being stigmatized and perceived by the community as lazy, weak, immoral, incapable of taking care of oneself, or having a mental illness. The emphasis on self-sufficiency deters an unknown number of needy families from reaching out for help.

Consequently, families in dire need may be overly concerned about their reputation, especially if relatives, neighbors, or friends find out that they are seeking charity. Some distrust or fear people who get paid to work in social service agencies. Threats to anonymity and confidentiality stemming from familiarity with agency personnel are another often cited deterrent for some rural families in seeking much needed assistance. Perhaps those who suffer the greatest consequences in these cases are the children (NRHA, 1996; Rosenheck et al., 1998; Walker, 1998).

Often, community decision makers are of higher socioeconomic status and hence are oblivious to the poor and needy amongst them. Further, local and regional services may not be coordinated due to turf guarding by agency personnel. In part, this behavior is an outcome of funding allocations that are based on the number of clients who are served. Because the client base is limited in less populated regions, losing even a few clients can lead to reduced revenues for the agency or, perhaps, staff positions being eliminated. Reimbursement structures, in turn, can result in fragmented and duplicated services. Charitable and nonprofit organizations generally function independently. Consequently, one agency may not be aware of what others in the community are able to offer. To create a continuum of care despite seemingly scarce resources, formal services must partner with informal resources (Chapter 4). The goal for all partners is creatively addressing the multiple needs of homeless people in their community. Nurses will assume a variety of roles in these partnerships, including advocate, activist, educator, counselor, collaborator, expert clinician, case manager, and researcher. Table 9.3 summarizes interventions associated with the various nursing roles in responding to the needs of homeless persons and families in rural communities.

PARTNERSHIPS FOR PREVENTION

With the downsizing of the federal government, greater responsibility is being placed at the state and local levels, and interventions for dealing with homelessness vary among communities. In rural areas, this may involve creating healthier economic infrastructures along with educational opportunities to make individuals competitive in the changing job market.

Financial Counseling

Prevention of rural homelessness may also entail counseling families in financial distress and facing business foreclosure. For example, advice on income management and debt restructuring might help some farmers and small business owners to stave off bankruptcy, eviction, and perhaps even a breakup of the family unit. Considering informal social dynamics, partnerships at the local level probably are the most effective approach to prevent homelessness and respond to the rural homeless. The faith community, for instance, might be able to assume a role in earlier recognition to help at-risk families in their congregation. Volunteers with a strong business or banking background could help these families access financial counseling to prevent them from becoming home-

TABLE 9.3 Nursing Roles and Interventions for Homeless Persons in Rural Communities

Nursing Roles	Intervention Strategies
Advocate and activist	Advocate with local, state, and national lawmakers for accessible health care and social services for the needy Create awareness and mobilize the community to assist the needy in the community Consult/partner with community leaders to write proposals for grants to develop/expand/enhance local resources
Educator and counselor	Recall Maslow's hierarchy of needs—do not make assumptions about what the client may or may not know Recognize that time may not be measured in a linear fashion (hours, days, etc.) Focus on prevention and health promotion education Be compassionate, respectful, and supportive to clients Be familiar with support groups that clients can be referred to (e.g., AA, AlAnon, parenting, anger management)
Partner and collaborator	Develop a network of providers, resources, and potential referral entities Create/disseminate a database of local and nearby resources
Expert clinician and case manager	Create a trusting environment Demonstrate nonjudgmental attitude Integrate client's lifestyle and resources when planning/prescribing interventions Develop cultural and linguistic competence
Researcher	Initiate independent research activities Partner/consult with other entities in collecting data and developing interventions Utilize research findings relevant to other roles (e.g., advocate, activist, partner, collaborator, clinician, case manager, educator, counselor) Measure outcomes of existing programs/interventions Publish findings from previous activities

less. Financial institutions are assuming a greater role in offering counseling services to prevent some families from becoming destitute and homeless due to economic failure.

Promoting Community Awareness

The stigma of seeking public assistance is a definite barrier for the rural homeless; thus, many are unaware of "that problem in our little town." Unlike the urban homeless, those in rural areas tend to be lost, invisible, and not featured on the national television networks' news reports. Nurses as activists, advocates, and educators have a role in creating awareness and sensitizing people to issues surrounding homelessness. Leaders in rural communities might benefit from seminars informing them of the public and private programs that could prevent homelessness or assist the homeless among them. Awareness could extend to identifying federal and state agencies that fund programs, writing competitive grant proposals, inviting philanthropic organizations to partner with the community, and designing initiatives that respond to particular community needs. Administrators of small health-related agencies often are not aware of these resources because they are overextended by heavy client caseloads and multiple responsibilities. Multiagency databases should be quickly and easily accessible to nurses and other types of health care providers who make referrals and coordinate client care. These must be kept up to date or they will be of little use to anyone.

Essentially, the activist, advocate, education, and counseling roles are at the core of a wide range of nursing interventions, in this case focusing on the rural homeless. Urgently needed are outcome data of existing programs to develop evidence-based nursing interventions targeting rural homelessness. Nurses in the researcher role can make important contributions to meeting this need and contribute to the theoretical foundations of rural nursing.

LEGAL AND ETHICAL CONSIDERATIONS

There are multiple complex and unresolved legal and ethical issues surrounding homelessness. Often cited are the real and potential threats to the health of the public, the personal safety of homeless persons, and the allocation of scarce resources. Safety issues, for example, center on how and where to house the homeless with highly infectious diseases such as HIV/AIDS or tuberculosis. How should a community deal with persons who refuse to take medications so that they do not pose a health risk to the public? Child safety and neglect are other issues that coexist with homelessness. Who determines if, or when, children should be taken from parents and placed in foster care? How should school truancy be monitored and attendance be enforced? There also are multifaceted concerns surrounding domestic violence, abuse, and motivating adults to leave situations that may become life threatening. With respect to welfare reform, over the short term most states report that the number of people on their public assistance program has declined. Though at first such reports seem encouraging, what is the long-term impact on poor people, and is homelessness being perpetuated? How is this affecting the children in these families now and their likelihood of becoming contributing members to our society? Do the outcomes differ among families in rural and urban settings? How do informal networks fit into this highly complex societal equation? (Chapter 17 expands on rural ethical issues.)

Because little is known about rural homelessness, a multitude of research questions emerge about this phenomenon. The most obvious question is whether rural homelessness merits particular treatment or whether it merely is part of a national problem. Considering features of the health care delivery, should policy developers make distinctions between rural and urban homelessness? Are certain interventions better suited for the rural or the urban homeless? There are no definitive answers to the many questions. Empirical data are needed to support the implementation of policy for rural homeless families and to formulate nursing interventions to meet their pressing health care needs. (Chapter 18 expands on nursing research related to the rural phenomenon.)

SUMMARY

This chapter highlighted issues associated with rural homelessness. The absence of data poses challenges to developing nursing interventions for this group that are ethically and legally sound. As partners, health care providers in general, nurses in particular, researchers, policy makers, and the rural community must deal with the many factors that contribute to homelessness.

DISCUSSION QUESTIONS

Interview a public nurse who works with the rural homeless.

➢ What referral services are most often used?
➢ What resources are most needed?
➢ Describe the rewards and challenges of working with homeless and very poor people.
➢ How does the nurse remain hopeful in the midst of despair and suffering?
➢ Elaborate on effective partnerships that have enhanced services for the homeless.
➢ Discuss real and potential legal and ethical issues.
➢ Describe welfare reform initiatives in your state.
➢ What has been the impact on rural communities?
➢ Has any group in particular been affected: for example, single mothers with children, displaced homemakers, single men?
➢ Are there data to indicate welfare reform's short-term outcome on homelessness and health care in the state?

SUGGESTED RESEARCH ACTIVITIES

Describe how rural faith-based communities assist needy congregation members.

➢ How are homeless families cared for? Identify common themes in comments of interviewees. How do these fit with the conceptual development of a rural nursing theory? Disseminate your findings.
➢ Describe rural homelessness in your county. What are the most common health problems of this targeted group? How do they describe their resources and the greatest challenges to overcoming their life situation? How does the family access health care services? Describe their most recent experience with the health care delivery system. Disseminate your findings.

The following are Internet sites that you can use to find out more about the homeless in America:

> Health Care for the Homeless Resource Center: http://www.nhchc.org
> Policy Research Associates, Inc.: http://www.prainc.com
> National Coalition for the Homeless: http://nch.ari.net
> National Institute of Mental Health: http://www.nimh.gov
> National Rural Health Association: http://nrharural.org

REFERENCES

Acquaviva, T., & Lancaster, J. (1999). Poverty and homelessness. In M. Stanhope & J. Lancaster (Eds.), *Community health nursing: Promoting health of aggregates, families and individuals*. St. Louis, MO: C. V. Mosby.

American Public Health Association (APHA). (1997). Featuring homelessness. *American Journal of Public Health, 87*(2), entire issue.

Bureau of the Census. (1994). *Statistical abstract for the United States: 1994*. Washington, DC: Author.

First, R., Toomey, G., & Rife, J. (1990). *Preliminary findings on rural homelessness in Ohio*. Columbus: Ohio State University Press.

Foster, C. (Ed.). (1993). *Homelessness in America*. Wylie, TX: Information Plus.

Gladden, J. (1991). Homelessness. A rural perspective. In A. Bushy (Ed.), *Rural nursing* (Vol. 1, pp. 375-393). Newbury Park, CA: Sage.

Johnson, N. (Ed.). (1997). Featuring homelessness [Special issue]. *American Journal of Public Health, 87*(2).

Lemal, C. (1998). *Access to prenatal care for immigrant women in Georgia: A study of the effect of welfare reform on eligibility for prenatal care services: A report to the State Office of Rural Health and Primary Care and the Georgia Mutual Assistance Association Consortium* (Pub. No. 9377). Augusta, GA: National Council for State Legislatures.

Loy, M. (1997). Rural veterans: Outreach and treatment. *Vet Center, 18*(2), 2-6.

Mooneyhan, R. (1997). Homeless veterans case study review. *Vet Center, 18*(1), 2-7.

National Coalition for the Homeless. (1987). *Rural homelessness in America: Appalachia and the South*. Washington, DC: Author.

National Coalition for the Homeless. (1989). *American nightmare: A decade of homelessness in the United States*. Washington, DC: Author.

National Institute of Mental Health. (1992). *Outcasts on main street: Report of the Federal Task Force on Homelessness and Severe Mental Illness* (Pub. No. ADM 92-1904). Washington, DC: U.S. Department of Health and Human Services, Interagency Council on the Homeless.

National Rural Health Association. (1996). *The rural homeless: America's lost population*. Kansas City, MO: Author.

Ohio Department of Health. (1985). *Homelessness in Ohio: A study of people in need*. Columbus, OH: Author.

Patton, L. (1988). The rural homeless. In National Academy of Sciences (Eds.), *Homelessness, health and human needs*. Washington, DC: Academy Press.

Preston, D., & Child, L. (1997). *Reliquary*. New York: Tom Doherty Associates, Inc.

Ratnesar, R. (1999, February 8). Not gone, but forgotten. *Time, 153*(5), 30-31.

Rosenheck, R., Morrissey, J., Lam, J., Calloway, M., Johnson., H., & Goldman, F. (1998). Service system integration: Access to services and housing outcomes in a program for homeless persons with severe mental illness. *American Journal of Public Health, 88,* 1610-1616.

Sobel, R. (1998, August 10). Fearsome madness. *U.S. News and World Report, 125*(6), 53-54.

Wagner, J., Menke, E., & Cicone, J. (1994). The health of rural homeless women with young children. *Journal of Rural Health, 10*(1), 49-57.

Walker, C. (1998). CE credit: Homeless people and mental health. *American Journal of Nursing, 98*(11), 26-35.

CHAPTER 10

HIV/AIDS

The Silent Enemy Within Rural Communities

KEY TERMS

➢ Faith community
➢ Volunteers
➢ Parish nursing
➢ Persons living with HIV/AIDS (PLWAs)
➢ TB-NET

OBJECTIVES

After reading this chapter, you will be able to

➢ Highlight trends related to HIV/AIDS in rural compared with urban communities.
➢ Analyze rural social and cultural factors that can affect a community's response to persons living with HIV/AIDS.
➢ Develop strategies to enhance services for persons living with HIV/AIDS in communities with scarce or nonexistent resources.
➢ Examine the role of the faith community in the prevention, treatment, and control of the HIV/AIDS epidemic.

ESSENTIAL POINTS TO REMEMBER

➢ Of all the HIV/AIDS cases in our nation, 64% are from major metropolitan areas and the other 36% are from nonmetro areas. Newly reported HIV/AIDS cases in the United States are increasing in the rural South among young people, African Americans, Hispanics, and women. The continued and rapid spread of HIV/AIDS in rural areas probably is due to the failure of current prevention efforts.
➢ Racism, homophobia, and stigmatization are detrimental to preventing HIV/AIDS and getting at-risk rural individuals tested and into treatment for it.

Nurses' attitudes about the disease often reflect community perspectives because they have similar values.

➢ It can be difficult for a specialist to keep up with the latest treatment for HIV/AIDS. Rural nurses must stay informed through newsletters, the Internet, and conferences to provide quality care to persons living with AIDS (PLWAs).

OVERVIEW

Human immunodeficiency virus (HIV) and the associated autoimmune deficiency syndrome (AIDS) are growing global concerns that are increasing the demands on health care providers. This chapter compares rural and urban epidemiologic trends of HIV/AIDS, highlights barriers to care, and presents nursing strategies to enhance care for rural persons living with AIDS (PLWAs). It is important to comment on the choice of terms in this chapter. Recently, at a national conference, one professional, in sharing his lived experiences, asked participants to consider using the term *persons living with AIDS* rather than *persons with AIDS* (PWAs) to emphasize that AIDS is now, with proper treatment, an illness that people can manage and live with over the long term. Hence, the use of his suggested term in this chapter.

EPIDEMIOLOGIC TRENDS

HIV/AIDS was first reported in the early 1980s and became an epidemic in major cities during the next decade. The epidemic is now spreading to rural areas. Though numbers seem relatively low, there is evidence that, compared with large standard metropolitan statistical areas (SMSAs, areas with a population of 50,000 or more; see Chapter 2), HIV/AIDS is more rapidly increasing in small SMSAs (population of 50,000 to 500,000) and non-SMSAs (population of less than 50,000). Between 1991 and 1992, there was a dramatic increase of AIDS in non-SMSAs (9.4%) compared with small SMSAs (3.3%) and large SMSAs (3.1%) (Centers for Disease Control [CDC], 1995a, 1995b, 1998a, 1998b). From 1982 to 1984, the 25 counties with the highest rates of newly diagnosed cases of HIV/AIDS had an average population of 1.1 million. That trend changed between 1988 and 1990, when the 25 counties with the highest rate of increase in newly diagnosed HIV/AIDS cases were primarily rural, with an average county population of 73,000 (CDC, 1998a, 1998b).

The South is experiencing the most rapid growth of HIV/AIDS cases. There were 86,462 AIDS cases reported in the South from 1993 to 1995, a 31% increase from the previously reported 65,926 cases. Of all adolescent and young adult PLWAs (ages 13-29 years), 27% were living in small SMSAs and non-SMSAs at the time of diagnosis. Residents of small SMSAs and non-SMSAs accounted for one third of the cases attributable to male-to-male sexual contact (Berry, 1993). This is an interesting statistic in light of the conservative religious belief system usually associated with the south's "Bible belt," which admonishes persons engaging in this behavior. The South also has a higher percentage of female PLWAs who come from rural areas. Specifically, in 1994, of all the female cases of newly diagnosed HIV/AIDS, women in the rural South accounted for 10% compared to a national rate of 6%. In the South, PLWAs are more likely to be female, heterosexual, and nonwhite (Bushy, 2000; Gwinn & Wortley, 1996; Holmes et al., 1997; National Rural Health Association [NRHA], 1997, 1998).

Incomplete data about rural populations again are a confounding factor when examining rural epidemiologic trends of HIV/AIDS. Other than cumulative totals for non-SMSAs, the CDC does not publish rural statistics in its surveillance reports. In fact, it was not until 1991 that the CDC first began differentiating by small SMSA and non-SMSA counties. The problem is compounded by individual states' reporting mechanisms of rural data on HIV/AIDS. Essentially, the manner in which data are reported is influenced by a state's testing policies (i.e., anonymous, confidential) and approaches to notifying partners and case finding. Furthermore, rural residents may be more likely to travel to urban areas for HIV testing due to community-related confidentiality issues. There also is evidence that rural residents are less likely to seek HIV testing (Berry, 1993; Berry, McKinney, & McLain, 1996; Davis, Cameron, & Stapelton, 1992; Dimick, Levenson, Manteuffel, & Donnellan, 1996; Fuszard, Sowell, Hoff, & Waters, 1991; Graham, Forester, Wysong, Rosenthal, & James, 1995; Mainous & Matheny, 1996; Mainous, Neill, & Matheny, 1995).

There are conflicting reports as to the actual number of PLWAs who become infected in cities and subsequently return to their rural homes of origin for care versus becoming infected in a rural area and traveling to an urban provider for state-of-the-art treatment. Some travel more than 2 hours to obtain medical care because they lack confidence in local providers or are unable to find a local physician who will see them. Many are fearful of the personal consequences associated with hometown social dynamics. Confidentiality issues can also hinder prevention programs. Testing for HIV, discussing sexual practices with a clinician, obtaining treatment for HIV/AIDS, or even buying condoms in a local store are all important HIV prevention activities. However, those infection prevention behaviors can be difficult to engage in *confidentially* when most of the local residents know each other (Hitt, 1998; Wislowski, Andrulis, & Martin, 1992).

Recently, substantial numbers of cases have come to the surface in rural America. However, it is very difficult to determine the exact number of persons who migrate to rural areas after they have been diagnosed elsewhere with the condition. Dr. Mark Colomb emphasizes that in-migration explains only part of the rural HIV/AIDS epidemic: "Not only do we see people coming home; it also is homegrown. You don't have to leave a place like Macon, Ga., or Tupelo, Miss., to get infected. You can be a lifelong resident and get it right here" (quoted in NRHA, 1998, p. 10).

Further, there is a strong association between rates of sexually transmitted diseases (STDs) and HIV seroprevalence. For example, Alabama, Georgia, Mississippi, North Carolina, and South Carolina rank among the top 10 states for both gonorrhea and primary and secondary syphilis rates. Many of the current HIV/AIDS cases in these states can be traced to the syphilis epidemic in the late 1980s. Therefore, prevention education about STDs also is important, as it is a comorbidity factor in HIV/AIDS (Bushy, 2000; NRHA, 1997, 1998).

AT-RISK GROUPS

All people are at some risk for the disease, but certain groups are especially vulnerable: minorities, women, men having sex with other men, and children. In rural areas, these groups often experience additional concerns in trying to access services to diagnose and treat the disease. Two groups pose particular problems in rural areas: recently released prisoners and migrant farmworkers with HIV/AIDS (Berry et al., 1996; Bushy, 2000; NRHA, 1997, 1998). The first group, prisoners on antiretroviral therapy, generally are released with a month's supply of medication. Upon discharge, they are not referred to another agency for follow-up care and medical management of the disease. Likewise, migrant farmworkers, upon being diagnosed with HIV/AIDS in a migrant health clinic, usually are started on antiretroviral therapy. As they migrate from one area to another, following seasonal crop production, they find that in another state they may not be eligible for medication assistance. Or it may take time to complete the extensive paperwork to become eligible, and by that time they have moved on. Both groups are difficult to track and monitor, and it is difficult to coordinate an array of essential and continuing health-related services. Life span for these two groups is much shorter than for others with HIV/AIDS because of challenges in managing its multitude of chronic opportunistic diseases.

One solution may be to develop a portable medical record system that ensures continuity follow-up care for the two groups. A tracking system for HIV/AIDS could be patterned after the National Tuberculosis Network (TB-NET) that is used with migrant workers who move from one state to another. The system monitors infected persons, their prescribed medications, and any resistance patterns (Nist, 1996). For ex-prisoners with HIV/AIDS, such a tracking system would need to be coordinated by correctional facilities with other public health agencies. For migrant workers, coordination efforts would be needed between migrant health clinics and homeless clinics. Needless to say, an array of ethical and legal issues surrounding confidentiality and anonymity would need to be addressed before implementing any kind of HIV/AIDS tracking system.

SOCIAL ISOLATION

Social isolation is a major concern among rural PLWAs. Traditionally, rural residents have relied on informal networks of family members, neighbors, and friends for transportation, financial assistance, temporary housing, and emotional support. Unfortunately, the stigma surrounding HIV/AIDS and the behaviors that put people at risk for the disease have prevented many who are infected from seeking care. Social norms in rural communities can make it extremely difficult for a PLWA to self-disclose, as reflected in this poignant remark:

> A small community can be a really wonderful thing, and it can be very supportive, but the opposite side of that is that if someone doesn't conform to their community [standards] it can be an incredibly terrible thing. In an urban area, there are places to hide. In

rural areas, there's no place to hide; so we need to understand what that means [to the PLWA] and how we can deliver services in that environment. (W. Goldstein, quoted in NRHA, 1998, p. 26)

The experience of social isolation is further illustrated by the case of a young male dance instructor in a smaller town in the South who hid his homosexuality and HIV/AIDS diagnoses for more than 5 years. Mostly, he was afraid of being fired, so he became isolated from his students, who were older women, a highly religious and conservative population. Eventually it became necessary to reveal his diagnosis and lifestyle to explain the frequent absences. Upon disclosure, he was overwhelmed by the unfailing support and expressions of love and concern provided by this unlikely group of adult students ([name withheld], personal communication, May 1997). Personally knowing an individual who is infected with HIV can change others' attitudes and behaviors. Rural communities across the country are being confronted with the fact that their sons, daughters, and parents are infected with HIV. Attitudes must change for support to be provided to loved ones with the disease, especially in small and conservative towns. The greatest challenge for rural nurses is to change negative attitudes and stereotypes about HIV/AIDS in their own community (Heckman, Somolai, Kelly, Stevenson, & Galdabini, 1996).

ACCESS TO SERVICES AND PROVIDERS

In the United States, health-related services for HIV/AIDS have evolved in relation to local circumstances. In frontier states, for instance—areas of Idaho, Montana, Wyoming, Colorado, and the Dakotas—PLWAs often must drive hundreds of miles for treatment. Here one finds few physicians who are trained or willing to offer those kinds of services. Communities in these regions are unable to establish cost-effective programs because the actual numbers of HIV/AIDS cases have been small. A seemingly low number of cases contributes to the social isolation experienced by rural PLWAs, especially in less populated frontier areas (Bushy, 2000; Carwei, Sabo, & Berry, 1993; NRHA, 1997, 1998). Transportation often is a problem because rural bus and taxi services are quite limited and many PLWAs do not own a vehicle or are unable to drive. This can pose challenges to someone who is very ill and weakened by a multitude of opportunistic diseases. To address these concerns, some rural health care providers are partnering with local service organizations and faith communities (religious congregations) to coordinate volunteer transportation. Yet providers report that if and when they can find volunteers, their clients are reluctant to ride along because they do not want other localities to know about their HIV/AIDS status. Transportation infrastructures also can hinder a PLWA from obtaining medications, and this can disrupt time-sensitive pharmacotherapeutic regimens. To help address client adherence issues, some states have a Drug Assistance Program that also subsidizes mailing prescriptions directly to a client's home—if he or she has an address ("Pill Burden," 1998; Sowell & Christensen, 1996). Urban-based nurses must know how to coordinate formal and informal resources for clients returning to homes in rural environments. But rural-based nurses may be in a better position to advocate for services to enhance care for PLWAs and to address their concerns about confidentiality and social isolation. Regardless of the setting, nurses should be knowledgeable about supplementary programs to prevent disruptions in care for PLWAs.

Outreach and case management services are being used on a wider scale to address the growing needs of PLWAs in rural communities and reduce fragmented care. Nurses often are involved in these activities, especially for administering and monitoring pharmacotherapeutic regimens. Working with PLWAs is a vocational calling requiring a high level of dedication and commitment on the part of the person doing it. Simply doing this job for the sake of a salary is not enough, as the emotional burnout rate is very high. Characteristics of successful caregivers of PLWAs include the ability to effectively inter-act with a population that often has a lifestyle and views that are quite different from those of the provider. Coordinating an array of core and supplementary services for rural clients in general requires case managers and outreach workers to show creativity, flexi-bility, and the ability to connect formal and informal systems of support (Bushy, in press; NRHA, 1997, 1998).

For example, outreach workers who work with men who have sex with other men face some rather unusual challenges in rural areas. Religious preferences that advocate behavior sanctions against persons having an alternative sexual orientation make it most difficult to identify individuals in this high-risk group. Yet on the basis of CDC reports, male-to-male sexual contact is a significant source of transmission of HIV in rural com-munities. When a behavior is not condoned, persons who engage in it are stigmatized. Epidemiologists speculate that a high proportion of HIV/AIDS-infected men in rural ar-eas may be bisexual: that is, married with children and engaging in secret homosexual activities. Subsequently, those behaviors are contributing to an increased incidence of heterosexual transmission of the virus in rural areas (Bushy, 2000; CDC, 1998a, 1998b; Health Resources Services Administration, 1997; NRHA, 1998).

Reaching gay and bisexual men in rural communities usually can be accomplished through their social network but may be difficult due to the secrecy associated with it. One of the more effective strategies is outreach activities to a bar or club where persons with this orientation congregate. Face-to-face activities can be augmented with leaving educational materials (brochures) in public places, such as gyms, laundromats, restrooms of a truck stop, restaurants, grain elevators, or service stations. The message is important, but so is the messenger. Some propose that the most effective educators, case managers, and advocates are PLWAs themselves. Even though community fit is impor-tant, nurses must be accepting and nonjudgmental when providing services to PLWAs, regardless of the setting. In rural areas, nurses must be especially sensitive to prejudicial community attitudes and the manner in which a PLWA responds.

The news is not all bad, however. Individuals with HIV/AIDS are living longer due to new kinds of drugs and treatment modalities. This means that an ever-increasing num-ber of PLWAs will need long-term treatment and nursing care. Correspondingly, there will be an increased demand for nurse case managers to care for these clients, and this will dramatically affect the rural health care delivery system (Bushy, 2000; NRHA, 1998). Of great concern are the excessive costs for the medications as well as for admin-istering and monitoring them. Providing care to one or two PLWAs who are indigent could bankrupt a small hospital that already was in a tenuous financial situation. Other rural health care service gaps are behavioral health counseling services and HIV medical specialties.

As for maintaining expertise, it can be difficult for an urban-based HIV medical specialist to keep up with the latest treatment protocols. The burden is even greater for general practitioners in a rural area, who must deal not only with treatment of the disease but also with a multitude of other chronic health problems. Pharmacotherapeutics for HIV/AIDS are becoming more complex and individual specific. Therefore, rural nurses must stay informed to provide quality care within the constraints of scarce resources. Sources of current information on HIV/AIDS include newsletters, journals, the Internet, and multidisciplinary continuing educational offerings.

Poverty limits access to an array of services and treatment options for PLWAs. More specifically, rural PLWAs are likely to be poor, be members of a minority group, not have public or private health insurance, and delay seeking care until the disease is in advanced stages. Therefore, when finally seeking treatment, they tend to be very ill. Hence, survival time of rural PLWAs is significantly shorter than for their urban counterparts (NRHA, 1997, 1998). Safe living arrangements are another concern for many PLWAs. The lack of transitional housing in rural communities forces some PLWAs to conceal their diagnosis in order to stay at local homeless shelters. A few live on the street, in vacant buildings, and on deserted farmsteads. Even though there are only a few homeless persons in most areas, many PLWAs in this environment live in housing that is substandard or totally inadequate (Chapter 9). To provide a continuum of ongoing care to PLWAs, partnership models of various types have been organized, such as lay volunteers and health care providers from the public and private sector (Chapter 4). Collaboration will become even more important as managed care gains a greater presence in rural America and as services become even more limited (Chapter 12).

EDUCATION

Epidemiologists speculate that the continued and rapid growth of HIV/AIDS in rural areas probably is due to failure of current education prevention efforts. The racism, homophobia, and stigmatization of persons with HIV/AIDS that prevail in many rural communities are particularly detrimental to prevention and to getting individuals tested and into treatment (Berry, 1993; Carwei et al., 1993; Hitt, 1998; Rounds, 1988; Rumley, Shappley, Waivers, & Esenhart, 1991; Sowell & Christensen, 1996). Religious barriers, homophobia, and "sex phobia" are attitudes that prevent open and candid discussions about HIV prevention in the home, school, and community. Education about HIV/AIDS must begin early on. Yet the low likelihood of offering HIV/STD education at home and in school reflects the conservatism of rural communities as a whole. The following comment by Dr. Mark Colomb reflects the experiences of many rural nurses who have attempted to provide educational offerings on STDs/HIV/AIDS to young people. "They [school administrators] say, 'I'll let you come in, but show me what you're going to talk about. Give me your entire presentation—word-for-word and *no condoms* mentioned. It has to be abstinence-based [content]'" (quoted in NRHA, 1998, p. 12).

Education on HIV/AIDS might be better accepted if content were integrated into school curricula and programs were developed by the faith community. For this reason, nurses should cultivate working relationships with school administrators, school boards, teachers, and pastors. If they know and trust the nurse, almost anything can be accomplished. Senior pastors often are gatekeepers in small communities. Moreover, members of the congregation often serve on the board and teach in local schools. It is prudent, therefore, to seek a pastor's sanction before making contact with women's and youth groups to educate about sensitive topics such as STDs/HIV/AIDS and family planning. Sometimes the minister's wife can assist in making the "right" connections to work within the community.

Health professionals in rural communities also must be educated about HIV/AIDS. Moreover, attitudes of rural health care providers concerning PLWAs often can reveal underlying attitudes of their community. In particular, nurses in a rural area, as members of the community, often share similar values and prejudices. Not being personally acquainted with a PLWA can contribute to negative and prejudicial attitudes. Continuing education can go a long way to reduce fear, anxiety, and resentment and bring about behavior changes among health professionals toward PLWAs. Guided clinical experiences and personally knowing a PLWA can lessen the fear of contagion and the perceived threat of becoming infected. Panel presentations and PLWAs sharing their stories can help to change attitudes among health professionals who previously had little if any exposure to clients with HIV/AIDS (Dimick et al., 1996).

Knowledge of the presence of a PLWA in a rural community may be the wake-up call and the first "real" opportunity for a nurse to educate the community. Before planning any HIV/AIDS education program, nurses should consider the sociocultural norms of the community (Sowell & Christensen, 1996). A wide variety of educational resources are available from government agencies and private foundations to help nurses develop the right message, in the right way, to the right group. This is reinforced by one HIV prevention coordinator in South Carolina:

> Many people are in denial. Because, if I drink a beer or get up in the morning and drink a six-pack or a case, I'm not an alcoholic and I don't have a problem. An alcoholic is the guy over on skid row who is not working and living off my tax dollars. That's the attitude that some people have. They don't perceive the person who works for one of our local industries and uses drugs on the weekend as a drug abuser. (quoted in NRHA, 1998, p. 21)

Community values affect sexual behaviors and can hinder progress of HIV/AIDS prevention education. For instance, the belief that condoms are a sign of distrust on the part of the woman is of particular concern among nurses and health educators who work with Haitian and Latino communities. For African Americans, the Tuskegee study of untreated syphilis in black males has left a lingering distrust of government and the public health system. Distrust, however, is not unique to rural areas, as African Americans in urban settings also are suspicious of the message and strategies being employed by HIV risk reduction programs (Thomas & Quinn, 1991). Less is known about Native American and Mexican American populations, but some experts report that these communities are still in denial about the occurrence of the disease in their communities (Bushy, in press; NRHA, 1998). Successful models of education efforts from urban areas simply do not work in rural populations, as these are not sensitive to and do not reflect local values:

> A poster with two very nice young men sort of kissing, with 15 earrings in their ears and a condom plastered in the middle, is not going to fly in southern Georgia. The Baptist minister will run you out of town in no time flat. Moreover, you can't do a mass media campaign when the television station that the people watch has so much snow on it [the screen] because it [transmission station] is [located] so far away. We've got cable; we've got satellite dishes, but you have to pay. Since a lot of us don't have what it takes to pay, we may not get the message. (S. Thurman, quoted in NRHA, 1998, p. 13)

Education and prevention programs for HIV/AIDS must target specific populations within rural communities. The message and intervention should be culturally appropriate for people of a different gender, race, ethnic and religious background, and sexual orientation. A nurse in the educator role must first learn about a targeted population's cultural beliefs: who the group members are and what they do. Representatives from the targeted group should be actively involved in program planning.

ENHANCING RESOURCES FOR PLWAs

The escalating numbers of PLWAs are placing great demands on national, state, and local health-related services, especially in rural communities. Volunteers are one strategy that is being used more and more often to expand staffing and resources for PLWAs. However, volunteer programs generally require extensive education, guidance, and oversight. Table 10.1 presents strategies for enhancing services for rural PLWAs. For example, for organizations having few resources, volunteers often are perceived as a way to augment scarce or nonexistent resources. Nurse managers should be aware, however, that volunteer programs can be incredibly staff and time intensive. In the long run, the payoff can be great after individuals have been trained and if they remain in the volunteer program. But reaching that level of proficiency can present significant challenges for a one- or two-person agency. The time that must be allocated by staff to start and subsequently manage volunteers can be as costly as hiring another employee. Using volunteers is not easier or cheaper. Essentially, one allocates time instead of paying someone to do a job (Aruffo, Thompson, Gottlieb, & Dobbins, 1995; Dimick et al., 1996; Djupi, 1995).

The following strategies may be useful to rural nurse administrators who are planning to use volunteers to enhance HIV/AIDS services. First, match a volunteer's interests and skills with the job to be done. Ideally, volunteers should be interviewed just as a manager would conduct an organizational employee search. Volunteers quickly become discouraged and burned out when trying to do too much and devoting extensive time to sick clients. The stress of caring for and working with PLWAs in the community is comparable to that of hospice care. Volunteers in both of these programs need ongoing emo-

TABLE 10.1 Enhancing Services for Rural PLWAs

➤ Determine which counties/areas will be served. Assess the site and immediacy of the nearest services that are similar or can augment existing services in the local region.

➤ Invite key players from these counties/areas to plan the primary care system (e.g., hospitals, public health departments, rural health clinics, primary physicians, nurse practitioners, HIV/AIDS service organizations/coalitions, other private and public entities).

➤ Determine what role(s) each member will have in the delivery model: for example, planning, implementing, financing, marketing, evaluating services.

➤ Ensure that core clinical services are supplemented by HIV/AIDS prevention education, continuing professional education, and maintenance and support services for PLWAs.

➤ Determine the cost of each service. Then decide if these can be provided at least at a breakeven rate. Consider other options, such as contracting with an urban-based provider for outreach services, purchasing a van, subcontracting with the Veterans Administration or Indian Health Service to transport clients to the clinic, or developing a volunteer or advocate program to enhance existing services.

➤ Develop and coordinate client care plans for both clinical and support services.

➤ Identify short-range and long-term funding mechanisms to continue operation of the clinic.

➤ Specify outcomes (short and long term) to assess program effectiveness and measure the quality of care and services.

➤ Delineate how professional staff will be able to maintain expertise in HIV/AIDS treatment. For example, if there is only one nurse practitioner or physician in the clinic, state what arrangements can be made for him or her to pursue continuing education that may be offered at a distant urban-based facility.

tional support, education, and debriefing sessions. If the job requirements are reasonable and there is a good fit between the person's skills and the job expectations, a volunteer is more likely to stay involved. Subsequently, satisfied volunteers often recruit friends to the program. Scheduling volunteers who also are friends at the same times is another effective retention strategy.

Acknowledge the contributions of volunteers in a manner that fits an individual's preferences. For example, some people need and prefer open and public acknowledgment in the local media or at a recognition ceremony; others prefer face-to-face feedback and dislike public accolades; and still others prefer not to have any recognition whatsoever, as they may be motivated by intrinsic spiritual beliefs. Volunteers must believe their work is valued! Clients (PLWAs), their significant others, and family members may be the best advocates for HIV/AIDS initiatives. Often they are willing to help a local organization if asked to do so and *if* their serostatus remains confidential.

Mobilize the Faith Community

With the rising incidence of HIV infection in minorities, more and more often religious congregations are assuming an active role in addressing the needs of their members and the community as a whole. Because pastors and congregational leaders often act as gatekeepers, their sanctioning a service, event, or program may be the key to gaining entrance into the community. Parish nursing programs are gaining a national prominence, and many of them are successful in disseminating prevention education for STDs/HIV/AIDS. In poor and rural areas, a congregation may not be able to afford that luxury. But volunteer nurses usually are warmly received by a parish to offer education on health promotion, illness (HIV/AIDS) prevention, blood pressure screening, and medication monitoring. To be accepted, a nurse must establish trust and rapport first with the congregation's leaders and subsequently with the membership.

Technology

Telecommunications technology also is being used to enhance services and support networks for PLWAs in remote and underserved regions. For nurses, technology is making HIV/AIDS-related information, consultation, and peer support more accessible at more convenient times. Technology also is helpful to overcome distance and transportation challenges. In instances where health professionals reflect negative or judgmental attitudes, technology cannot replace the human experience of actually knowing and working with a PLWA. Despite its convenience and even if it is more cost-effective, the Internet and other distributive-teaching learning [outreach] offerings may not be the best option for HIV/AIDS education (Hitt, 1998; NRHA, 1997, 1998).

For PLWAs in rural environments, telehealth/telemedicine technology can improve and even offer immediate access to an urban-based HIV/AIDS medical specialist. For example, some tertiary health care facilities and specialists in HIV/AIDS provide 24-hour toll-free phone service or access on the Internet. This enables clients with telephone access to have almost immediate responses to their questions regarding medications, laboratory diagnostics, or disease processes or to deal with an emotional crisis.

Toll-free telephone conferencing has been coordinated with rural clients. With this initiative, PLWAs participate in regularly scheduled support groups that are facilitated by a professional counselor. Outcomes have been favorable in helping to overcome confidentiality, geographic, and transportation barriers and also in reducing participants' sense of isolation. Another strategy to reduce social isolation for rural PLWAs is the "buddy" model. In general, this involves "buddying" two or more people to assist and provide support to each other: for example, HIV-positive African American women buddying with grandparents who are caring for grandchildren whose parent(s) died of AIDS. Such models generally are successful if clients have telephones, transportation, and the physical resources to maintain contact with their buddy.

SUMMARY

This chapter described issues surrounding the growing HIV/AIDS epidemic in rural America. Even as new drug therapies become available, PLWAs in rural and frontier areas face serious access and treatment issues. Rural health care providers in general and nurses in particular must have access to current information on preventing, diagnosing, and treating this pervasive infection. Nurses' voices must be heard by policy makers regarding this silent epidemic and the resources needed to meet the expanding needs of PLWAs in rural environments.

DISCUSSION QUESTIONS

➢ What are underlying factors for the dramatic increase of HIV/AIDS cases in rural areas? Describe strategies that are being used in your state to prevent HIV/AIDS and to enhance services for rural PLWAs. How effective are these initiatives?

➢ Partner with a rural nurse and work on one or more of these activities. Participate in or organize an HIV/AIDS fund-raising event. Organize a workshop to educate rural nurses and other health professionals about the ethical issues surrounding HIV/AIDS (education, financing services, allocation of scarce resources, experimental/trial drugs). Invite (coordinate) regional HIV/AIDS organizations that serve ethnic and racial groups to make presentations to your group. Coordinate a panel presentation on cultural competence in caring for rural PLWAs. Publish an article describing your program.

SUGGESTED RESEARCH ACTIVITIES

➢ Describe the care-seeking experiences of rural PLWAs. What happens when clients in a rural area don't want to use the local provider? What reasons do they cite for their health care-seeking behaviors (i.e., out-shopping for health care)? What health-related services do they believe are necessary to meet their needs? Identify common themes that emerge in these interviews. Disseminate the findings.

➢ Compile a listing of formal and informal HIV/AIDS-related support resources in your catchment area. Develop and then pilot-test an evaluation tool or tools to measure program and client outcomes of existing services.

REFERENCES

Aruffo, J., Thompson, R., Gottlieb, A., & Dobbins, W. (1995). An AIDS training program for rural mental health providers. *Psychiatric Services, 46,* 79-81.

Berry, D., McKinney, M., & McLain, M. (1996). Rural HIV services networks: Pattern of care and policy issues. *AIDS and Public Policy Journal, 11*(1), 35-45.

Berry, J. (1993). The emerging epidemiology of rural AIDS. *Journal of Rural Health, 9,* 293-304.

Bushy, A. (Ed.). (2000). *Rural minority health in the 21st century: Eliminating disparities. Conference proceedings for the Fourth Annual NRHA Rural Minority Conference.* Kansas City, MO: National Rural Health Association.

Carwei, V., Sabo, C., & Berry, D. (1993). HIV in traditional rural communities. *Nursing Clinics of North America, 28,* 231-239.

Centers for Disease Control and Prevention. (1995a). First 500,000 AIDS cases: United States, 1995. *Morbidity and Mortality Weekly Report, 44,* 849-853.

Centers for Disease Control and Prevention. (1995b). Update trends in AIDS among men who have sex with men: United States, 1989-1994. *Morbidity and Mortality Weekly Report, 44,* 401-404.

Centers for Disease Control and Prevention. (1998a). *HIV/AIDS surveillance report: Through June 1998.* Atlanta, GA: Author.

Centers for Disease Control and Prevention. (1998b). *Sexually transmitted disease surveillance, 1997.* Atlanta, GA: Author.

Davis, K., Cameron, B., & Stapelton, J. (1992). The impact of HIV migration to rural areas. *AIDS Patient Care, 6,* 225-228.

Dimick, L., Levenson, R., Manteuffel, B., & Donnellan, M. (1996). Nurse practitioners' reaction to persons with HIV/AIDS: The role of patient contact and education. *Journal of the American Academy of Nurse Practitioners, 8,* 419-426.

Djupi, A. (1995). Parish nursing. In E. Cohen (Ed.), *Case management in the 21st century.* St. Louis, MO: C. V. Mosby.

Fuszard, B., Sowell, R., Hoff, P., & Waters, M. (1991). Rural nurses join forces for AIDS care. *Nursing Connections, 4*(3), 51-61.

Graham, R., Forester, M., Wysong, J., Rosenthal, C., & James, P. (1995). *HIV/AIDS in the rural United States: Epidemiology and health services delivery.* Buffalo: New York Rural Health Research Center.

Gwinn, M., & Wortley, P. (1996). Epidemiology of HIV infection in women and newborns. *Clinical Obstetrics and Gynecology, 39,* 292-304.

Health Resources Services Administration. (1997, March). *AIDS Program Office: Fact sheet.* Washington, DC: Author.

Heckman, T., Somolai, A., Kelly, J., Stevenson, L., & Galdabini, K. (1996). Reducing barriers to care and improving quality of life for rural persons with HIV. *AIDS Patient Care and STDs, 10*(1), 37-43.

Hitt, S. (1998). HIV/AIDS: A growing concern for rural America. *Rural Health: FYI, 20*(3), 20-22.

Holmes, R., Fawal, H., Moon, T., Checks, J., Coleman, J., Woernle, C., & Vermund, S. H. (1997). Acquired immunodeficiency syndrome in Alabama: Special concerns for black women. *Southern Medical Journal, 90,* 697-701.

Mainous, A., & Matheny, S. (1996). Rural human immunodeficiency virus health service provision: Indications of rural-urban travel for care. *Archives of Family Medicine, 5,* 469-472.

Mainous, A., Neill, R., & Matheny, S. (1995). Frequency of human immunodeficiency virus testing among rural U.S. residents and why it is done. *Archives of Family Medicine, 4*(1), 41-45.

National Rural Health Association. (1997). *HIV/AIDS in rural America: An issue paper—November 1997.* Kansas City, MO: Author.

National Rural Health Association. (Ed.). (1998). *Southeastern Conference on Rural HIV/AIDS: Issues in prevention and treatment.* Kansas City, MO: Author.

Nist, A. (1996). Tuberculosis in farm workers. *Journal of the International Association of Physicians in AIDS Care, 2*(8), 12-19.

"Pill burden" often cause of AIDS treatment failure. (1998, July 3). *Bismarck Tribune,* p. 5A.

Rounds, K. (1988). AIDS in rural areas: Challenges in providing care. *Social Work, 33,* 257-261.

Rumley, R., Shappley, N., Waivers, L., & Esenhart, J. (1991). AIDS in rural eastern North Carolina: Patient migration: A rural AIDS burden. *AIDS, 5,* 1373-1378.

Sowell, R., & Christensen, P. (1996). HIV infection in rural communities. *Nursing Clinics of North America, 31*(1), 107-121.

Thomas, S., & Quinn, S. (1991). The Tuskegee syphilis study, 1932 to 1972: Implications for HIV education and AIDS risk education programs in the black community. *American Journal of Public Health, 8,* 1498-1505.

Wislowski, V., Andrulis, D., & Martin, V. (1992). *AIDS in rural America.* Baltimore: National Public Health and Hospital Institute.

CHAPTER 11

Rural Occupational Safety, Health, and Nursing

KEY TERMS

- ➢ Occupational Safety and Health Administration (OSHA)
- ➢ National Institute of Occupational Safety and Health (NIOSH)
- ➢ Epidemiologic triangle
- ➢ Surveillance
- ➢ Emergency medical services (EMS)
- ➢ First responder
- ➢ Agricultural health nursing
- ➢ Chemical exposure
- ➢ Pesticide drift
- ➢ Restricted entry (time interval)
- ➢ Sentinel event
- ➢ Postexposure symptoms
- ➢ Personal protective measures
- ➢ Health professional shortage areas (HPSAs)

OBJECTIVES

After reading this chapter, you will be able to

- ➢ Compare and contrast occupational morbidity and mortality rates among industries that predominate in rural settings.
- ➢ Analyze features that contribute to accidents and injuries in agricultural settings.
- ➢ Describe the roles of agricultural health nurses.
- ➢ Discuss the need for culturally appropriate educational programs that target at-risk rural occupational groups.

ESSENTIAL POINTS TO REMEMBER

➤ An initiative by the Centers for Disease Control (CDC) and the National Institute of Occupational Safety and Health (NIOSH) in 1991 led to the establishment of nine regional Centers for Agricultural Disease and Injury Research, Education and Prevention Programs. Their mission is to be responsive to the most pressing agricultural health and safety problems in their area.

➤ The etiology of diseases in rural environments fits with the *epidemiologic triangle* of agent, host, and environmental factors. A disability or serious illness directly affects the affected person and every family member, and all must adjust to it in their own way.

➤ Agricultural health nursing uses principles from community health and occupational health nursing to identify and prevent agriculturally related illnesses and injuries. Surveillance data are used to design nursing interventions that target agricultural illnesses and injuries.

OVERVIEW

This chapter examines occupational health and safety issues that occur in rural environments, primarily the agriculture industry because it does not fall under the auspices of the Occupational Safety and Health Administration (OSHA). The role and scope of an emerging occupational health specialty, agricultural health nursing, also is examined.

EPIDEMIOLOGY OF RURAL OCCUPATIONAL HAZARDS AND INJURIES

Exceedingly high-risk occupations of mining, forestry, commercial fishing, and agriculture predominantly exist in more remote regions of the nation. Mining and lumbering are highly regulated by OSHA. The regulations delineate who can, and cannot, be employed at the worksite, along with safety measures that must be in place to operate. Should an accident occur due to negligence or noncompliance, an employer can be penalized for infractions. Increasingly, the fishing industry is coming under the jurisdiction of OSHA. However, the agriculture industry is not regulated by that agency because farms and ranches tend to be family-operated enterprises with fewer than 11 paid employees (National Safety Council, 1998; Taylor, 1998). Rural communities often are financially dependent on one, perhaps two, major industries. Hence, successes and failures in the predominant industry affect the health of an entire community. Other residents provide services involving food, clothing, fuel, education, church, health care, and entertainment for persons directly engaged in the extractive industries. Consequently, in a one- or two-industry town, a special sense of community develops among residents. Likewise, an entire community is affected when one member is injured or dies in an occupation-related accident (Bull & Boyle, 1998).

Occupational injuries are a tragedy of enormous proportions in the United States. Annually, more than 2 million occupation-related injuries result in more than 75 million lost days of work. Of the 2 million injuries, from 7,000 to 11,000 result in death. Premature death results in the loss of at least 250,000 productive years of life. As compared to the death rate for all the major industrial groups (9 per 100,000), the agricultural industry rate is almost five times higher (42 per 100,000 workers). The rate for the commercial fishing industry is estimated to be from 20 to 30 times greater than for all occupations. The death rate from 1992 to 1996 was estimated to be *at least* 140 fatalities per 100,000 workers. During the last 10 years, death rates per 100,000 declined significantly in mining (78%) and construction (50%) but less so in agriculture (17%). The rate probably increased in the fishing industry due to economic forces, but data are not available on this occupational group (National Institute of Occupational Safety and Health [NIOSH], 1996, 1998a, 1998b, 1998c, 1998d).

Mining and lumbering are highly regulated by OSHA. For example, the equipment must meet rigid operation standards. As in many manufacturing plants, a safety officer is on site to deal with potential hazards. Also, there usually is someone to provide emergency care to injured employees. Individuals under or over specified ages cannot be at the worksite, and air and water quality must be monitored. Conversely, fishing and agriculture (farming/ranching) were recently listed as NIOSH priorities because of the high morbidity and mortality rates among workers in these industries. Due to space constraints, this chapter will discuss only occupational risks in agriculture.

NATIONAL INSTITUTE OF OCCUPATIONAL SAFETY AND HEALTH (NIOSH) RURAL INITIATIVE

According to NIOSH (1998a, 1998b), there are about 2 million farmers, 3 million farmworkers, and at least 6 million family members. In other words, between 10 and 11 million persons are directly or indirectly involved in agriculture. *Healthy People 2010: National Health Promotion and Disease Prevention Objectives* (U. S. Department of Health and Human Services [USDHHS], 1999) addresses farmworkers in its goals for occupational safety and health, targeting unintentional and traumatic injuries, occupational asthma, and hearing loss due to noise. An initiative by NIOSH (1991) established nine regional Centers for Agricultural Disease and Injury Research, Education and Prevention Programs to conduct research, education, and prevention projects that are responsive to their region's most pressing health and safety problems (Table 11.1) (Gerberich, Robertson, Gibson, & Renier, 1996; Jenkins & Marlenga, 1998; Jones, 1993; Petrea & Aherin, 1998).

Working with crops and animals of various types is for some a rewarding life and is an important source of employment in many communities. Of all U.S. workers, 2% work on farms; this includes both full-time and part-time farmers (13.1 million persons), farm families (6 million persons), and full-time farmworkers (3.4 million persons). Of the total agriculture workforce, approximately 2.5 million work for wages, and the majority declare nonfarm residence (80%). In other words, the farmer lives in an urban area and may hold another job besides working in agriculture. Of the total agriculture labor force, 5% are migrant workers. As for their gender and age, the majority are males (77%) who are over the age of 25 (55%), but children and women also are involved in farm-related work. With respect to the racial/ethnic composition of the agricultural labor pool, the

TABLE 11.1 NIOSH Agriculture Centers, Sites, and Program Objectives

Title and Site	Program Objectives
Pacific Northwest Agricultural Center at Seattle, Washington	Develop and conduct research related to the prevention of occupational disease and injury of agricultural workers and their families.
U.C. Davis Agricultural Health and Safety Center at Davis, California	Develop and implement model educational outreach and intervention programs promoting agricultural health and safety for agricultural workers and their families.
High Plains Intermountain Agricultural Center at Fort Collins, Colorado	Develop and evaluate control technologies to prevent illness and injuries among agricultural workers and their families.
Midwest Agricultural Center at Marshfield, Wisconsin	Develop and implement model programs for the prevention of illness among agricultural workers and their families.
Great Plains Agricultural Center at Iowa City, Iowa	Evaluate agricultural injury and disease prevention and educational materials and programs implemented by the center.
Southwest Agricultural Center at Tyler, Texas	Provide consultation and/or training to researchers, health and safety professionals, graduate/professional students, and agricultural extension agents and others in a position to improve the health and safety of agricultural workers.
Northeast Agricultural Center at Cooperstown, New York	
Southeast Agricultural Center at Lexington, Kentucky	Develop linkages and communication with other governmental and nongovernmental bodies involved in agricultural health and safety, with special emphasis on communications with CDC/NIOSH-sponsored agricultural health and safety programs.
Deep-South Agricultural Center at Tampa, Florida	

majority are white (73%), followed by Hispanics (13%) and blacks and persons of other backgrounds (14%). Regionally, the southern states have the highest percentage (40%) of farmworkers, followed by the north central states (28%) and other U.S. regions (32%). The validity of these workforce statistics is questionable, however. Demographers speculate that these data reflect only those who are employed year round and exclude casual and seasonal agricultural workers. If that is true, two thirds of all farmworkers are not included in USDA or NIOSH surveys, and high numbers of the uncounted are minorities, undocumented workers, women, and children. Few agribusiness owners or managers are of an ethnic or racial minority, but the reverse is true for hired farmworkers. Employees (farmworkers) experience additional occupational hazards because of their lack of education, limited understanding of the English language, and inadequate job safety training (NIOSH, 1998a, 1998b, 1998c, 1998d) (Table 11.2).

Accidents and Injuries

Agriculture can be an extremely dangerous occupation posing deadly risks to those involved with it. Agricultural workers are at high risk for chronic and acute conditions, including leukemia; Hodgkin's and non-Hodgkin's lymphoma, multiple myeloma and

TABLE 11.2 Common Health Problems in the Agriculture Industry

Respiratory conditions	Upper respiratory infections
	Hypersensitivity pneumonitis/bronchitis
	Pulmonary mycotoxicosis
	Occupational asthma
	Sinusitis
	Bronchitis
	Organic dust toxic syndrome
	Chemical toxicity (NO_x; H_2S; NH_3)
Agricultural chemicals toxicity (pesticides, herbicides, fungicides, fertilizers, other)	Dermatitis
	Other symptoms, dependent on chemical type; weather; duration of exposure; cost, availability, and fit of personal protective equipment (PPE); other
Mechanical trauma-induced injuries	Fractures
	Musculoskeletal disorders
	Hearing loss
	Heat/cold stress disorders
	Frostbite/burns
	Amputations
	Hypothermia
	Hyperthermia, other
Infectious diseases	Fungal, viral, bacterial, other
	Diarrheal diseases
	Tuberculosis
	Worm infestations
	HIV/AIDS
	Hepatitis
	STDs, other
Psychosocial conditions	Stress-related conditions
	Depression
	Suicide, other

cancers of the lip, skin, stomach, prostate, and brain; hearing loss; acute and chronic chemical poisoning; arthritis; respiratory infections; dermatitis; degenerative musculoskeletal syndromes; hearing loss; and a variety of stress-induced dysfunctions. Amputations and lacerations are common, especially among women, children, and the elderly. Tuberculosis, sexually transmitted diseases (STDs), and HIV/AIDS are of epidemic proportions among some migrant and seasonal farmworker communities. There also is a persistent incidence of depression in farming communities along with other behavioral health disorders.

Unlike other industries, agriculture is one of the few occupations where age does not limit participation. Still, a family-operated farm has an organizational structure similar to that of conventional industries, except that the players are of different ages. There are, however, profound risks that contribute to the occupational epidemiology in the agriculture industry. For example, children often perform the work of an adult, and senior adults (over the age of 55 years) remain actively involved in the physical labor of the farm.

These two groups are especially vulnerable and frequently fall victim to fatal accidents, serious injuries, and chronic and acute illnesses. Tragically, documented agriculture-related fatalities include children as young as 1 year of age and seniors as old as 93 years of age.

The etiology of diseases in rural environments fits with the epidemiologic triangle of agent, host, and environmental factors. *Agents* are the biological, chemical, physical, psychosocial, nutritional, and ergonomic factors that cause or contribute to occupation-related sentinel events (i.e., occurrences that are out of the ordinary or harmful in nature). *Host* factors include demographic, biological, and social traits that predispose a worker to the sentinel event or an untoward health outcome. *Environmental* factors include physical, biological, and social features that facilitate occurrence of a sentinel event (Table 11.3).

A disability or serious illness directly influences the affected person in many ways, psychologically, financially, and physically. The situation affects the entire family, and all family members must adjust in their own ways. Adjustment to a disability parallels the grief process. That is, shortly after the event there is denial, anger, and anxiety about the event and its consequences. This progresses to depression and bargaining with health professionals, family, friends, and even a Higher Power. There is no predetermined time frame for adjusting to a loss. Rather, each family progresses at its own rate, and some individuals can remain fixed in one stage for a very long time. Ultimately, healthy clients are able to integrate the event into their worldview.

The adjustment process can affect an individual's ability to safely perform activities of daily living and work. For instance, chronic depression and denial as to the seriousness of a physical or psychological limitation can cloud a farmer's judgment, leading to carelessness and risk for additional accidents. Medications taken to manage symptoms such as pain or muscle stiffness can help the person to "feel better" or even "good." Because farm activities must be done, the affected farmer may work with animals and around machinery and sometimes even drive vehicles. Impaired mental capacity increases the risks for further injury to the afflicted person as well as others in the area, often women, children, and elderly family members. Returning to work without appropriate safety or supportive devices exposes all of them to even greater occupational hazards (Boyd et al., 1997; Casey et al., 1997a, 1997b).

When an accident occurs, the person who is disabled may not be able to complete routine tasks that must be done, such as caring for animals, maintaining machinery, and performing routine activities associated with seasonal crop production. Hence, the responsibilities fall on a spouse or children. Children, in particular, often are expected to perform tasks that they never have done before, exposing them to additional hazards. The stress placed on individuals due to family role changes can be extreme. Farmers who are unable to return to work because of a disability usually experience depression, which typically accompanies unemployment. Family members are subsequently confronted with additional financial worries exacerbated by the parent's inability to work and hence to provide a stable income. Isolation, inherent in the rural lifestyle, can be aggravated because the family lives some distance from neighbors or extended family. Another dimen-

TABLE 11.3 Epidemiologic Triangle: Factors and Dimensions in Rural
Occupational Safety and Health

Factors	*Dimensions*	*Examples in Agriculture*
Agent: etiologic factor needed to cause disease or adverse health outcomes	Biological	Living organisms or their properties that can cause an adverse response in humans, such as bacteria, fungi, viruses, microorganisms and their toxins, anthropoids (crustaceans, arachnids, insects), allergens from higher plants, protein allergens from vertebrate animals (urine, feces, dander, saliva)
	Chemical	Arise from excessive airborne concentration from mists, vapors, gases, solids in the form of dust or fumes (e.g., pesticides, fertilizers)
	Physical	Include excessive levels of nonionizing radiation, noise, vibration, extremes of temperature/pressure
	Ergonomic	Include improperly designed equipment, tools, machinery, work areas, procedure; improper lifting, poor visual conditions, repetitive motions
Host: an individual, group, or population at risk for disease or adverse health outcomes	Demographic factors	Age, ethnicity, gender, level of education, literacy, occupation type, marital status, residence
	Biological traits	Health status, genetics, susceptibility, other
	Socioeconomic factors	Health habits, lifestyle, diet, exercise, smoking, not having the money to purchase safety devices for machinery
Environmental: influences the existence of the agent, exposure, or degree of susceptibility to the agent	Physical	Climate, setting, type of crop, pollution
	Biological	Factors needed for transmission/infection to occur, including wind, humidity, temperature, vector, foamite
	Social	Political, accessibility of information, government regulations

sion of isolation and avoidance for the afflicted is not having contact with others who have a similar disability. This does not allow the injured person to learn others' perspective on coping and dealing with the disability.

Farm operators usually are self-employed or part of a family operation; hence, many do not have health insurance coverage. If they have it, their policy may be inadequate. For example, there may be limited or no coverage for home health, rehabilitation, mental health services, a prosthesis, or durable medical equipment. Being uninsured or underinsured definitely affects a family's care-seeking behaviors and the ability to deal with their loved one's disability. Age of the labor force (children and elderly), coupled with limited access and availability of health care services, exacerbates the risk of poorer health outcomes among persons having agriculture-related injuries (Harper & Poling, 1998; Kelsey, May, & Jenkins, 1996; Keninger, 1998; Kululka, Cheek, & Jenkins, 1998; May, 1998a, 1998b).

Exposure to Chemicals

Use of and exposure to chemicals is an ever-increasing health problem in the agriculture industry. Each year, about 300,000 farmworkers are poisoned by chemicals used in agricultural production. Migrant and seasonal farmworkers and their families are at continuous risk for exposure to agricultural chemicals. Children in particular are highly susceptible to toxicity because lower dosages are needed to cause serious health consequences. Studies conducted in Florida and Washington (Grimes, 1998; Taylor, 1998) revealed that of all farmworkers, 40% had been sprayed either directly or by pesticide drift (droplets of the substance being carried in the air before settling on the ground or on vegetation). Of these, almost all (89%) did not know the name of the chemical to which they had been exposed. That is not surprising, given that very few farmworkers are knowledgeable about agricultural chemicals. They do not understand the concept of restricted entry interval into a field that has recently been sprayed with a chemical. Nor have most of them received training in how to protect themselves from these highly toxic chemicals. For that matter, most health professionals, even those in rural practice, are not knowledgeable about the symptoms associated with exposure to toxic agricultural chemicals. In particular, advanced practice nurses do not know about chemical toxicity; hence, they do not consider that in the differential diagnosis of a sick farmworker or a family member. Symptoms can vary depending on the chemical and are easily confused with common illnesses such as influenza, gastroenteritis, or the common cold. Health professionals as well as farmworkers should be educated on postexposure symptoms and the use of personal protective measures to avoid exposures (Chapter 6).

Stress

Agriculture is a demanding and technically complex occupation with marginal economic rewards for the remarkably long hours and hard work that are required from the entire family. In addition to the previously cited occupational hazards leading to death, farming has been included on the NIOSH list of the 10 most stressful occupations. Distressed farmers and their spouses commonly experience sleep disturbances, family conflict, concentration problems, depressive symptoms, and suicide (Dunbar, 1992; Elliott, Heaney, Wilkins, Mitchell, & Bean, 1995; Elkind, Carlson, & Shnable, 1998; Nordstrom et al., 1996). Even though stress is acknowledged to have potentially serious outcomes, farmers are unlikely to utilize existing community resources that might help them alleviate the problem. Hence, they may be increasing the risk of poor health outcomes for themselves as well as other family members (Chapter 8).

A number of programs have addressed stress among agricultural families. One of the more successful emerged from a partnership between the W. K. Kellogg Foundation and the New York Center of Health and Occupational Medicine (NYCHOM), the Farm Partners (FP) initiative (Jenkins & Marlenga, 1998; May, 1998a, 1998b). An objective of the FP program was increasing farm families' awareness and use of community resources to help them deal with their stress. The program recruited volunteers from within the farming community who worked as "case finders." The FP model parallels "peer counselor" programs implemented in some secondary schools. The volunteers are trained to recognize families in their community who are dealing poorly with emotional stress. Subsequently, they make a referral to an FP social worker, who then visits the family *on their farm.* The FP program has been widely lauded and could serve as a model for other communities dealing with economic strife and high levels of stress. An unexpected outcome has been that other farmer families have vicariously learned about community resources from their friends and neighbors who participated in FP. Increasingly, these are being accessed by farm families who need help, even *before* contacting staff at FP.

OCCUPATIONAL SAFETY AND HEALTH PROMOTION EDUCATION

Obviously, there is an urgent and ongoing need for occupational safety and health promotion education to reduce injuries and illnesses in the agriculture industry. The scattered nature of the workplace in agriculture makes prevention programs difficult to implement. Moreover, in most health and accident control campaigns, men are targeted. Yet rural women traditionally make most of the decisions about the family's health and preventive behaviors. Nurses therefore should take this dynamic into consideration when developing interventions. Short- and long-term outcomes must be measured to determine whether such interventions are making a difference in the targeted audience.

EMERGENCY MEDICAL SERVICES (EMS)

Occupation-related injuries can never be completely controlled, regardless of the industry. Therefore, emergency medical services (EMS) are needed to respond to the afflicted. Logistically, in remote areas EMS will be organized differently than in the inner city because of such factors as isolation and geographic distances. Traditionally, when an injury is severe, neighbors and extended family assist the affected family in their routine and seasonal work while the family deals with the crisis. Sometimes the crisis extends beyond natural support networks, as in the case of serious motor vehicle and farm implement accidents. In these cases, volunteers often become "first responders" in the local EMS. First responders (paraprofessionals and sometimes professionals) arrive on the scene of an accident to stabilize and then transport victims to an emergency department in a hospital (Frumkin & Mason, 1998; Keninger, 1998; Maningas, 1991; Rivara, 1997).

Becoming a first responder entails successfully completing an approved EMS course, which includes class attendance, field experiences, and passing the National Registry Examination. Individual state EMS councils may have additional requirements for EMS first responders. Dedicated rural volunteers often complete these courses on their own time and at their own expense so that emergency services will be available in their community. There are challenges in implementing and sustaining viable EMS programs in remote and health professional shortage areas (HPSAs). Financial viability always seems to be a consideration due to low client volume along with maintaining and sustaining emergency vehicles. Establishing a communication system that links physicians in emergency departments with the volunteers (first responders) who are riding in EMS vehicles (ambulances) often is another hurdle for some small towns to overcome. The education, certification, and assurance of clinical proficiency of an adequate number of EMS personnel can be an ongoing effort. Despite the real and potential obstacles, rural communities meet the challenge to develop an EMS response system. Partnerships are the underlying feature of successful rural EMS programs between federal, state, and county governments and local health care providers and community volunteers. Nurses should become knowledgeable about their local EMS program and be active in sustaining it. In the role of educator, a nurse can instruct residents on how to prevent accidents and treat victims prior to the arrival of EMS personnel. Some nurses work with the director of the local EMS to prepare and credential volunteers and first responders. Rural nurses have an important role in developing, implementing, and sustaining the EMS so that volunteers are prepared to safely stabilize and transport trauma victims to the nearest emergency department.

AGRICULTURE HEALTH NURSING

Along with the NIOSH initiative, agriculture health nursing (AHN) is emerging as a subspecialty with occupational health nursing (OHN) and community health nursing (CHN). Using an epidemiologic framework and drawing on principles from both CHN and OHN, the AHN has a pivotal role in meeting the nursing needs of farmers, farmworkers, and farm families ("Farmers' Journals," 1998; Jones, 1993; Keninger, 1998; Lee, 1998; Migliozzi & Randolph, 1993; Petrea & Aherin, 1998; Randolph & Migliozzi, 1993; Widtfeldt & Rooney, 1993; Wright, 1993). In many ways, AHN is not a new phenomenon. Almost a century ago, Clement (1914) described the skills needed by a nurse to care for families who lived and worked in agriculture enterprises:

> love of open country, good judgement, patience, a sense of humor, discreet and silent tongue, a knowledge of country traditions, sympathy with country people, willingness to give up city comforts when necessary, ability to teach, country breeding and a never-ending charity for the shortcomings of human beings. (p. 520)

Agriculture has not been considered an "industry" per se because farms do not have four walls or a well-defined workforce. Further, family members, including young children, are the workers. The rural environment is the AHN's practice domain, and the nursing focus is occupational risks and injuries occurring in agriculture. The client is a particular farming community. The AHN enters the worker's environment, going to the farm, which also may be the family's home, workplace, and recreational areas. The AHN's scope of practice consists of assessing and formulating a nursing diagnosis and then planning, intervening, and evaluating occupational risks and injuries of persons in the agriculture environment. Usually, the AHN does not provide hands-on primary health care but manages a client's case; some, however, are also APRNs. Because it is a rather new area of practice, AHNs must actively promote their role and services. One AHN stated that early in her practice, when she introduced herself to the clients by saying, "I'm Susie Jones, the ag nurse," it was not unusual for the family to report that they did not have any sick animals. In other words, these farming clients thought she worked with the veterinarian. These misperceptions are less evident with several years of public education about AHNs' role and scope of practice.

Surveillance is an important activity of the AHN, specifically identifying real and potential hazards, monitoring morbidity and mortality rates, and collecting epidemiological data regarding sentinel events (accidents, injuries, death). Anecdotal data are useful when speaking to farming audiences on agricultural health and safety. Surveillance data also support primary, secondary, and tertiary interventions targeting the agriculture community (Boyd et al., 1997; Casey et al., 1997a, 1997b; Randolph & Migliozzi, 1993).

Primary prevention can entail grassroots lobbying to inform elected state and federal lawmakers, health policy developers, and leaders in the agriculture industry about potential occupational risks to workers. In turn, these groups may require safety devices for machinery, personal protective equipment (PPE), and educational requirements for users of agricultural chemicals. Another important dimension of primary prevention is targeting the right group, with the right message: in this instance, the farm family.

Rural women, who may be labeled as "farmers' wives," are rarely viewed as active participants in farm labor by policy makers and financiers. But in reality, many of these women work alongside male family members in the day-to-day labor of operating the farm (Hibbard & Pope, 1987; Jenkins & Marlenga, 1998; Jones, 1993; Jones, Luchok, & McKnight, 1998; Keninger, 1998; Osterud & Jones, 1989; Rosenfeld, 1995; Sachs, 1993). However, there is a growing interest in the roles women have in agriculture and in maintaining their families' health. One reason for targeting women in the agriculture community is that they usually are part of established social networks that can facilitate the dissemination of health and safety messages. Because they are decision makers, it is reasonable to assume that agriculture safety is within their domain. The need for occupational health and safety education is greatest for the most vulnerable in the agriculture industry, namely the young and seniors. Farm wives may be the most effective in reaching these two groups as well.

Secondary prevention activities for the AHN include providing rapid and appropriate treatment of work-related injuries and illnesses: for instance, being actively involved with the local EMS as a first responder or providing consultation to them on common and unusual accidents such as farm implement amputations and injuries caused by animals. Such information prepares the EMS to treat victims and purchase essential lifesaving and extracting equipment (e.g., Jaws of Life) to access, stabilize, and transport patients.

Tertiary prevention for the AHN means helping affected individuals to return to their previous level of performance insofar as this is possible, through case managing and coordinating a continuum of care for them. The agriculture industry may have other considerations, such as assisting a farmer to find someone to care for animals or crop production (e.g., plowing, harvesting, thinning). For many, agriculture is the only work they know. An AHN can help access resources and encourage the family during career and lifestyle transitions.

NURSING RESEARCH NEEDS

Most of the information about health and safety risks in the agriculture industry has been gathered by other disciplines. Because AHN is evolving as a focus area, there is an urgent need for research on this high-risk occupational group, which includes males and females of all ages. There also is a need to design and evaluate nursing interventions that target the agriculture workforce, especially children and the very old. Previous studies have mostly addressed the utilization of services, but data are needed about determinants of care-seeking behaviors. Nurse researchers may find Dunkin's framework useful to identify specific factors that contribute to health-related activities of an agricultural family or even a community. Educational interventions have not been measured in terms of behavior changes in the agricultural workforce. Nor are there studies on whether the environment was modified to reduce hazards and risks to the farmer, farmworkers, and their families. Even though this chapter has focused on the agriculture industry, nursing research is sparse on other rural occupations, such as fishing, mining, and logging. Obviously, there is a need for a balance of quantitative, qualitative, and anecdotal evidence on phenomena relevant to nurses (Kululka et al., 1998). These are but a few of the multiple needs for research that will enhance the theoretical base for rural nursing.

SUMMARY

This chapter focused on risks and injuries in rural environments, primarily the agriculture industry. Regardless of the occupation, in a rural area the entire community is affected when one member is injured or dies in an occupation-related incident. As a subspecialty of CHN and OHN, AHN is a newly emerging nursing specialty area of practice and research.

DISCUSSION QUESTIONS

Interview an occupational health nurse or an agricultural health nurse.

➢ Have the person describe his or her professional roles, scope of practice, responsibilities, rewards, and challenges.

➢ What surveillance activities are occurring?

➢ How are the data used to implement primary, secondary, and tertiary interventions with agriculture workers and their families?

➢ Identify chemicals that are used for agriculture production in your state.

➢ How and when are these to be used?

➢ What safety precautions must be taken when these are used, such as personal protective equipment or drift management?

➢ What requirements must be met by the person who purchases and/or uses these products? Who enforces these?

➢ List the symptoms of chemical exposure for each.

➢ How should exposures be treated, immediately (in the field) and several hours later (in the emergency room)?

➢ What educational materials are available to inform farmworkers and their families about chemical exposure?

SUGGESTED RESEARCH ACTIVITIES

➢ Develop a nursing care plan to treat a person who has been exposed to agricultural chemicals that are used in surrounding rural areas.

➢ Undertake a literature review on agricultural health nursing. Write an integrated analysis based on your readings about this emergency specialty. Describe how the roles of the agriculture health nurse interface with community health nursing and occupational health nursing.

REFERENCES

Boyd, J., Hill, M., Pollock, G., Gelberg, K., Roerig, S., & Grant, A. (1997). Epidemiologic characteristics of reported hand injuries: New York State 1991-1995. *Journal of Agricultural Safety and Health, 3*(2), 101-107.

Bull, R., & Boyle, A. (1998). The maritime environment: A comparison with land-based remote area health care. *Australian Journal of Rural Health, 6*(2), 83-88.

Casey, G., Grant, A., Roerig, D., Boyd, J., Hill, M., & London, M. (1997a). Farm worker injuries associated with bulls. *American Association Occupational Health Nursing, 45,* 393-396.

Casey, G., Grant, A., Roerig, D., Boyd, J., Hill, M., & London, M. (1997b). Farm worker injuries associated with cows. *American Association Occupational Health Nursing, 45,* 447-450.

Clement, T. (1914). American Red Cross Town and Country Nursing Services. *American Journal of Nursing, 14,* 520.

Dunbar, E. (1992). Rural mental health administration. In M. Austin & W. Hersey (Eds.), *Handbook of mental health administration: The middle management perspective.* San Francisco: Jossey-Bass.

Elkind, P., Carlson, J., & Schnable, B. (1998). Agricultural hazards reduction through stress management. *Journal of Agromedicine, 5*(2), 23-32.

Elliott, M., Heaney, C., Wilkins, J., Mitchell, G., & Bean, T. (1995). Depression and perceived stress among cash grain farmers in Ohio. *Journal of Agriculture Safety and Health, 1,* 177-184.

Farmers' journals provide an ag history lesson. (1998, December 20). *Bismarck Tribune,* p. 6A.

Frumkin, H., & Mason, S. (1998). Physician training in agricultural safety and health: The Emory Agromedicine training project. *Journal of Agromedicine, 5*(2), 49-68.

Gerberich, S., Robertson, L., Gibson, R., & Renier, C. (1996). An epidemiological study of roadway fatalities related to farm vehicles, 1988-1993. *American College of Occupational and Environmental Health, 38,* 1135-1140.

Grimes, G. (1998). The Farm Worker Health and Safety Institute (FHSI). *Journal of Agromedicine, 5*(2), 33-38.

Harper, J., & Poling, R. (1998). The South Carolina Farm Leaders for Agricultural Safety and Health Education Program. *Journal of Agromedicine, 5*(2), 9-17.

Hibbard, J., & Pope, C. (1987). Women's roles, interest in health and health behavior. *Women and Health, 12*(2), 67-84.

Jenkins, S., & Marlenga, B. (1998). Introduction to the W. K. Kellogg's Agricultural Safety and Health (ASH) Initiative. *Journal of Agromedicine, 5*(2), 1-3.

Jones, M., Luchok, K., & McKnight, R. (1998). Empowering farm women to reduce hazards to family health and safety on the farm. *Journal of Agromedicine, 5*(2), 91-99.

Jones, S. (1993). Agricultural injury surveillance: Occupational health nurses' role. *Journal of the American Association of Occupational Health Nursing, 41,* 434-436.

Kelsey, T., May, J., & Jenkins, P. (1996). Farm tractors, and the use of seat belts and roll-over protective structures. *American Journal of Industrial Medicine, 30,* 447-451.

Keninger, T. (1998). Prevention of secondary injuries/disabilities: A consumer responsive approach. *Journal of Agromedicine, 5*(2), 17-23.

Kululka, G., Cheek, H., & Jenkins, S. (1998). The agricultural safety and health external evaluation summary. *Journal of Agromedicine, 5*(2), 107-112.

Lee, H. (1998). *Conceptual basis for rural nursing.* New York: Springer.

Maningas, P. (1991). *Emergency medical services in rural America: New solutions to urgent needs.* Washington, DC: Federal Office of Rural Health Policy.

May, J. (1998a). Clinically significant occupational stressors in New York farmers and farm families. *Journal of Agricultural Safety and Health, 4*(1), 9-14.

May, J. (1998b). The Farm Partners (FP) Program: Addressing the problem of occupational stress in agriculture. *Journal of Agromedicine, 5*(2), 39-48.

Migliozzi, A., & Randolph, S. (1993). Agricultural health and safety [Editorial]. *Journal of the American Association of Occupational Health Nursing, 41,* 413.

National Institute of Occupational Safety and Health. (1996). *National Occupational Research Agenda (NORA)* (Pub. No. 96-115). Washington, DC: U.S. Department of Health and Human Services.

National Institute for Occupational Safety and Health. (1998a). *Centers for agricultural disease and injury research, education, and prevention: Program descriptions.* Washington, DC: U.S. Department of Health and Human Services.

National Institute for Occupational Safety and Health. (1998b). *Centers for agricultural disease and injury research, education, and prevention: Regional agricultural profiles. Prepared by the Agricultural Centers.* Washington, DC: U.S. Department of Health and Human Services.

National Institute of Occupational Safety and Health. (1998c). *Helicopter logging safety: Alaska Interagency Working Group for the Prevention of Occupational Injuries.* Washington, DC: U.S. Department of Health and Human Services.

National Institute for Occupational Safety and Health. (1998d). *Injuries among farm workers in the United States, 1994.* Washington, DC: U.S. Department of Health and Human Services.

National Safety Council. (1998). *Accident facts.* Chicago: Author.

Nordstrom, D., Layde, P., Olson, K., Stueland, D., Follen, M., & Brand, L. (1996). Fall-related occupational injuries on farms. *American Journal of Industrial Medicine, 29,* 509-515.

Osterud, N., & Jones, L. (1989). If I must say so myself: Oral histories of rural women. *Rural History Review, 17,* 1-23.

Petrea, R., & Aherin, R. (1998). Evaluation finding of an agricultural health and safety community leadership development process. *Journal of Agromedicine, 5*(2), 77-90.

Randolph, S. A., & Migliozzi, A. A. (1993). The role of the agricultural health nurse. *Journal of the American Association of Occupational Health Nursing, 41,* 429-433.

Rivara, F. P. (1997). Fatal and non-fatal farm injuries to children and adolescents in the United States, 1990-93. *Injury Prevention, 3,* 190-194.

Rosenfeld, R. (1995). *Farm women: Work, farm and family in the United States.* Chapel Hill: University of North Carolina Press.

Sachs, C. (1993). *The invisible farmers: Women in agricultural production.* Totowa, NJ: Rowman & Allanheld.

Taylor, C. (1998, October). *Practical considerations for agricultural assessments versus conventional industry.* Paper presented at the Fourth Annual International Symposium, Rural Health and Safety in a Changing World, Saskatoon, Saskatchewan, Canada.

U.S. Department of Health and Human Services. (1999). *Healthy people 2010: National health promotion and disease prevention objectives.* Washington, DC: Government Printing Office.

Widtfeldt, A., & Rooney, E. (1993). Continuous quality improvement in occupational health nursing. *Journal of the American Association of Occupational Health Nursing, 41,* 456-459.

Wright, K. (1993). Management of agricultural injuries and illness. *Nursing Clinics of North America, 28,* 253-266.

PART III
———

NATIONAL AND GLOBAL
FUTURISTIC PERSPECTIVES

Part III presents national and global futuristic perspectives and builds on the chapters that were included in the two preceding parts. It begins with Chapter 12, which examines managed care in rural America. Highlighted are stimulating forces and some impeding forces to development of integrated managed care organizations (MCOs) in rural markets.

The next four chapters focus specifically on rural nursing from a global perspective. Chapter 13 focuses on rural nursing in the United States. In Chapter 14, Dr. Desley Hegney presents the Australian perspective. Chapter 15, by Dr. Donna Rennie, Kathy Baird-Crooks, Gail Remus, and Joyce Engel, offers the Canadian perspective. Chapter 16 synthesizes the information in the three preceding chapters on rural nursing in Australia, Canada, and the United States, identifying commonalities and variances in the features of rural nursing practice from a global perspective. Chapter 17 discusses ethical situations and what nurses in rural practice should know about preventing and dealing with such events.

This part, and of course the book, concludes with Chapter 18, which examines rural nursing research. This research is the link between rural theory and evidence-based practice. Methodological issues are examined relative to the rural environment, and nursing research agendas are identified.

CHAPTER 12

The Meaning of Managed Care for Rural America

KEY TERMS

- ➤ Capitation
- ➤ Comprehensive span of services
- ➤ Fee for service
- ➤ Managed care
- ➤ Managed care organization (MCO)
- ➤ Prepayment
- ➤ Risk sharing
- ➤ Third-party payer
- ➤ Marginalizing providers
- ➤ Gatekeeping
- ➤ Critical access hospital (CAH)
- ➤ Covered lives
- ➤ Utilization review
- ➤ Quality assurance assessment/measures

OBJECTIVES

After reading this chapter, you will be able to

- ➤ Identify factors that can affect penetration of managed care into rural market areas.
- ➤ Compare and contrast characteristics of rural counties included in managed care organization services areas with those that are not in managed care organization service areas.
- ➤ Discuss the roles of nurses in rural managed health care organizations.

ESSENTIAL POINTS TO REMEMBER

➤ Managed care is expanding in rural areas, but enrollment rates still are relatively low. The number of rural counties in the service area of a managed care organization (MCO) has been increasing since 1991 and grew dramatically between 1994 and 1995.

➤ Rural counties located in an MCO service area differ from rural counties not in an MCO service area on demographic, socioeconomic, and health system characteristics. The average population density of rural counties located in an MCO service area is almost twice that of rural counties without an MCO. Most likely that is because there are not enough people to ensure a certain level of profits.

➤ Rural counties in MCO service areas have higher percentages of population employed in manufacturing, white-collar, construction, and health services and a lower percentage of population employed in agriculture.

OVERVIEW

Rural America, despite the low population density, has not been neglected in the nation's move to managed health care. This chapter examines a few of the complex issues facing rural communities as the health care system consolidates and moves from fee-for-service to a capitated model. The implications for rural nurses are highlighted within the discussion.

EVOLUTION OF THE U.S. HEALTH CARE DELIVERY SYSTEM

Managed care is not new to rural America. More than 150 years ago, miners paid a fee to secure medical care from salaried physicians. However, the care provided by "camp doctors" was not uniform in quality. Some states passed laws that restricted physicians from being employed on a salaried basis to practice medicine. Difficulties identified in those early models of health maintenance organizations (HMOs) are the same challenges that exist in the current market-driven health care industry, particularly in rural communities.

Major changes are occurring in where care is delivered: that is, from acute care hospitals to community-based facilities. These were fueled by the phenomenal growth in health care costs, technological advances, and growing numbers of elderly and poor people who need financial support for health care. Over the past decade, nearly 1,000 acute care hospitals closed, the average daily inpatient census dropped by 21%, and patient length of stay decreased by 7%. As for the impact on rural delivery systems, since 1980 more than 20% of all rural hospitals have closed. Experts state that existing hospital beds still outnumber the demand; hence, they project that even more closures are anticipated before the end of this decade (American Hospital Association [AHA], 1997; Cooper, 1995; Gorman, 1999). Table 12.1 highlights the evolution of health care delivery from a fee-for-service model, to the capitation model, to the projected model. To survive, even thrive, nurses must be flexible and adapt along with the health care delivery system as a whole, regardless of whether the setting is urban or rural (Agency for Health Care Policy and Research [AHCPR], 1995, 1996; Office of Rural Health Policy [ORHP], 1997a, 1997b, 1998).

TABLE 12.1 Evolution of U.S. Health Care System

	1990	*1995*	*2000*
Reimbursement	Prospective payment (1983) and some fee for service (pre-1983)	Mix of discounted fee for service and capitation	Capitation
Organizational structure	Acute care hospital	Integrated delivery system	Delivery system with integrated financing
System purpose	Treating disease	Defining appropriate treatment setting	Preventing and treating disease, maintaining health
Economic function	Stabilizing rural economy	Maintaining practitioner supply	Protecting rural resources from urban predators
Investment bias	Bricks and mortar (build buildings)	Physician practices	Health plan development
Economic incentive	Hospitalization	Outpatient treatment	Profit Prevention
Scope of services defined by:	Practitioners	Competitive market forces Focus on price and quality	Normative population-based data

SOURCE: Adapted from University of Minnesota (1997).

Managed care is expanding into rural areas. In 1995, more than 80% of all rural countries were in the service area of at least one MCO. Of all MCOs, about 75% include at least one rural county in their service area. However, of all MCOs serving rural counties, only 14 (2.4%) had their headquarters in a rural county. Rural counties in MCO service areas differ from those not in MCO service areas on several characteristics. Specifically, the average population and population density of rural counties located in an MCO service area are almost twice those of counties without an MCO service area. Employment patterns also differ. Most notably, rural counties in an MCO service area have a higher percentage of the population employed in manufacturing and lower percentages employed in agriculture than counties not in such an area. Health systems characteristics vary as well: Rural counties outside of MCO service areas have more hospital beds per capita but lower occupancy rates and fewer physicians (Maine Rural Health Research Center, 1997; National Rural Health Association [NRHA], 1998; North Carolina Rural Health Research and Policy Analysis Center [NCRHRPAC], 1997; Office of Technology Assessment [OTA], 1995).

State governments also are turning to managed care to insure their employees. In 1993, of the 3.6 million active state employees, more than 1 million were enrolled in MCOs. Medicare and Medicaid programs also are developing managed care options for enrollees. The rural population is older, poorer, and less healthy than its urban counterpart. Consequently, these demographic factors have implications for developing prepaid capitated managed care plans that enroll Medicare and Medicaid recipients in rural counties. The seemingly low number of rural Medicare and Medicaid recipients who are enrolled in managed care leaves some rural providers feeling immune to its effects. This situation is projected to change, however, as Congress takes measures to control Medicare costs and as states develop ways to reduce Medicaid expenditures (James, Wysong, Rosenthal, & Crawford, 1993; NCRHRPAC, 1997; University of Minnesota Rural Health Research Center [UMRHRC], 1997).

DEFINING MANAGED CARE

The term *managed care,* though widely used, does not have a commonly accepted definition and can mean different things to different people. For instance, to the chief executive officer (CEO) of an MCO, the term probably means a system that integrates financing and delivery of health care to a population of covered lives by a selected group of providers, using a formal program to ensure quality. To many physicians and nurses, managed care means more government regulations and paperwork with less control over their own practice. To many consumers, managed care is equated with rationing, lack of choice of provider, and poor quality. The latter perspective stems from MCOs' approaches to control (manage) their enrollees' use of health care services (NRHA, 1998).

Ideally, the goal of all MCOs should be to curtail costs but not at the expense of quality. An MCO can be profitable *if* it is able to provide all of the needed services for members enrolled in a health plan but at a lower cost than the aggregated *capitated payment.* Essentially, this is the premium paid by an employer or individual to the MCO for services. Another feature of managed care is that both the providers and the MCO share the *financial risk.* That is to say, they must absorb any costs for delivered care (services) that exceeded capitated payments for enrollees in the managed care plan. The incentive is for providers to prevent illness and minimize the use of more costly services. Four common techniques are used to achieve this goal. But due to geographic, demographic, and economic features that differentiate rural from urban areas, these techniques may not yield similar outcomes in the two settings.

Limiting Provider Panels

The principal mechanism for managing costs by MCOs is to limit their number of contracted providers. For example, for inpatient care, an MCO may contract with only one hospital in a given area. Essentially, the MCO contracts for discounted rates from a facility in return for increased patient volume. For medical care, the MCO contracts with a limited number of primary care physicians (provider panel) from whom enrollees (covered lives) in a given service area are required to receive care. The MCO also contracts with selected specialists for a 'discounted' fee-for-service rate. If necessary, primary care physicians refer their patients to the specialists who also are on the MCO's panel of providers. Typically, the MCO pays a capitated (per-member/per-month) rate to physicians on its provider panel. A basic tenet of managed care is increasing profitability through competition. Further, high volume is a dimension of successful competition. This economic model does not work in rural areas, where MCOs cannot get a high enough volume (critical mass) of enrollees and where there may be a very low number of providers. Hence, there can be no competition between providers either. The nursing community continues to express concern about some MCOs' pattern of excluding APRNs from provider panels. In effect, this prevents APRNs from caring for patients who are enrolled in those MCOs (American Nurses Association, 1992). In some areas, APRNs became providers by educating MCO administrators and consumers. However, state nurse practice can be a disincentive to hiring APRNs.

A community must be actively involved in determining local needs and preferences rather than simply having the urban-based MCO make those decisions when it enters a rural service area. Ensuring local access with an appropriate supply and mix of providers depends on demographic, epidemiologic, and geographic characteristics of a particular community. For example, if a community has a greater proportion of elderly people but low numbers of children and women, the community leaders in partnership with administrators of the MCO may agree that it is not realistic to have local obstetrical services. Conversely, it may be prudent to have a cardiologist readily available. Likewise, the predominant industry in a region influences the type of emergency and primary care services that are needed. For example, if the county's economy is tourist dependent, emergency services and ambulatory clinics may need to have 24-hour availability. Or if a county's economy is agriculture driven, there may be a need for emergency, trauma, and surgical capability, with air transport capability to a tertiary medical center. The community must also determine the boundaries for its delivery system, and geographic features may be a factor.

For example, if the travel time to an urban area is relatively short and transportation is relatively easy, most health care services can be available outside the community. In such cases, there probably is room for competition between several urban-based managed care plans that serve rural consumers in the market area (Chapter 2). Conversely, if a community is geographically remote and isolated, it may be necessary to make a wider array of health care services available locally (Chapter 1).

Distributing Risk

Another cost management strategy used by MCOs is to place financial risk on their panel of providers in caring for enrollees. Capitated payments (per member/per month) to primary care physicians usually cover ambulatory care, preventive services, and related ancillary services. Theoretically, capitated payments encourage a physician to control the volume and array of services provided to individual patients. The MCO also may reserve (hold back) a portion of the prepaid capitated premium to ensure that any other expenditures originating with the physician are within the parameters of the plan. This strategy disperses the fiscal risk among the provider panel in the MCO. In other words, there is an incentive to primary care providers to keep people healthy and to not use costly diagnostic and specialty services.

Anecdotal reports from physicians in rural areas indicate that because their clients tend to be less healthy, the cost for treating chronic health problems often surpasses their allocated capitated fee to enroll in the plan. This fiscal model is of special concern with vulnerable populations, including minorities, the elderly, and the poor, who often require more intensive treatment and more services. Incurring excessive costs has resulted in some MCOs' severing contracts with rural providers. This strategy is forcing patients to seek care from another primary care provider who may be located outside the local community or even in another state. This phenomenon, sometimes referred to as *marginalizing* a health care provider, seems to be occurring with greater frequency among physicians who care for rural minority populations.

Because enrollment in rural managed care plans tends to be quite low, how APRNs fare in this environment remains to be seen. This is an area for nurse researchers to examine, along with obtaining an accurate account of what really is occurring with underserved populations and nursing's impact (Idaho Rural Health Coalition [IRHC], 1995; OTA, 1995; Rosenberg & Associates, 1995, 1997).

Reviewing Utilization and Ensuring Quality

Utilization review and quality assurance measures are two other strategies used by MCOs to control costs and enrolled members' use of health care services. With utilization review, all services (other than primary care) must be authorized by a primary care provider to ensure that the care provided to an enrollee (beneficiary) is medically necessary and delivered in the least costly manner. Many physicians cynically refer to this process as "1-800-May I." Should a beneficiary use services that are deemed to be inappropriate by the utilization review board (team, case manager), the provider or the patient may be required to pay for that care. Who pays will depend on the locus of control for decision making in the MCO. To minimize the possibility of denying needed care, MCOs use a variety of quality assurance standards. Generally, these are measured on three dimensions: qualifications of providers, the review process for appropriateness of interventions rendered by providers on its panel, and outcome measures. The National Committee for Quality Assurance (NCQA, 1993) has developed quality review standards for accrediting MCOs that are becoming widely accepted in the managed care industry.

Gatekeeping

In highly regulated MCOs where physicians adhere to established protocols to control utilization of services, the three previously described measures usually are sufficient. However, when physicians can continue to practice in the private sector, often the MCO uses primary care physicians and sometimes nurse practitioners as gatekeepers for its enrollees. Gatekeepers must authorize all care that enrollees receive as well as specify who can provide it. Generally, rural physicians are uncomfortable with all of the demands placed on them in the role of gatekeeper. This is partly attributable to the requirement that all services must be preapproved. This mandate is time consuming, sometimes requiring 24-hour physician availability. Of concern in rural areas, too, is that the only clients who enroll in a managed care plan are those who are in need of medical services.

The cost of providing care to a "less healthy" population greatly outweighs the capitation rate. Hence, the profit margin for the MCO is consistently low or showing a loss. This perception raises concern among consumers regarding MCOs' motives for not approving care, especially in vulnerable rural populations.

MCOs AND THE RURAL MARKET

Nationally, the growth of MCOs has been significant, but the penetration in rural areas continues to be relatively small. A number of stimulating and impeding factors affect the development of integrated rural MCOs (NRHA, 1998; UMRHRC, 1997).

Stimulating Forces

Locally Driven Forces

More and more, rural communities are organizing their own local health care services or participating in MCO plans to preserve the availability of those services. In addition, increasing numbers of community-based agencies in rural areas are participating in managed care plans as well as maintaining the traditional fee-for-service option. Most often, this means that local residents or health care providers seek to work with an urban-based MCO to provide or enhance services in their community.

Expansion of Urban-Based MCOs

Another driving force is that more and more urban-based MCOs are providing rural services to meet the needs of their beneficiaries. For an MCO to acquire a contract with an urban-based business corporation, such as a textile or automotive manufacturer or national fast food franchise, it must provide health care for employees wherever the company operates. Often, the employees include those living in small towns where manufacturing and the service industries are gaining prominence. Consequently, MCOs are contracting with predominantly urban-based corporations having rural suboperations to provide health care to their employees.

Reduction of Government Expenditures

Development of managed care also is stimulated by the pressure being placed on state government to control the cost of Medicaid expenditures. Most states are trying to increase the number of Medicaid recipients by enrolling them in managed care plans. Again, some states have been more successful than others. Likewise, state-sponsored employee health benefit plans are purchasing services from MCOs. These trends rein-

force the need for making managed care plans available to state employees who work in
state agencies in rural as well as urban communities.

Impeding Forces

A number of reasons are given for why managed care is growing more slowly in rural settings. The most often cited barriers are discussed below (AHA, 1997; AHCPR,
1995, 1996; IRHC, 1995; Slifkin, Ricketts, & Howard, 1996).

Shortages of Providers

Even though nearly one fourth of all Americans live in rural areas, less than 12% of
all physicians practice there. It is estimated that of all rural physicians, about 25% will retire by the year 2000. From these figures, one can infer that rural physicians are not recent
graduates. Not only is there an insufficient physician supply, but there are not enough
nurses, psychologists, social workers, physical therapists, occupational therapists, and
medical technicians. The crucial step in developing an integrated health care system is
determining a community's need for essential and ancillary services. Subsequently, an
appropriate mix of health professionals must be available to deliver those services.

Increasingly, fewer physicians are willing to spend all of their working lives in rural
areas. This is due to the limited income potential, perceived limitations for professional
growth, less collegial interaction, and fewer spousal employment opportunities. These
same quality-of-life factors contribute to the recruitment and retention of nonphysician
primary care providers such as nurse practitioners, nurse midwives, and physician assistants (PAs). Access to primary health care in rural areas can be greatly enhanced through
collaboration among physician and nonphysician providers. The ability of MCOs to ensure adequate primary and preventive care, however, could be dependent on the responsibilities given to APRNs and other nonphysician providers (AHA 1997; Cheh &
Thompson, 1997).

In a rural area, APRNs and PAs often make up for the lack of physicians, especially
in underserved regions. The availability of other kinds of providers, especially psychologists, pharmacists, social workers, and physical therapists, as well as specialized technical staff such as radiology and laboratory personnel, also is important in ensuring access
to a continuum of care (i.e., a comprehensive span of services). Though willingness to
work in a rural area may not be based only on monetary factors, practitioners are not
likely to stay unless they receive a reasonable income, especially if salaries are higher in
urban areas (Chapters 13 through 16).

Lack of an Integrated System

To successfully enter into managed care arrangements, infrastructures must be in
place to render care to MCO beneficiaries. Especially needed are information systems
that can perform clinical coordination and measure outcomes. In most rural markets, integrated systems of this type either have not yet begun or are in the earliest stages of development. The financial viability of an MCO ultimately depends on effective case man-

agement. In urban areas, case management usually is carried out by primary care providers who have at their disposal a variety of support services and personnel. In rural areas, information or case management systems are seldom in place to assist primary care providers to case-manage enrollees' use of services. Consequently, creating these resources often becomes part of the responsibility of MCOs entering rural service areas.

Inadequate Technology

Many rural hospitals do not have the biomedical and communication technology that urban hospitals often take for granted. In fact, their current technology could be considered outdated and in need of replacement. Lack of capital also makes biotechnology upgrades unattainable for struggling rural hospitals. Thus, MCOs usually are not eager to contract with facilities having outdated equipment and low patient volumes to be on their provider panel. Consequently, when small rural hospitals are purchased by a large health care system, they often are closed. Sometimes the facility is used for other community-based or outreach services. This trend has had varying health outcomes for a community as a whole and its access to essential and ancillary services. To address these concerns, legislative initiatives have been implemented to support rural hospitals that are not profitable yet may be critically important because there are no other hospitals in the particular area.

The Rural Hospital Flexibility Program, created under Section 4201 of the Balanced Budget Act of 1997, allocated funds to states to help them address such rural access issues (Weisgrau, 1999). The designation of critical access hospitals (CAHs) is the most recent effort by the federal government to respond to the emergency and health care needs of remote and isolated areas (Table 12.2). Essentially, the program offers flexible alternatives for small rural hospitals that are financially struggling and are highly dependent on Medicare revenues. The legislative intent is to match a rural community's emergency care needs with its provider capabilities. The act acknowledges that health care is a critical dimension of rural economic sustainability and development; the two are intricately intertwined (Chapter 2). It allows for mid-level practitioners to be remotely supervised by an off-site physician, as well as for minimum staffing requirements. The bed size is absolutely limited to no more than 15 acute care beds; length of stay is limited to no more than 96 hours. There is a swing-bed option (a certain number of beds that can be used for nonacute extended care) for up to 25 beds, but there can never be more than 15 occupied acute care beds at a given time. A critical access hospital will be reimbursed by Medicare on a fee-for-service rate. Each state must define critical access hospitals out of the ones already in operation. It is not yet known how this initiative will play out in the various states or what the long-range impact will be on nursing practice and the health of rural communities as a whole.

Resistance by Providers

Physicians are key to managing care, and there can be disincentives for MCOs to enter rural areas. MCOs are built around group practices where physicians collectively

TABLE 12.2 Medicare Rural Hospital Flexibility Program (Critical Access Hospital [CAH])

Extent of Program	50 States
Eligibility	Current hospital Not for profit
Service limit (length of stay)	96 hours
Service limit (size)	15 beds (maximum) or 25 beds with swing beds
Location criteria	Rural and 35+ mile drive to hospital or CAH (15 miles in mountains or areas with secondary roads or state certificates as a "Necessary Provider"
Medicare payment	Cost based
Services	Inpatient Emergency Laboratory Radiology Some ancillary and support services may be provided part time, off site
Emergency services	Available 24 hours Staff has emergency service training or experience Staff is on call and available within 30 minutes
Medical staff	At least one physician (need not be on site) May include mid-level practitioners
Nursing staff	RN, CNS, or LPN on duty when there is an inpatient in the facility
Hours of operation	24 hours if occupied If not occupied, emergency services made available
Network	Network = At least 1 CAH and 1 hospital If a member of network, agreements maintained with network hospital(s) for ➢ Referral and transfer ➢ Transportation services ➢ Communications Agreement with network hospital, PRO, or equivalent for ➢ Credentialing ➢ Quality assurance
Legislative intent, rationale, philosophy, and goals	Provide alternative to financially failing rural hospital Match community need to provider capabilities Provide regulatory relief to underserved rural communities Provide foundation for rural networks Allow mid-level practitioner with remote supervision Recognize hospital as part of community economic viability (often is one of the largest local employers) Provide safety net at fee-for-service reimbursement Make emergency services more flexible but accessible

share the risk and implement standards to control utilization of services. The majority of physicians in rural areas are not in group practice, and most are nearing retirement age. A high proportion are independent entrepreneurs who do not like having outside parties intrude into their clinical practice. Overall, rural physicians are reluctant to become part of an entity that could require them to follow guidelines that they feel may or may not be in their or the community's best interests and that are handed down from what they perceive to be a "faceless" entity. In addition to clinical concerns, there are serious financial issues for rural practitioners associated with third-party reimbursement rates' being significantly lower than in metropolitan areas.

Antitrust Regulations

Collaboration among rural providers has been a double-edged sword for federal and state policy makers. On the one hand, organizing networks of health care providers has permitted enormous cost savings and has often improved the quality of care. On the other hand, consolidated provider networks evoke the potential for illegal price fixing, group boycotts, or market divisions. Unfortunately, antitrust enforcement agencies leave many rural providers unsure of the fine line between a procooperative network and an anticooperative network. Health professionals, rural and urban alike, question the extent to which competing providers can come together without risking the threat of an antitrust investigation or lawsuit. Antitrust issues are being studied by Congress, but legislation focusing on health care has not been enacted. Other than being indirectly affected, nurses have not been involved in antitrust legal actions. Whether that will continue remains to be seen as new nursing models of care delivery emerge (ORHP, 1998).

Few or No Larger Employers

In urban areas, large employers are among the first to embrace managed care and the potential cost savings associated with such plans. But rural areas are characterized by small and family business enterprises and employers who hire seasonal and part-time employees. Consequently, without large employers, there are no major players to facilitate involvement in MCOs at the local level. Interestingly, counties with manufacturers, service-related industries, and construction have a significantly higher proportion of their residents enrolled in managed care plans. Conversely, counties in which agriculture predominates have lower numbers enrolled in MCO plans.

Low-Volume Market

MCOs are significantly deterred from entering rural areas whose population is below a critical population density (i.e., critical mass). Managed care strategies are volume based. In many rural areas, the population base is viewed by MCOs as inadequate to spread the financial risk that is an inherent aspect of managed care. A rural primary care provider who treats a low volume of patients can be more expensive on a per-case basis than an urban-based specialist having a higher patient volume. For example, access to prenatal and obstetrical care may be locally available through a nurse midwife and a family practitioner in a rural county. But an MCO having a rural service area may expect its enrollees to travel 50 miles or further to see an urban-based obstetrician on its panel who has a more profitable, volume-based contractual agreement. A rural enrollee, in this case a pregnant woman, who does not wish to travel the extra distance either will not receive adequate prenatal care or will choose to pay out of pocket to obtain care from the local physician or nurse midwife.

Other concerns arise when an MCO is the primary insurance source in a rural community and chooses not to contract with the only obstetrician in the area. In this scenario, a major segment of an already limited patient supply (low volume) may disappear, with the result that the local obstetrician is no longer able to maintain a viable practice in the community and has to move away. Consequently, local residents who are not enrolled in the only MCO are left without any obstetrical care other than by traveling many miles for that service. These examples illustrate some of the unresolved economic, social, legal, and ethical issues associated with access to care that must be carefully analyzed prior to the expansion of an MCO into a rural market area.

High Numbers of Uninsured Persons

The number of uninsured rural Americans is at least 15% higher than the national average and 24% higher than in urban areas. This rural-urban disparity is attributable to many factors, including fewer large employers who provide health care benefits, lower socioeconomic status, and the overall poorer health status of rural persons. Managed care is volume based; therefore, an MCO must have an adequate number of enrollees to disperse the financial risk. If there are fewer enrollees, who also are less healthy, the potential for adverse membership selection increases. In other words, there are efforts to exclude persons with preexisting conditions by increasing premiums significantly and/or by varying premiums on the basis of age and gender. Strategies to manage costs and disperse financial risk have serious health ramifications for vulnerable populations who have no or inadequate health care coverage. Adverse selection strategies should be of particular concern to nurses because of the ethical issues associated with such cost-managing efforts.

Community Understanding

Increasingly, managed care is becoming the principal care reimbursement modality in our nation. Many rural citizens view the arrival of MCOs as an unwanted encroachment of urban predators. Some propose that MCOs will drive out physicians and nurses who currently are in the community, further narrowing their freedom of choice. To develop an integrated health care system, the community must be educated about the ensuing changes in health care delivery. The community must thus become competent to make decisions in its best interest. If the community does not assume responsibility for its own health, outsiders will do it for the community. Nurses in rural communities have a responsibility to become active participants in community educational efforts.

SUMMARY

This chapter examined issues relevant to nursing within MCOs. Managed care is rapidly expanding in the rural market area. Yet most MCOs have had little experience in rural America and the approaches that are needed to ensure financial viability. Rural nurses must assume an active role in shaping the future of health care at federal, state, local, and institutional levels.

DISCUSSION QUESTIONS

➤ Managed care is gaining a greater presence across the nation, and the prevalence of enrollment varies from state to state. How prevalent is managed care in your state compared to the nation as a whole? In rural areas compared to urban areas? In your community? Describe nurses' roles in regional MCOs. Interview APRNs employed in a rural MCO. How do their observations fit with the ideas presented in this chapter?

➤ Discuss the scope of practice and reimbursement practices in your state for APRNs who are on provider panels of MCOs in your state. What are the MCO enrollment patterns of Medicare/Medicaid beneficiaries in your state?

SUGGESTED RESEARCH ACTIVITIES

➤ What are the perceived benefits and problems of managed care plans, as described by consumers in a selected rural community?

➤ Explore the role, function, and reimbursement practices for APRNs in managed care plans in a rural MCO plan, compared to those for nurses who practice in an urban-based MCO.

➤ Compare the health outcomes of those enrolled in rural-based MCOs with those enrolled in urban-based MCOs.

➤ Complete a cost-benefit analysis of services rendered with treatment outcomes, comparing physicians' and APRNs' practice patterns.

REFERENCES

Agency for Health Care Policy and Research. (1995, November). *Managed care and rural America* (Pub. No. 95-R011). Rockville, MD: U.S. Department of Health and Human Services.

Agency for Health Care Policy and Research. (1996, September). *Accessing roles and responsibilities in a managed care environment: A workbook for local health officials* (Pub. No. 96-0057). Rockville, MD: U.S. Department of Health and Human Services.

American Hospital Association. (1997). *Profile of nonmetropolitan hospitals, 1991-1995.* Chicago: Author.

American Nurses Association. (1992). *America's agenda for health care reform.* Washington, DC: Author.

Cheh, V., & Thompson, R. (1997). *Rural health clinics: Improved access at a cost* (MPR Ref. No. 8293). Baltimore: Health Care Financing Administration.

Cooper, J. (1995). Managed care in rural America. *Journal of Family Practice, 41*(2), 115-117.

Gorman, C. (1999, February 8). Bleak days for doctors. *Time, 153,* 53.

Idaho Rural Health Coalition. (1995). *Managed care: Risks and opportunities, or (almost) everything you wanted to know about managed care but were afraid to ask.* Pocatello, ID: Author.

James, P., Wysong, J., Rosenthal, T., & Crawford, M. (1993). *Medicaid managed care for underserved populations: The rural perspective.* Buffalo: New York Rural Health Research Center, Office of Rural Health.

Maine Rural Health Research Center. (1997). Ready or not: Rural hospitals are changing. *Rural Health News (Portland, ME), 4*(1), 1, 3-4.

National Committee for Quality Assurance. (1993). *Health Plan Employer Data Set.* Washington, DC: Author.

National Rural Health Association. (1998, February). *A vision for health reform models for America's rural communities: Issue paper.* Kansas City, MO: Author.

North Carolina Rural Health Research and Policy Analysis Center. (1997). Study examines preparedness of rural community-based practices to move to managed care. *Rural Gazette (Chapel Hill, NC), 7*(1), 1, 4.

Office of Rural Health Policy. (1997a, February). Achieving equity in rural Medicare capitation payment: Reforms of the AAPCC methodology. *Rural Policy Brief, 1*(1). Rockville, MD: U.S. Department of Health and Human Services.

Office of Rural Health Policy. (1997b, April). *Market reform and managed care: Implications for rural communities* (Pub. No. 96-0057). Rockville, MD: U.S. Department of Health and Human Services.

Office of Rural Health Policy. (1998, January). *Rural health: A vision for 2010.* Rockville, MD: U.S. Department of Health and Human Services.

Office of Technology Assessment. (1995). *Impact of health reform on rural areas: Lessons from the states.* Washington, DC: Author.

Rosenberg & Associates. (1995). *Issues and options facing rural communities under managed care: A report provided to the California Institute for Rural Health.* Oakland, CA: Author.

Rosenberg & Associates. (1997). *Health care antitrust enforcement in rural America: A recommended safety zone.* Bethesda, MD: Office of Rural Health Policy.

Slifkin, R., Ricketts, T., & Howard, H. (1996). Potential effects of managed competition in rural areas. *Health Care Financing Review, 17*(4), 143-156.

University of Minnesota Rural Health Research Center. (1997, April). *Rural managed care: Patterns and prospects.* Minneapolis, MN: Author.

Weisgrau, S. (1999). *Description of critical access hospitals (CAH).* Lawrence, KS: Rural Health Consultants.

CHAPTER 13

Rural Nursing in the United States

KEY TERMS

> ➤ Urban bias
> ➤ Swing beds
> ➤ Advanced practice registered nurse (APRN)
> ➤ Clinical specialist (CS)
> ➤ Nurse practitioner (NP)
> ➤ Certified nurse midwife (CNM)
> ➤ Nurse anesthetist
> ➤ Direct caregiver
> ➤ Indirect caregiver
> ➤ Swing-bed facility
> ➤ Rural health clinic (RHC)
> ➤ Student payback loans

OBJECTIVES

After reading this chapter, you will be able to

> ➤ Analyze current trends affecting the supply and demand in the rural nursing workforce.
> ➤ Describe the role and scope of nursing in the rural U.S. health care system.
> ➤ List federal initiatives that were designed to improve access to care in rural areas.
> ➤ Examine rural social, cultural, and economic factors that can influence nursing practice.

ESSENTIAL POINTS TO REMEMBER

> ➤ Workforce projections indicate that the U.S. health care delivery system will require an additional 100,000 primary care providers in the next decade; of these, 70,000 should be APRNs. The unmet health care needs of rural clients offer a

plethora of professional and research opportunities for nurses who choose to practice in this environment.

➤ Nurses in advanced practice roles need to have a strong community health background, to be expert generalists, and to be able to provide primary health care to diverse clients.

➤ Nationally, rural nurses are older than their urban counterparts. Many live and work in the same community for decades.

➤ Technology is changing the way health care is delivered in rural areas and is being used to improve access to nursing educational offerings.

OVERVIEW

This chapter describes rural nursing in the United States. Political, social, cultural, and economic factors are examined that affect nurses' practice, education, recruitment, and retention in rural areas (see also Bushy, 1998).

BACKGROUND

Almost a decade ago, the American Association of Colleges of Nursing (AACN, 1994) and the American Nurses Association (ANA, 1991, 1996) recommended that Congress pass legislation that would support the following initiatives to help improve rural consumers' access to care:

➤ Provide direct reimbursements to nurse practitioners (NPs) and clinical nurse specialists (CNSs) for services rendered in rural and underserved areas of the country.

➤ Allocate federal and state funds for telecommunication infrastructures to educate and recruit nurses.

➤ Encourage collaboration among hospitals, professional nursing schools, and communities to create rural practice.

Progress has been made in implementing these nursing initiatives, and some states have had greater success than others. Other changes in health care delivery are affecting nursing education and rural practice too. Primary care is assuming greater prominence, whereas acute care, traditionally provided in hospitals, is declining and community-based services have shown exponential growth. Reimbursement has changed from fee for service to capitated managed care. Accompanying these changes is the need for nurses to have more sophisticated skills and an ability to function in expanded roles. In the United States, there is an increasing need for advanced practice registered nurses (APRNs), especially NPs, clinical specialists (CSs), certified nurse midwives (CNMs), and certified registered nurse anesthetists (CRNAs). The title *APRN* sometimes is used in reference to nurses prepared at the master's level in a specialty or functional area, such as education, informatics, or administration. In this chapter, the term specifically refers to the four clinical specialties (direct care providers), but that is not to diminish the importance of "nonclinical" specialties (indirect care providers). Rather, the narrower definition is to help focus the discussion. It cannot be overemphasized that nurses with advanced education in nonclinical as well as clinical specialties are in short supply in most rural practice settings. All of these specialties are needed to refine nursing's infrastructure in rural health care delivery systems and to develop the theoretical underpinnings for rural practice (Barger, 1996; National Institute for Nursing Research [NINR], 1995; Pickard, 1996; Salmon, 1999).

NURSING WORKFORCE TRENDS

A shortage of nurses across all settings, rural and urban alike, is a growing concern in the U.S. health care system. The nursing profession has always had ebbs and flows in the workforce, but the current shortage is different from the earlier ones. For example, the critical shortage in the late 1980s was of significant concern for the public, policy makers, and the nursing profession. During that time, the number of registered nurses (RNs) who practiced in their discipline increased by 10%. Of the 2 million nurses in the United States, about 80% were actively filling a position that required an RN. The current shortage is associated with the "graying" (aging) of the nursing profession. Young men and women are not entering the profession as they have in the past. Of even greater concern is that far too few students of minority origins are enrolling in and completing nursing educational programs. Rural nurses are older than their urban counterparts. Partly this is related to the fact that rural nurses in many cases live in the same community and have worked in the same institution for decades (Duncan, Coward, & Gilbert, 1997; Dunkin, Stratton, Movassaghi, & Kindig, 1994; Hanson, 1997; Dunkin, Stratton, & Juhl, 1996; Stratton, Dunkin, Muse, Harris, & Geller, 1995).

Nurses in advanced practice roles are in especially short supply nationwide (Hanson, 1999; Office of Technology Assessment, 1994). Health professional workforce projections indicate that the U.S. health care delivery system will require an additional 100,000 primary care providers in the next decade. Of these, 70% (70,000) should be APRNs. The Pew Health Professions Commission (1994) recommends doubling the number of NPs by the year 2000. Further, these kinds of nurses are underused, resulting in an annual cost of about $60 billion to the U.S. health care system. Underuse (not using APRNs where such providers are appropriate) partly is attributable to the restrictions imposed by state nurse practice acts and partly to reimbursement preferences of third-party payers (Medicaid, Medicare, insurance companies). Some states permit a broader scope of practice for APRNs, and this has helped to improve access to care in health professional shortage areas (HPSAs). Across the nation, efforts are underway to deal with state practice restrictions so that APRNs can function in roles for which they are prepared (Marchione & Garland, 1997).

Affecting the current nursing shortage, too, are changes in the delivery and utilization patterns of health care. The largest segment of nurses work in hospitals, but increasingly more are working in a wide array of community-based health care settings. In rural areas, the percentage of nurses employed by hospitals declines with the number of people who reside in a county. In other words, counties having the fewest people also have lower numbers of nurses who work in an acute care institution. Perhaps there no longer is a functioning hospital in which nurses can work, or it has a very low patient census, so that only a few nurses are needed to staff it. Anecdotal reports by residents living in HPSAs describe herculean efforts to access care (Davis & Droes, 1993). Those care-seeking behaviors underscore the reality that many rural communities still do not have an adequate number or an appropriate mix of health professionals, specifically RNs and APRNs (Chapter 5).

Another change in the delivery and utilization of health care is the declining number of hospital beds and decreasing patient length of stay (LOS; in-hospital days). Beds designated for critical care, however, are increasing in response to the number of patients who are admitted with extremely acute conditions. In other words, hospitalized patients are sicker than ever and are subsequently discharged faster—and sicker. In the hospital and after discharge, clients, now more than ever, require highly skilled nurses to manage their complex care. Emphasis in the new health care paradigm is shifting from "cure" to "care." Biotechnology advances that preserve and sustain life also are changing care-seeking behaviors and the delivery of care. For example, remote telemetry and telehealth systems now allow for urban-based experts to consult with NPs and their patients in a rural clinic.

Nurses are needed to provide primary health care within managed care organizations (MCOs). Greater numbers of elderly persons and persons suffering from chronic and disabling conditions are present in schools and in the workplace. Increasingly, nurses are involved in planning, implementing, and evaluating services in all types of health care settings, as well as participating in the development of health policy. Unlike previous shortages, the current one stems from increased demand by the changing system rather than an inadequate supply of nurses. Supply-demand factors affect the nursing workforce even more profoundly in HPSAs. Registered nurses are prepared to deal with many different clinical and management functions, an ability that makes them extremely cost-effective providers of high-quality care. Policy developers continue to look to nurses to provide vital health care services to U.S. citizens, and APRNs specifically are cited as potential providers of primary care in HPSAs (Edwards, Lenz, & East, 1993).

In the past decade, several hundred rural hospitals closed, most often because of financial failure. Subsequently, physicians and nurses who worked there also departed, either by moving away from the community or by commuting to work in another facility. The domino effect left many counties without any providers and with even less access to care. To fill the void, outreach services sometimes are provided by tertiary health care institutions to consumers in rural catchments. In other cases, community hospitals have been transformed into expanded primary and ambulatory care units with emergency capabilities. In other states, "swing-bed" facilities were implemented: that is, hospitals in which a designated number of beds can be used for either acute care or long-term care patients. This state-sponsored initiative helped some small hospitals in remote geographical regions to sustain fiscal viability and continue providing care to consumers in the area. Anecdotal reports from across the nation reveal that there are tremendous needs for primary care, health promotion, and preventive services (e.g., farm safety, screening clinics, nutrition, stress management, wellness education, child care, immunizations). Overall, these unmet needs offer a plethora of professional and research opportunities for nurses who choose rural practice, especially those in advanced practice roles (Bureau of Health Professions, 1990; U.S. Department of Health and Human Services, 1997).

INITIATIVES TO IMPROVE ACCESS TO CARE

Over the decades, a variety of initiatives have focused on improving health care accessibility in rural areas, primarily through education, recruitment, and retention of health professionals (Appendix D). One particular initiative of significance to APRNs is Public Law No. 95-210 (1977), which led to the development of the Rural Health Clinics Service Act and subsequent amendments that mandated utilization of mid-level practitioners (midwives, NPs, physician's assistants) in these types of clinics (Kolimaga, Konrad, & Ricketts, 1994; Rural Information Center Health Services [RICHS], 1994). Educational incentives in the form of student work-payback loans and sign-on bonuses are designed to entice providers to work in underserved areas for the National Health Service Corps, state offices of rural health, and local health care organizations. Most of these stipulate that a student sign a contract to work in an underserved area after graduation, for a specified period of time that is based on the dollar amount awarded.

Increased emphasis is placed on accountability to educational programs that receive federal money, and their outcomes are closely monitored. Institutions receiving federal health professional training grants are required to provide student clinical rotations in underserved communities. Graduates must be able and willing to improve access to care for underserved populations in rural areas. Rural nurses should be aware of federal and state initiatives targeting the education, recruitment, and retention of health personnel. Often they are consulted by a community member with an interest in becoming a nurse, and this kind of information may help in that decision. In turn, that person may decide to return to the community to work upon graduating from the program.

EXPANDED ROLE OPPORTUNITIES FOR RURAL NURSES

For many Americans who choose to live in a sparsely populated or remote geographical area, APRNs (NPs, CNMs, CSs, CRNAs) are vital to improving their access to care. Accompanying community-based care is an expanding demand for CSs who can focus on community as the client. Rural nurses holding these credentials (master's degree in community health or public or occupational health nursing and certification as a CS) function in a variety of roles on a daily basis, including advocate, educator, consultant, administrator, case manager, direct care provider, and researcher. In rural areas, the CS may be an occupational health nurse, parish nurse, school nurse, and agricultural health nurse to provide cost-effective preventive services in the community. CSs are armed with knowledge about community resources, and their area of expertise is knowing how to access these. Services planned and coordinated by a CS tend to be less fragmented and usually are well accepted by residents in rural settings (Case, 1991). Increasingly, CSs are seeking additional education to become an NP or CNM to better meet the practice demands that exist in underserved rural regions.

NPs and CNMs provide primary care. But they may also be able to help hospital-based nurses define nursing care requirements for inpatients, coordinate discharge plans, and provide case management services. CNMs often help address the critical void in maternal and women's health, especially where there are limited or nonexistent obstetrical services. Some CNMs are prepared to provide health care to women across the age spectrum as well as maternity care (Fenton, Rounds, & Anderson, 1991; Hanson, 1997; Jenkins & Marx, 1994; Pearson, 1997). The essence of rural nursing is being an "expert generalist." NPs and CNMs in rural practice settings must be generalists who have developed expert skills in physical assessment, clinical decision making, and working with community resources. Rural-based NPs and CNMs need a strong community and public health orientation. In other words, they must first be community health nurses who have added skills to their repertoire, specifically preventive care, primary care diagnosis, and treatment. Preventing illness poses particular challenges to APRNs because health promotion programs are severely lacking in many rural parts of the nation.

The focus for NPs in rural environments usually is community-based primary care. Family nurse practitioners (FNPs) in particular are prepared to care for families and individuals across the life span. They are able to interface with other kinds of health care professionals and thus provide a continuum of preventive and primary care services. In addition, NPs and CNMs can make client referrals to specialty or support services within the community or, if needed, to urban-based tertiary medical centers. They work in rural health clinics, private practice, or outreach clinics, with a physician in a solo practice arrangement, and in health departments, and they are projected to have a major role in critical access hospitals (Chapter 12, Table 12.2). It is not unusual to find an NP or a CNM functioning as a principal primary health care provider in these communities with remote physician supervision. These nurses are the vital link between urban-based tertiary health providers and clients receiving care in a rural outreach clinic. Essentially, their generalist nursing skills coupled with a strong community background contribute to favorable health outcomes for their clients and the community as a whole.

For decades, certified registered nurse anesthetists (CRNAs) have been the mainstay of America's rural hospitals ("The Nurse Anesthetist," 1997; Turner & Gunn, 1991). Anesthesiologists tend to practice in urban-based acute care facilities. Consequently, CRNAs have had an important role in supporting and sustaining emergency, obstetric, and surgical services in small hospitals for decades in more remote areas across the 50 states. Unlike NPs and CNMs, CRNAs tend to remain in practice for a longer time, often in the same community. Attrition from anesthesia practice is relatively low compared with that from nursing in general. This trend may be due to men's making up nearly half of all CRNAs. Comparatively, of the total nursing workforce, men represent less than 5%. Nurse anesthetists are the principal, often sole, anesthesia provider in rural communities. Emergency room nurses, operating room nurses, and CRNAs are essential to the emergency capability of rural hospitals. Along with physicians, these teams stabilize injured persons prior to transportation to an urban-based tertiary care center. They also care for emergencies that, once stabilized, may not necessitate transfer outside of the community. In recent years, there has been a trend for urban-based CRNAs to provide outreach services to small hospitals: for example, on one particular day each week or perhaps twice each month. Consequently, rural patients who need more immediate or emergency surgery must be transported to another tertiary site for nonelective surgical procedures. This trend of out-shopping for health care by the more affluent has dramatically reduced access to essential services for other rural residents, especially the poor, the elderly, and those with limited transportation capabilities.

The ideal mix of providers in a rural setting is an interdisciplinary team composed of the physician, an NP, a midwife, and a social worker (RICHS, 1994). Other members can be added depending on a community's needs, preferences, and available health care facilities. For example, communities that have a hospital are more likely to have an extended-care facility, behavioral health services, and perhaps other specialty services. Communities vary in the type of essential health care providers they are able to recruit and retain. Factors that can hinder or enhance recruitment and retention of health professionals are local and regional lifestyle features, spousal employment opportunities, and adequacy of schools and shopping facilities (Ramsbottom-Lucier, Emmett, Rich, & Wilson, 1996). Likewise, each community has a unique blend of leaders from various disciplines, resources, and subgroups who set the tone for health care delivery in that region. For example, a physician in a given county may be the primary referral source for tertiary outreach teams who work in adjacent counties.

Camaraderie between health professionals from various disciplines is described by many APRNs as one of the most positive aspects of rural practice. For them, geographical isolation and less immediate accessibility to peers may actually encourage professionals to work as partners, regardless of hierarchy or turf. Nurses who choose rural practice must become involved in the local culture to be accepted and trusted by residents. Obviously, casting off the label of "community outsider" requires nurses' emotional investment and time, and some nurses will be better accepted than others. Nurses in general, and APRNs in particular, having community roots are more apt to be accepted, as they tend to be familiar with the realities of rural life and a community's social dynamics and power structures.

RURAL NURSING: REWARDS AND CHALLENGES

It is not prudent to generalize about rural practice, for each community and health care facility is unique, as are the nurses who work there. But in the literature, several salient themes emerge regarding rural nursing practice: great distances between places, scarce resources, multiple practice roles ("wearing several hats on the job"), and the need for generalist skills with less opportunity to specialize. This kind of practice allows for greater autonomy and independence because of geographic and professional isolation. Rural nurses have high community visibility; this can be highly rewarding, but it can also present some challenges in maintaining anonymity and confidentiality. Likewise, boundaries between personal and public life usually are less clearly delineated than in more populated settings. In turn, these rural features can pose some unusual legal and ethical dimensions to nurses' roles and scope of practice. These features of rural practice can be viewed as either good or not so good, depending on a given situation (Barger, 1996; Lee, 1998).

The Generalist Specialist

Rural nurses provide care to patients of all ages with a broad range of conditions. Consequently, nurses in these practice settings must be flexible, creative, and able to think critically. On a given day, for example, a nurse who is employed in a small rural hospital may care for patients in the emergency department, in labor and delivery, and on the medical unit, which may have one or two surgical and pediatric patients as well. Often their clients are personal acquaintances—friends, neighbors, and relatives. Nursing care continues after the person's discharge from the hospital because the nurse lives in the same community with patients and their families. Informal, sometimes frequent, encounters are apt to occur in various community sites, allowing for further discussion about the health condition. Nurses may be expected to make difficult decisions with insufficient or nonexistent resources and without immediate access to peers and other health professionals with whom to consult. Long after some events have taken place, nurses may contemplate the legal and ethical ramifications of painful decisions. Rural nurses tend to be highly professional, dedicated, and committed to keeping up with current developments in nursing despite limited access to education. A significant number work at the same job and reside in the same community for decades (Dunkin et al., 1994, 1996; Stratton, Dunkin, & Juhl, 1995; Stratton, Dunkin, Muse, et al., 1995).

Unfortunately, that is not the case for all nurses who choose a rural practice site. Some report that they accepted a position in a remote health care facility because, initially, they perceived rural life to be idyllic and free from urban lifestyle stressors. A small number even say they "had no idea what they were getting into" when deciding on a rural community. In part, their misperceptions (in some cases, ignorance) can be attributed to professional education programs, nursing in particular, that do not expose students to the rural practice environment. In other cases, the nurse may have participated in an educational payback loan program, such as the National Health Services Corps. Upon graduation, the individual may have selected or been assigned to a remote HPSA without knowing anything about rural life and even less about nursing in an underserved remote setting. Hopefully, the revisited initiatives to educate, recruit, and retain nurses that include student exposure to the rural environment will help to alleviate less favorable outcomes.

Urban-Biased Educational Programs

Generally, professionals are educated in urban settings and have their clinical experiences there as well. Until quite recently, nursing students had little, if any, exposure to rural practice; hence, they probably had an urban educational bias after graduation (NINR, 1995). Experiential deficits can lead to insensitivity that exacerbates rural clients' mistrust of urban-oriented health care professionals. Lack of exposure also deters students from practicing in a rural community. The aforementioned federal and state-sponsored educational incentive programs have helped some communities to recruit and retain nurses, but shortages remain in HPSAs, especially shortages of APRNs. Even though the job market is good for nurses, only a few nursing texts examine rural practice issues.

High Visibility

Generally, nurses who live and work in small rural communities have high public visibility. In part, this is attributable to most residents' having had someone in their family, at one time or another, use the local health care system. Thus, clients and their families continue to interact in many settings with nurses who are their neighbors, personal friends, friends of friends, or extended family. Local residents tend to see nurses in rural communities as their "personal" caregivers. Hence, nurses usually are well known and highly regarded by the townsfolk. Nurses who have resided in the area for many years often are given great esteem in their localities, sometimes even more than is given to physicians, especially those who provide only outreach services to the community (Lee, 1998; Winstead-Fry, Tiffany, & Shippee-Rice, 1992). Visibility may be appealing and gratifying to some. However, maintaining anonymity and confidentiality can become a concern, even among nurses who enjoy being personally acquainted with most locals. Nonanonymity has both advantages and disadvantages, as illustrated by the following remark:

> Personally knowing a person helps me plan holistic nursing care. After the patient leaves the hospital, I can follow his or her progress when we meet in a store, at church, or at community events. For home-bound patients, I receive word-of-mouth reports from relatives, friends, neighbors, and church members. People tell me about their health problems and recovery progress, whether or not I ask them. I have learned to always act interested and show concern. Sometimes the conversations become embarrassing, time consuming, and disruptive for my family, though. ([Name withheld], personal communication, 1997)

High visibility has implications for recruiting and retaining nurses as well as for planning, delivering, and evaluating nursing services in a rural community. Nurses in rural practice often are able to provide useful insights to students on ways to effectively deal with less formal interpersonal dynamics. Their suggestions also may help less seasoned nurses who are just entering the community to work more effectively within the local culture.

Community Dynamics

A community's cultural values and social dynamics also affect nursing practice patterns. For example, some rural communities are reported to be more conservative in their beliefs on gender roles. That is, certain residents have more definitive ideas as to what constitutes "men's work" as opposed to "women's work." Traditionally, this implies that women's work is given less importance because of the lack of compensation for domestic activities, care of the sick, and child care. Inherent in this frame of reference is that women's work should be volunteered for the well-being of the family and the community. Herein lies somewhat of a dilemma for nurses.

On the one hand, nursing is a predominantly female profession and hence is often viewed as women's work. On the other hand, a nurse's skills are a highly valued health care resource in the rural community. For example, in small communities, a nurse often is consulted by local people who drop by her home for advice on a health problem before going to the doctor, is called upon to respond to traffic accidents and check out the victims, or is invited to give health-related talks in schools and local service, civic, and church organizations. The more willing the nurse and the more effective his or her speaking ability, usually the greater the number of such invitations. These requests generally come with an expectation that the service will be volunteered, without reimbursement for the nurse's time and expertise. These incidents further blur the already nebulous distinction between the nurse's professional and personal life. Some nurses find these claims on their time to be a stressor in their rural practice. But many others find them to be a highly rewarding dimension of rural practice.

Another example of the social dynamics in very small communities is that the identity of a woman often stems from her relationship to someone else—usually a male. That is, a woman is identified as the wife, sister, daughter, or mother of another. Also, even though a woman has been married for decades—all the while using her husband's surname (e.g., Sue Jones) some longtime residents will continue to use her maiden name (e.g., Sue Smith). (Of course, they "remember when she was born and knew her all through school.") Consequently, a recent graduate who wants to work in a small town will have no identity of her own, even as a nurse. This can have professional implications for APRNs and female physicians who choose to work there. Advertently or inadvertently, all these community dynamics can contribute to the retention or attrition of nurses in rural health care facilities, sometimes for the good and sometimes to the detriment of the local health care system.

Salaries

Even though the disparities are lessening in the United States, salaries continue to show inequities based on gender. That is, in similar positions women are paid less than their male counterparts in urban as well as rural settings. Furthermore, like urban-based nurses, rural nurses have wide salary ranges. A recent study, however, offers some interesting, perhaps disturbing, insights on rural nurses' salaries. On average, baccalaureate-prepared registered nurses (RNs) practicing in rural areas receive about $5,000 less per year than those in nonrural areas (Pan & Straub, 1997). The financial return on additional years of experience also is reported to be lower for RNs practicing in rural areas than elsewhere in the nation. This finding, coupled with relatively lower bonuses for those with graduate degrees, reflects weaker earning power for rural nurses. Some speculate, however, that nurses' "real earnings" may be comparable when the differences in cost of living (reported to be lower in rural areas) are considered. And as with the cost of living, there are regional differences in the salaries of nurses. Individuals considering rural practice must assess the entire situation, including the value they place on quality-of-life factors, before making any kind of career decision. (See the Discussion Questions at the end of this chapter.)

Workforce estimates project that the demand for nurses with baccalaureate degrees will increase with the expansion of MCOs. The trend to use less prepared auxiliary and licensed personnel is not proving to be cost-effective because such personnel lack the wide range of skills that nurses have as well as nurses' ability to respond to the many un-anticipated events that occur daily in health care institutions providing care to patients. The greatest nursing needs will be in ambulatory care settings, public health, home health and mental health agencies, and nursing education programs. At stake is whether rural facilities will be able to compete financially for the inadequate supply of nurses having higher levels of professional education. If rural providers do not reward the productivity and human capital investment of nurses, the distribution of nurses will continue to favor other employment locations, specifically urban-based settings serving a higher client market volume.

For NPs, financial returns are reported to be higher in both settings but more so in rural areas. One explanation offered for this finding is that APRNs may be offsetting shortages of primary care physicians in rural areas. The APRN role is highly legitimized and favorably viewed by most U.S. consumers but not necessarily by third-party payers (insurance companies) or physicians. Whether the financial premium for APRNs, specifically NPs, continues will depend on how rapidly changes occur in demand and supply. Ultimately, economic factors affect the education, recruitment, and retention of nurses in rural environments.

Isolation and Scarce Resources

Isolation, geographic and professional, and scarce resources are other salient characteristics of rural environments that ultimately affect recruitment and retention of nurses. Geographic isolation often is a critical factor in rural clients' access to services. Distance and isolation are not always understood by those who are responsible for discharge planning of rural-resident patients from an urban-based hospital. Lack of understanding about the effect of distances on the availability and accessibility of services also is evident among policy makers at all levels, local, county, state, and federal.

For example, county commissioners sometimes consider nursing positions in the health department to be less essential services than other types of public infrastructures, such as communication systems, roads and bridges, law enforcement, schools, and welfare and social services. Obviously all these public services are critical to sustaining the economic viability and overall health of a small community. Moreover, rural areas tend to have a lower tax base and hence less revenue to support a full array of essential public services. Given the lack of fiscal resources, some who are involved in budget preparation may rationalize that there are insufficient people to warrant a full-time equivalent (FTE) county nursing position. Consequently, in more remote rural areas it is not unusual to find two or more counties combining resources to hire a district nurse. This can be a win-win arrangement for all, especially when the combined population is low, fairly healthy, and concentrated in the same geographical region. But problems can arise for these nurses when distances between communities are great or there are natural barriers such as mountains, rivers, forests, and inclement weather conditions. These factors can hinder nurses from getting to certain populations in the multicounty catchment area.

The scarcity of resources in many instances is made even more problematic by distance. Rural areas tend to have fewer health care providers of all types, whether physician specialists; respiratory, physical, enteral, occupational, or nutrition therapists; social workers; psychologists; or APRNs of various backgrounds. Consequently, rural nurses describe how they often are expected in their facility to "pick up the slack" and cover those services. In addition, they are expected to participate in the activities mandated by external regulating agencies, in particular continuous quality improvement and in-service education. Many report that they enjoy the independence, autonomy, and diversity of work. Others, however, find the multiple responsibilities overwhelming, especially without peer support and access to consultation from other disciplines. Establishing rapport with other providers in the community offers nurses a convenient backup and referral network should unanticipated practice situations arise.

Challenges and Benefits of Technology

Technology is changing the way health care is delivered in both rural and urban areas. Technology can enhance the ability to educate, recruit, and retain health care providers in more remote areas as well. Federal initiatives to get every U.S. community connected to the Internet have resulted in many small towns' having better access to telecommunications technology than some urban residents. Technology can facilitate communication between rural-based providers and urban-based specialists or between remotely connected APRNs and precepting physicians in another small community in the region, and it can link university-based academicians with students at rural practice sites located in the far corners of the state. Technology is enabling nurse scholars to partner with rural clinicians to implement studies that previously were not feasible. Face-to-face discussions are taking new forms: Health care personnel can communicate by video screens without having to be physically present in the same building. The interactions can be real time (synchronous) or at a time that is more convenient for all the participants (asynchronous) (Health Resources Services Administration [HRSA], 1997; NINR, 1995; Penney, Gibbons, & Bushy, 1996; Pew, 1994; Whitener, 1996).

Geographic remoteness requires nurses to have outstanding ability to be flexible and creative, to evaluate clients' needs, and to prioritize the services that are available in a community. Technology is overcoming distance factors that formerly restricted rural nurses' access to continuing and advanced education offerings (BSN, MSN, APRN). For instance, fax machines, overnight mail service, and computers (e-mail, World Wide Web, mobile cellular telephones) are being used for instantaneous consultation with nursing faculty and international experts at large medical centers. Distributive teaching-learning technology (teacher and student areas located at separate sites) is making courses available to rural nurses desiring additional education. On a less sophisticated level, consumers and health professionals are using videotapes, audiotapes, and the Internet, at their convenience, to learn about relevant health topics. Some rural APRNs have citizens'-band radios (CBs) or cellular telephones, if necessary, providing almost immediate, though remote, access to physicians, hospitals, emergency services, or even the county sheriff.

Significant federal monies have been appropriated for the development of telecommunications and telehealth infrastructures. However, outcome data are lacking or inconclusive. The information deficit is of concern to federal agencies that sponsor grants. Currently, efforts are underway to measure technology-related outcomes. Nurses should be aware that formative (process assessment) and summative (outcome measures) evaluations are important considerations when developing and writing proposals to seek grant monies for a rural technology initiative. Therefore, appropriate program evaluation methods should always be included in proposals for rural technology and telehealth-related initiatives.

SUMMARY

This chapter emphasized that nurses are a vital link in rural health care systems. Despite the apparent lack of many resources that urban-based nurses may take for granted, historically, most rural residents and rural nurses have fared quite well with self-care, neighborliness, and community support. To better address rural health care needs, nursing organizations along with policy makers have offered initiatives so that nurses can function in expanded roles for which they are prepared.

DISCUSSION QUESTIONS

The following questionnaire can be used to determine whether rural practice is for you. Assess your level of agreement with each statement, rating each item as *strongly agree, doesn't matter,* or *strongly disagree.* Discuss your answers with peers.

➢ Nurses who practice in rural communities have few opportunities for professional development.
➢ The nursing care that is delivered in rural ambulatory clinics is less complex than that provided in urban settings.
➢ Adequate primary care and urgent care require immediate access to specialty services.
➢ When a client has a serious health problem, coordination of care should be done through a medical specialist.
➢ A community-based ambulatory clinic with APRNs can address a broad range of health needs in a rural area.
➢ Practicing in a rural setting isolates nurses from professional peers.

> ➢ Referring clients for care outside the home community makes it difficult to maintain continuity of care.

> ➢ I personally plan to practice in a rural setting after completing this program or at some other time in the future.

> ➢ I feel that safe nursing practice requires immediate access to a broad array of health resources and personnel.

> ➢ I would be quite comfortable having one of my neighbors or relatives as a client/patient.

> ➢ NPs (CNMs, CRNAs) *really need* to have a physician in the health care facility when they see clients/patients.

> ➢ The social and cultural atmosphere that is available in an urban setting is very important to me.

> ➢ The financial rewards for nursing practice are greater in urban settings.

> ➢ Nurses who practice in rural settings see a greater variety of common health problems than nurses in urban settings do.

> ➢ I would enjoy the challenge of being one of only a few health care providers in a small community-based clinic.

> ➢ Small-town life is appealing to me.

> ➢ Rural residency fits with my family's lifestyle and preference.

SUGGESTED RESEARCH ACTIVITIES

Compile a demographic profile of rural nurses in your geographical area on the following factors: age, gender, marital status, years of education, area of specialization, experience, length of time employed in their current worksite, personal history in/with rural communities.

> ➢ How do rural and urban nurses compare on the demographic factors?

> ➢ What are the self-described reasons for selecting and/or remaining in rural practice?

> ➢ What are rural nurses' self-described roles and scope of nursing practice?

> ➢ Compare rural nurses' responses with those of nurses who practice in a large urban-based facility.

> ➢ What suggestions do nurses in rural practice have for others who are considering or planning to live and work in a rural community?

> ➢ What are the self-reported educational needs of nurses in rural practice? Compare the nurses' self-reported needs with their nursing administrators' perceptions and expectations.

REFERENCES

American Association of Colleges of Nursing. (1994). *Position statement: Certification and regulation of advanced practice nurses.* Washington, DC: Author.

American Nurses Association. (1991). *Council of Community Health Nurses' community-based nursing services: Innovative models.* Washington, DC: Author.

American Nurses Association, Rural/Frontier Health Care Task Force. (1996). *Rural/frontier nursing: The challenge to grow.* Washington, DC: Author.

Barger, S. (1996). Rural nurses: Here today and gone tomorrow? *Rural Clinician Quarterly, 6*(3), 3-4.

Bureau of Health Professions. (1990). *Report to the president and Congress on the status of health personnel in the U.S.* (DHHS Pub. No. HRS-OD-90-3). Washington, DC: Author.

Bushy, A. (1998). Rural nursing in the United States: Where do we stand as we enter the new millennium. *Australian Journal of Rural Health, 6,* 65-71.

Case, T. (1991). Work stresses of community health nurses in Oklahoma. In A. Bushy (Ed.), *Rural nursing* (Vol. 2). Newbury Park, CA: Sage.

Davis, D., & Droes, N. (1993). Community health nursing in rural and frontier counties. *Nursing Clinics of North America, 28,* 159-169.

Duncan, P., Coward, R., & Gilbert, G. (1997). Rural-urban comparisons of age and health at the time of nursing home admission. *Journal of Rural Health, 13,* 6-18.

Dunkin, J., Stratton, T., & Juhl, N. (1996). Why rural practice. *Nursing Management, 27*(2), 26-28.

Dunkin, J., Stratton, T., Movassaghi, H., & Kindig, D. (1994). Characteristics of metropolitan and nonmetropolitan community health nurses. *Texas Journal of Rural Health, 7*(1), 18-27.

Edwards, J., Lenz, C., & East, J. (1993). Nurse-managed primary care: Serving a rural Appalachian population. *Family and Community Health, 16*(2), 52-57.

Fenton, M., Rounds, L., & Anderson, E. (1991). Combining the role of the nurse practitioner and the community health nurse: An educational model for implementing community-based primary care. *Journal of the American Academy of Nurse Practitioners, 3*(3), 99-105.

Hanson, C. (1999). Rural nurse practitioner. In J. Hickey, R. Ouimette, & S. Venegoni (Eds.), *Advanced practice nursing.* Philadelphia: J. B. Lippincott.

Hanson, M. (1997, September 24). Rural nurses scarce. *Bismarck Tribune,* pp. 1A, 12A.

Health Resources Services Administration. (1997). *Exploratory evaluation of rural applications of telemedicine.* Rockville, MD: Author.

Jenkins, M., & Marx, E. (1994). Nurse practitioners and community health nurses: Clinical partnerships and future visions. *Nursing Clinics of North America, 29,* 459-470.

Kolimaga, J., Konrad, T., & Ricketts, T. (1994). Does subsidizing rural community health centers hurt private practice physicians? *Journal of Health Care of the Poor Underserved, 5,* 124-141.

Lee, H. (1998). *Conceptual basis for rural nursing.* New York: Springer.

Marchione, J., & Garland, T. (1997). An emerging profession? The case of the nurse practitioner. *Image: Journal of Nursing Scholarship, 29,* 335-349.

National Institute for Nursing Research. (1995). *Community-based health care: Nursing strategies* (Pub. No. 95-3917). Bethesda, MD: Author.

The nurse anesthetist: Issues in rural health care. (1997). *Today's Surgical Nurse, 9*(1), 41-42.

Office of Technology Assessment. (1994). *Health care in rural America.* Washington, DC: Government Printing Office.

Pan, S., & Straub, L. (1997). Education for rural health professionals. *Journal of Rural Health, 13*(1), 78-85.

Pearson, L. (1997). Annual update of how each state stands on legislative issues affecting advanced nursing practice. *Nurse Practitioner, 22*(1), 18-86.

Penney, N., Gibbons, B., & Bushy, A. (1996). Partners in distance learning: Project outreach. *Journal of Nursing Administration, 26*(7), 27-36.

Pew Health Professions Commission. (1994). *Resource book for health professions, education strategies, planning and policy development.* San Francisco: University of California San Francisco Center for Health Professions.

Pickard, M. (1996). Rural nursing: A decade in review. *Rural Clinician Quarterly, 6*(3), 1-2.

Ramsbottom-Lucier, M., Emmett, K., Rich, E., & Wilson, J. (1996). Hills, ridges, mountains and roads: Geographical factors and access to care in a rural state. *Journal of Rural Health, 12,* 386-394.

Rural Information Center Health Services. (1994). *Rural health in brief: Nurse practitioners, physician assistants, and certified nurse-midwives: Primary care providers in rural areas.* Washington, DC: U.S. Department of Agriculture.

Salmon, M. (1999). Thoughts on nursing: Where it has been and where it is going. *Nursing Health Care Perspectives, 20*(1), 20-25.

Stratton, T., Dunkin, J., & Juhl, N. (1995). Redefining the nursing shortage. A rural perspective. *Nursing Outlook, 43*(2), 71-77.

Stratton, T., Dunkin, J., Muse, K., Harris, T., & Geller, J. (1995). Retainment incentives in three rural practice settings: Influence on the job satisfaction of registered nurses. *Applied Nursing Research, 8*(2), 73-80.

Turner, T., & Gunn, I. (1991). Issues in rural health nursing. In A. Bushy (Ed.), *Rural nursing* (Vol. 2, pp. 105-127). Newbury Park, CA: Sage.

U.S. Department of Health and Human Services. (1997). *Facts about rural physicians and primary care providers.* Hyattsville, MD: Author.

Whitener, L. (1996). Telecommunications and rural health care. *Journal of Rural Health, 12*(1), 67-71.

Winstead-Fry, P., Tiffany, J. C., & Shippee-Rice, R. V. (1992). *Rural health nursing: Stories of creativity, commitment, and connectedness* (NLN Pub. No. 21-2408). New York: National League of Nursing.

CHAPTER 14

Rural Nursing in Australia

DESLEY HEGNEY

KEY TERMS

- ➤ Advanced nurse practitioner
- ➤ Rural nurse
- ➤ Remote nurse
- ➤ Enrolled nurse workforce
- ➤ Allied health professional
- ➤ Spatially inequitable
- ➤ Case mix funding
- ➤ User-pays system
- ➤ Staff locums

OBJECTIVES

After reading this chapter, you will be able to

- ➤ Compare and contrast the Australian rural nursing issues to those of the United States and Canada
- ➤ Discuss the impact of interdisciplinary relationships on the role and function of rural nurses in Australia.
- ➤ Analyze the impact of rurality on rural nursing practice in Australia.
- ➤ Propose solutions to overcome the barriers identified with regard to rural nursing in Australia.

ESSENTIAL POINTS TO REMEMBER

➢ Rural nurses in Australia have a different role than metropolitan nurses. There is a lack of recognition of the difference of the expanded role of rural nursing practice. The need for a medical practitioner to be employed in each rural community has dominated the recruitment and retention debate in Australia. The high turnover rate and shortage of rural nurses have been ignored because the nursing workforce is seen to be expendable.

➢ Though health care is provided equally to all Australians under a universal-taxation-funded model, rural Australians have fewer services than those in metropolitan areas.

➢ The education and training of rural nurses, both in preparation for practice and continuing after employment, are problematic in that the majority of nurses are denied access to affordable and appropriate programs.

OVERVIEW

This chapter describes rural nursing in Australia. Political, social, cultural, and economic factors are examined that affect nurses' practice, education, recruitment, and retention in rural areas (Hegney, 1996, 1997a, 1997b, 1997c).

INTRODUCTION

Australia is the driest continent in the world. It is a land of contrasts with fertile tropical rainforests, green rolling hills cloaked in gum trees, snow-covered alps, desert, and a coastline that is teeming with life. This ancient land (at least 4.3 billion years old) has been changed forever by the introduction of European farming practices and the needs of early settlers to recreate England in Australia. As the population grew, settlement predominated in the coastal areas of Australia, which have a superior environment to the harsher inlands. Approximately 80% of Australia's 20 million people live close to the eastern and southern coast, which is the country's most gentle and fertile crescent (Beale & Fray, 1990).

Rural Australia is diverse in its economic base, its demographic attributes, and its future prospects. Distance, which has influenced the development of rural Australia, has shaped its past and is likely to shape its future. During the last 200 years, rural Australia has experienced the growth and decline of towns, mostly associated with the growth and decline of economically viable primary production. Many of the hospitals that were established to serve these populations, along with the health practitioners who moved into rural areas to provide health care to rural people, are no longer justified as viable or efficient. During the last 200 years, the reality of rural life has seldom overcome the myths that have been incorporated into the discourse of Australians. Possibly, the recent agricultural crisis and long drought have brought the hardships faced by rural Australians closer to those in the metropolitan areas and provincial cities. Yet rural Australia is still seen as a place where the myths of "mateship," "battlers," and "stoicism" remain, and as a healthy place to live.

THE AUSTRALIAN HEALTH CARE SYSTEM

Australia has a health care system similar to that of Canada, with a universal, taxation-funded health insurance (Medicare) that ensures that all Australians receive free hospital treatment (Palmer & Short, 1994). Visits to medical practitioners are either fully or partly subsidized by Medicare. Australians also have the option of private insurance that allows them to elect to be admitted to a public or private hospital as a private-paying patient. Hospitals, nursing homes, mental health, and community nursing services have two types of service delivery—public (government funded) and private (for-profit and not-for-profit). Australia has three tiers of health service delivery: the federal government, state and territory governments, and local government levels. Each tier of government has various powers and responsibilities concerning health care determined by the Australian Constitution. For example, the federal government is responsible for funding health services (through Medicare) and directs these payments to the state and territory governments. The state and territory governments are responsible for the direct provision of health care (through public hospitals, community health services, and so on), with local government having a relatively minor role. State and territory governments also administer registration of health professionals (nurses, medical practitioners) and licensing and regulation of private hospitals and private nursing homes. The majority of funding for health services is targeted toward "cure" rather than prevention. In 1989-90, for example, only 4.4% of all recurrent health expenditure was allocated to community and public health (Australian Institute of Health and Welfare [AIHW], 1993). Sixty percent of the budget was spent on institutional care. This expenditure reflects the dominance of the medical profession in Australia in health expenditure and policy, which has a strong historical origin.

HEALTH STATUS OF RURAL AUSTRALIANS

The health status of Australia's rural population varies enormously. Several studies indicate that Australia's rural communities have differing health problems and therefore health needs. However, there are specific diseases that have a high morbidity and mortality rate in rural areas (Department of Community Services and Health, 1991; Humphreys & Rolley, 1993; Western Australian Department of Health, 1994). More specifically, there are high levels of stress-related illnesses such as hypertension and psychiatric disorders among farming families due to the close connection of business and personal life on the farm (Lawrence, 1987; Titulaer, Trickett, & Bhatia, 1997). In addition, farm suicides among male 15- to 24-year-olds are higher than in metropolitan areas. Rural male suicides in this age group accounted for 38 deaths per 100,000 compared to 27 deaths per

100,000 in urban areas in 1988. Domestic violence, youth suicide, chronic illness, and the consumption of alcohol and tobacco are higher among rural people (Lawrence & Williams, 1990). Rural residents display an above-average incidence of endocrine and nutritional disorders; metabolic diseases; immunity disorders; respiratory, musculo-skeletal, genitourinary, skin, and subcutaneous tissue diseases; and motor vehicle accidents than urban residents (Fitzwarryne & Fitzwarryne, 1982; Humphreys & Rolley, 1991, 1993). Although this higher incidence of disease and injury may be related to aspects of the rural environment and rural lifestyle, there is also evidence to suggest that the shortage of health services contributes to the problems.

RURAL HEALTH SERVICES

The provision of health services to rural areas is complex in that the problems of distance and sparsely populated areas have to be overcome. Until the recent introduction of case mix funding, most health services in rural areas were funded on historical "wants" rather than actual needs. An examination of the discourses surrounding health service provision in rural areas reveals three features. First, there is ample evidence that health services are inadequately provided. Second, the pattern of provision is spatially inequitable. Third, there has been no integrated policy for the delivery of health services to rural areas, so provision and planning have been largely an ad hoc effort.

INITIATIVES TO RESTRUCTURE SERVICES

In the 1990s, there have been attempts by state, territory, and federal governments to restructure health services. Rolley and Humphreys (1993) identified three broad categories of restructuring: geographical restructuring, privatization of functions, and changes in the form of service provision.

Geographical Restructuring

To achieve economies of scale and to maximize local efficiencies, changes have occurred that have resulted in the redistribution of existing services. This has meant the rationalization and centralization of many services into larger units, the closure and/or reduction of smaller units, and the spatial relocation of services and offices due to population shifts. Political considerations have also influenced the provision of centralized or regionalized health services. Due to the policy of centralization and regionalization, many country people now have to travel further for health care. The decision to provide services is increasingly being made on the grounds of expenditure, not of effectiveness of the service.

Privatization of Functions

Changes that have occurred have affected labor and employment. There is an increasing discourse surrounding privatization and individuals meeting their own needs. The "user-pays" system is now being applied to rural health services. An example is the privatization of health services at Port Macquarie in New South Wales and La Trobe Regional Hospital in Victoria (Rolley & Humphreys, 1993; Walmsley, 1993). The trend toward a "user-pays" system and the delivery of health care through private practitioners could mean fewer services in small or isolated areas to which private medical practitioners are not attracted.

Changes in Service Provision

The advent of technology has benefited some rural people while disadvantaging others. For example, the Computer Aided Livestock Marketing system means that farmers can now sell livestock direct. Teleconferencing, videoconferencing, and distance learning have decreased isolation for some rural residents, but for some they have meant the loss of employment. The high-technology trend in health care has meant that expensive specialist services (e.g., CAT scanners) are available only in larger regional or metropolitan centers (Rolley & Humphreys, 1993; Walmsley, 1993). The net result of all these changes has been a transfer of costs to the user of the health service and the depopulation of small rural communities as local services are downgraded or closed. Another add-on effect of the downgrading of services in rural areas is that these smaller towns become less attractive to new settlers as they have fewer services available.

All is not negative, however, as service providers have become aware that the geographical diversity of rural areas dictates that health services be locally relevant. In addition, the development of policies on rural health by some state governments (Western Australia, Queensland, and South Australia) and the development of the National Rural Health Strategy (1994) by the federal government are beginning to have some impact on the previously metropolitan-driven health policies of the past. Regardless of the rhetoric of these policies (federal, state, or territory), they have resulted in consideration of the different needs of rural residents.

DEFINING *RURAL* IN THE AUSTRALIAN CONTEXT

As in the United States, in Australia there is no common definition of *rural*. Federal and state government departments employ different definitions. This can be explained by economic factors (e.g., remote-area nurses are paid more than nurses employed in the more populated rural areas) and political factors (state/federal relations). Despite the lack of a standard definition, there is a recognition that rural areas are diverse in economic base, population characteristics (age, ethnicity, gender balances), and health status.

Similarly, there is no one definition of rural nursing in Australia. The most recent definition describes rural nursing as the practice of nurses who are employed in a rural health facility where there are no full-time medical practitioners on duty or of nurses who are employed in community health in a rural area (Hegney, 1996, 1997a, 1997b, 1997c). This definition recognizes that it is the rural environment that determines the context of rural nursing practice (distance from support services) and therefore the advanced practice nature of the rural nurse's role.

RURAL NURSES: DEMOGRAPHICS

In Australia, two types of nurses work in rural areas—rural nurses and remote-area nurses. Remote-area nurses have long been recognized as having a different role than nurses in metropolitan areas because of their isolation from medical practitioners, whereas rural nurses have until relatively recently not voiced their perception of having a different role than metropolitan nurses. Though discussion continues in Australia as to whether rural and remote-area nurses should be discussed separately, as they have different roles, McMurray et al. (1998) have argued that their roles have more in common than has previously been acknowledged. That is, their practice is relatively autonomous and is determined by the needs of each individual rural community.

In 1994, rural and remote-area nurses (both registered and enrolled) constituted 28.3% of the total nursing workforce (AIHW, 1997). This is similar to the distribution of the overall rural population, with 27.8% living in rural and remote areas. There is, however, unequal distribution of nurses in rural and remote areas, with 959.6 remote-area nurses per 100,000 population, 1,262.1 metropolitan nurses per 100,000 population, and 1,702.2 rural nurses per 100,000 population. Similarly, the enrolled nurse workforce is disproportionate, with approximately twice as many enrolled nurses in rural areas (488.1 per 100,000 population) as in metropolitan areas (241.6 per 100,000 population).

Rural nurses are predominantly female. It appears, however, that the smaller the health service, the more female the population. The average age of rural nurses is higher than that of remote-area and metropolitan-area nurses. For example, in 1994 over 16% of rural nurses were aged 50 years and over (AIHW, 1997). Also, rural nurses are more likely to be employed part time than either remote-area or metropolitan nurses. Remote-area nurses worked an average of 33.2 hours per week, which contrasted with 29.8 hours per week in rural areas and 32.6 hours per week in metropolitan areas. Approximately 89% of rural nurses are hospital rather than university prepared. In addition, rural nurses who have trained in rural hospitals are more likely to be employed in medium-sized health facilities (11-50 acute beds). In contrast, nurses who trained in a metropolitan area are more likely to work in larger rural health facilities (over 50 acute beds). Like the medical workforce in Australia and overseas, Australian rural nurses are more likely to be working in a rural area if they grew up in a rural area. With the increased age of the rural nursing workforce and the reluctance of university-prepared nurses to work in rural areas, the current shortage will worsen (Kamien & Buttfield, 1990; Smith, 1996).

THE SCOPE OF NURSING PRACTICE

Nursing roles in rural Australia differ and are affected by several factors. Geographical location, the population density of the area, the type of employing health institution, and the health needs of the community are examples of factors that define the context in which a rural nurse works. The context of practice, it has been argued, determines the role and function of the rural nurse (Australian Health Ministers' Advisory Council, 1993; Hegney, 1996). The level of responsibility accepted by rural nurses is described as high in comparison to that of metropolitan nurses (King, 1994). This level of responsibility has been linked to the reportedly high job satisfaction level of rural nurses. Research in Australia on the role and function of rural nurses has revealed that the majority of the community believe that rural nurses are competent in a vast array of nursing skills. These are acquired by education and daily practice, and nurses possess skills that are highly valued by the community in which they work (Burley & Harvey, 1993; Thornton, 1992).

Rural nurses' role, often described as "jack of all trades" or "extended," "expanded," or "multiskilled," is not new to rural nurses. Rather, this diverse scope of practice has been the norm for rural and remote-area nursing practice since their inception (Biacca, 1993; Cooke & Jones, 1994; Coxhead, 1993; Dawson, 1992; Tonna, 1991). In small rural and remote nursing health facilities, the generalist (broad) role means that the nurse is providing care as well as dealing with situations external to the health environment, including the well-being, development, and safety of the local community in which he or she works (New South Wales Health, 1998). It is argued, therefore, that the role is one of an advanced nurse practitioner and that rural nurses must have skills and knowledge

> beyond that acquired in basic nursing education, as well as the advanced knowledge and skills to meet the needs of the population that is unserved, or underserved, by medical services which normally are available to residents in more populated urban communities. (McMurray et al., 1998, p. 9)

Unlike other similarly developed countries, such as the United States and Canada, Australia does not recognize or legitimize this advanced nursing practice role in law. Several studies, however, have made recommendations that an advanced practice nursing role be legitimized in Australia (Hegney, 1997a, 1997b, 1997c). As in the United States, the United Kingdom, and Canada, it is recognized that the medical and pharmaceutical professions will oppose this legitimization (Baker & Napthine, 1994; Coxhead, 1993).

RURAL PRACTICE ISSUES

Before advanced nurse practitioners can practice in Australia, other aspects of rural nursing practice need to be addressed, such as educational preparation, access to continuing professional education, recruitment and retention issues, personal and professional isolation, anonymity issues, marketing of rural nursing as a desirable career, and strengthening of intersectorial communication. The next section presents a brief discussion on factors that affect nursing practice in rural Australia.

Anonymity

In small towns, people know each other and are often related. Because of the relative stability of the rural nursing workforce, the majority of nurses practice in one health service for long periods of time. As well as being members of a small community, rural nurses can provide health care to several generations of the same family (Martin, 1993, 1994). This aspect of their role has been described as "womb to tomb care." Being known by the community and knowing the community have been described as distinguishing features of rural nursing practice. Some suggest that rural nurses have a unique insight into their community and its needs. In addition, rural communities also have the expectation that the nurse will be an integral member of the community. Some suggest that rural nurses lose their anonymity by virtue of their rural practice, as they never are off duty (Sturmey & Edwards, 1991; Thornton, 1992).

For some rural nurses, never being off duty is a negative aspect of their practice; for others, it is a positive aspect. Leaving the community or "getting out" is for some nurses an important coping mechanism. To do this, however, nurses must have access to relief staff *locums* (i.e., health professionals who are not employed in the health facility and who come from an outside agency to replace a permanent staff member when the member is on leave). The lack of locum relief is a barrier that has been identified as affecting nurses' ability to leave the community not only for "time out" but for continuing professional education. Knowing the community also means that the nurse often has to provide care to relatives and friends. When the crisis is over, the loss belongs to the nurse as well as the patient and/or family (Buckley & Gray, 1993; Harris, 1992; Siegloff & Hegney, 1996; Sigsby, 1991).

Professional Isolation

Distance does not necessarily mean isolation. Nurses can feel isolated in metropolitan settings, especially if they are working as a sole practitioner, such as a nurse midwife or occupational health nurse. But the literature suggests that rural nurses do feel isolated in their practice. A major reason for the sense of isolation is the distances between health services and thus among nursing, medical, and allied health support services and personnel. (An allied health professional is a member of a related health discipline but not a medical practitioner or nurse. Allied health professionals include pharmacists, physiotherapists, occupational therapists, dentists, speech therapists, and so on.) A major concern to rural nurses is their ability to form peer network support groups. Such networks need not be confined to nursing but should be formed with other health professionals. The formation of network groups can decrease feelings of isolation and assist nurses in the verbal sharing of knowledge that is such an integral part of nursing (Hart, Albrecht, Bull, & Marshall, 1992; Hill & Alexander, 1994; Stevens & Allan, 1992). Networks that facilitate education and training offerings also decrease rural nurses' feelings of isolation (Blue & Howe-Adams, 1992; Knox, 1992; Lampshire & Rolfe, 1993, 1996). The ability to form networking groups is influenced by nurses' access to modern technology (i.e., e-mail and Internet capabilities) along with their interpersonal skills. However, the ability of nurses to establish formal and informal networks also requires employer support. Presence of such support correlates with job satisfaction and the recruitment and retention of nurses in rural areas (Hegney, 1997a, 1997b, 1997c).

Recruitment and Retention

Though much has been written about the shortage of medical practitioners in rural areas, very little attention has been paid to the increasing shortage of rural nurses and midwives in Australia. The top 10 specialties for which positions were being actively recruited were "generalist, mental health, intensive care, midwifery, operating theatre, emergency department, orthopaedic, community health and paediatrics" (New South Wales Health, 1998, p. 4). In Northern Queensland, the turnover rate of nurses is as high as 600% per annum (Hegney, 1997b). Factors that have been linked to retention include poor accommodation, the lack of a career pathway, few or no child care facilities, a lack of access to education and training, a lack of employer support, the level of stress, legal aspects of role relationships with medical officers, and inadequate locum relief. Factors that do not appear to be linked to job satisfaction include the type of employment, the years worked in the health service, the level of employment, and having undertaken education and training in the last 12 months.

Recruitment of rural nurses is becoming problematic in Australia. Factors that influence nurses' decision to work in rural areas include the lack of marketing of rural nursing as a desirable career option, the low number of clinical placements currently available for preregistration undergraduate nursing students, and the lack of graduate-year placements in rural facilities (Hegney, 1996, 1997a, 1997c). Many of the factors affecting recruitment and retention have already been mentioned or will be mentioned later in this chapter. The factor of relationships of the nurse with medical practitioners, however, deserves some discussion.

Relationships With Medical Practitioners

One factor that often influences the level of responsibility of rural nurses is the number of medical officers and allied health workers employed by or appointed to the health service. This varies from different-sized health services with nurses working alone who rely on off-site medical services (Royal Flying Doctor Service, general practitioner in neighboring town, visiting health teams such as mental health and aged care) to hospitals that have resident medical officers, medical specialists, and a wide range of allied health workers.

In small rural hospitals, the first patient contact in an emergency is the nurse. General practitioners employed in the town can be unavailable for periods ranging from 30 minutes to 1 hour or, in some cases, not available at all—as is all too frequently the case in towns that do not have a medical practitioner and are trying to recruit another. This lack of on-site medical input is the main difference between the role and function of rural nurses and those of nurses employed in urban settings. Further, in many small rural hospitals there is no pharmacist, radiographer, physiotherapist, occupational therapist, and so on. In these health facilities, nurses dispense medications on a telephone order from an off-site medical practitioner, take x-rays, and provide allied health services to rural residents.

Despite the rhetoric of interdisciplinary teams in rural areas, there is often role conflict between the nurse and the medical officer (Pearson, 1993). This conflict can be a cause of stress and a reason for poor retention rates in some areas. Conflicts often arise when the off-site medical officer is required to attend the hospital. During the day, the medical officer may be conducting a consulting session with private patients. During the night, often the nurse, having assessed the patient, must discuss the client with the medical officer. These telephone conversations are reported to be a source of stress to many nurses, as often the medical practitioner does not wish to attend the patient in the hospital. Community nurses also report that they need to ensure good working relationships with the medical practitioners.

Many general practitioners underestimate the skills of rural hospital and community nurses, not recognizing their experience and expertise. This may lead to a situation in which medical practitioners limit nurses' ability to deliver holistic care and allow them only to deliver fragmented care. For example, they request that the nurse check on a client's blood pressure without giving a concise picture of the client's condition or without prescribing medication or even making a formal referral to the nurse for follow-up care (Lampshire & Rolfe, 1993). The poor relationship between the medical practitioner and the nurse also affects the level of care available to a client. Hegney (1997b) argued that legitimizing the role of the rural nurse by allowing the advanced practitioner role will increase the job satisfaction of rural nurses, decrease the high caseload of rural medical practitioners, and result in a quality service to rural consumers.

Education and Training

Since 1990, all undergraduate registered nurse programs in Australia have been conducted in higher education institutions. Each higher education institution has an individual curriculum, though one that has been accredited by the state registering authority. Also, from 1999, all enrolled nursing programs will be conducted at Colleges of Technical and Further Education. This transfer of nursing programs at the undergraduate level to tertiary providers has meant that all rural hospital undergraduate programs have closed. Postgraduate continuing and formal education is less clear-cut, with a mixture of education and training providers offering programs (universities, rural health training units, university departments of rural health, hospitals). A major criticism of the transfer of nursing education to the tertiary sector (at undergraduate and postgraduate levels) is the cost to the student. Excessive cost affects a nurse's ability to enroll in a course as well as temporary clinical placements. In addition, there is a lack of rural clinical placements and a lack of graduate courses for the newly graduated registered nurse (Hegney, 1997b, 1997c; New South Wales Health, 1998). In contrast to the funding that has been made available for the preparation and continuing education of medical practitioners, little if any funding has been provided for nursing.

The Australian literature contains a wealth of information on the lack of access to education and training of rural and remote-area nurses. It particularly focuses on the need for appropriate, accessible, and flexible programs, preferably delivered within the rural clinical environment. Barriers to education and training that have been identified include family commitments, inability to afford unpaid leave, lack of locum relief staff, lack of finance, lack of information on what courses are available, lack of employer support, and the unsuitability of many courses for rural nursing practice (Blue, 1992, 1993; Buckley & Gray, 1993; Hanley, 1996; Jones & Blue, 1998; Keyzer, 1994; Spencer, 1997).

The recent report by McMurray et al. (1998) recommends that a single practice credential should be introduced that prepares the rural and remote-area nurse as an advanced nurse practitioner (rural and remote). A master's-level nursing degree should incorporate the principles of flexibility in access and delivery, recognition of prior learning, and articulation. Further, curricula should be based upon advanced nursing competencies and should focus on clinical applications. Rural nurses must be educationally prepared for their role before they are employed. They need access to continuing education and training. Finally, employers must be partners in the preparation and continuing education of rural nurses.

SUMMARY

Australia's changing health care system means better informed consumers and primary health care services that are tailored to meet the needs of a particular community. This chapter described nurses' roles in rural parts of Australia. Nurses, in turn, must become proactive in educating rural communities about the capabilities of advanced nurse practitioners. Consumers also must be informed about how these nurses fit in the changing system and how they can improve access to primary health care.

DISCUSSION QUESTIONS

Discuss how the concepts of rural and rural nursing are defined in the Australian context.

➢ What are the historical bases of rural nursing practice in Australia?

➢ How does rural nursing practice fit with the theories put forth in Chapter 3?

➢ Is it possible to apply the information provided in this chapter on Australia to Dunkin's (American) exemplar presented in Chapter 5 of this text? Compare and contrast the geographic and demographic makeup of Australia with that of the United States and Canada.

SUGGESTED RESEARCH ACTIVITIES

Collaborate with an international scholar(s) to examine the following questions.

➢ Describe and compare rural communities' perceptions of nurses' role and scope of practice.

➢ Examine the nursing and non-nursing skill mix required for small rural health facilities (with regard to enrolled and registered nurses).

➢ What models of nursing services are the most appropriate for small rural communities (fewer than 5,000 people)? Are there differences among nations (i.e., Canada, Australia, and the United States)?

➢ What are the roles and scope of practice of nurses in remote areas? How cost-effective are visiting nurses in sparsely populated rural regions?

➢ Investigate strategies that are effective in improving the health status of residents in rural areas.

REFERENCES

Australian Health Ministers' Advisory Council. (1993). *Proposals for a revised national rural health strategy.* Canberra: Australian Government Publishing Service.

Australian Institute of Health and Welfare. (1993). *Australian health expenditure to 1991-1992* (Health Expenditure Bull. No. 8). Canberra: Author.

Australian Institute of Health and Welfare. (1997). *National nurse labourforce collection: 1994.* Canberra: Australian Government Printing Service.

Baker, H., & Napthine, R. (1994). *Nurses and medications: A literature review.* Melbourne: Australian Nursing Federation.

Beale, B., & Fray, P. (1990). *The vanishing continent: Australia's degraded environment.* Sydney, Australia: Hodder & Stoughton.

Biacca, S. (1993). Rural mental health nursing: A forgotten frontier? In Association for Australian Rural Nurses (Ed.), *Nursing the country: Conference proceedings of the Association for Australian Rural Nurses Inc.* (pp. 121-127). Warrnambool: Association for Australian Rural Nurses.

Blue, I. (1992). Take Mohammed to the mountain. In *Infront: Outback. Conference proceedings of the Australian Rural Health Conference* (pp. 21-28). Toowoomba, Australia: Toowoomba Health Services.

Blue, I. (1993). *A critical analysis of postgraduate education opportunities for rural nurses practising in the northern and western regions of South Australia.* Whyalla: University of South Australia.

Blue, I., & Howe-Adams, J. (1992). Educational choices: A program of educational support for multidisciplinary health professionals in rural and remote areas. In M. Courtney (Ed.), *Issues in rural nursing* (pp. 133-144). Armidale, Australia: University of New England.

Buckley, P., & Gray, G. (1993). *Across the spinifex: Registered nurses working in rural and remote South Australia.* Adelaide: Flinders University of South Australia.

Burley, M., & Harvey, D. (1993). Nurses and their small rural communities. In Association for Australian Rural Nurses (Ed.), *Nursing the country: Conference proceedings of the Association for Australian Rural Nurses Inc.* (pp. 149-158). Warrnambool: Association for Australian Rural Nurses.

Cooke, T., & Jones, J. (1994). Advanced life support: A rural clinician's perspective. In Association for Australian Rural Nurses (Ed.), *Windmills, wisdom and wonderment: Conference proceedings of the Association for Australian Rural Nurses Inc.* Roseworthy: Association for Australian Rural Nurses.

Coxhead, J. (1993). United we stand—divided we fall. *Australian Journal of Rural Health, 1,* 13-18.

Dawson, J. (1992). Anecdotal evidence: Driving force for rural nursing practice. In *Infront: Outback. Conference proceedings of the Australian Rural Health Conference* (pp. 83-88). Toowoomba, Australia: Toowoomba Health Services.

Department of Community Services and Health. (1991). *National Rural Health Conference: A fair go for rural health: A national rural health strategy.* Canberra, Australia: Author.

Fitzwarryne, P., & Fitzwarryne, C. (1982). *Health education promotion program (rural areas): Evaluation of a demonstration project.* Canberra, Australia: Health Research Association.

Hanley, A. (1996). *Australian rural nurses' education, training and support.* Whyalla: Association for Australian Rural Nurses.

Harris, R. (1992). *Australian rural health: A national survey of education needs.* Wollongong, Australia: University of Wollongong.

Hart, G., Albrecht, M., Bull, R., & Marshall, L. (1992). Peer consultation: A professional development opportunity for nurses employed in rural settings. In *Infront: Outback. Conference proceedings of the National Rural Health Conference* (pp. 143-148). Toowoomba, Australia: Toowoomba Health Services.

Hegney, D. (1996). *The windmill of rural health: A Foucauldian analysis of the discourses of rural nursing in Australia, 1991-1994.* Unpublished doctoral dissertation, Southern Cross University, Lismore, Australia.

Hegney, D. (1997a). Defining rural and rural nursing. In L. Siegloff (Ed.), *Rural nursing in the Australian context* (pp. 25-44). Canberra, Australia: Royal College of Nursing.

Hegney, D. (1997b). Extended, expanded, multi-skilled or advanced practice? *Collegian, 4,* 22-27.

Hegney, D. (1997c). Rural nursing practice. In L. Siegloff (Ed.), *Rural nursing in the Australian context* (pp. 25-44). Canberra: Royal College of Nursing, Australia.

Hill, P., & Alexander, T. (1994). Beyond the bounds of distance. In Association for Australian Rural Nurses (Ed.), *Windmills, wisdom and wonderment: Conference proceedings of the Association for Australian Rural Nurses Inc.* Roseworthy: Association for Australian Rural Nurses.

Humphreys, J., & Rolley, F. (1991). *Health and health care in rural Australia.* Armidale, Australia: University of New England.

Humphreys, J., & Rolley, F. (1993). Neglected factors in planning rural health services. In K. Malko (Ed.), *A fair go for rural health: Forward together* (pp. 47-54). Armidale, Australia: University of New England.

Jones, J., & Blue, I. (1998). *Education, training and professional support for rural nurses: A national survey of rural health training units.* Whyalla: Association for Australian Rural Nurses.

Kamien, M., & Buttfield, I. (1990). Some solutions to the shortage of general practitioners in rural Australia. Part 1. Selection of medical students. *Medical Journal of Australia, 15,* 105-107.

Keyzer, D. (1994). Expanding the role of the nurse: Nurse practitioners and case managers. *Australian Journal of Rural Health, 2,* 5-11.

King, J. (1994). Windmills, wisdom and wonderment: Can you find it all in nursing? In *Windmills, wisdom and wonderment: Conference proceedings of the Association for Australian Rural Nurses Inc.,* Roseworthy: Association for Australian Rural Nurses.

Knox, C. (1992). An historical perspective of continuing education in rural South Australia. *Australian Journal of Rural Health, 1,* 11-16.

Lampshire & Rolfe. (1993). *The realities of rural district nursing: A study of practice issues and education needs—Loddon-Mallee region.* Victoria, Australia: Victorian In-Service Nurse Education and Department of Health and Community Services.

Lampshire & Rolfe. (1996). *Postgraduate and continuing education for Victorian rural nurses: Issues and further directions.* Melbourne, Australia: CURHEV (Co-ordinating Unit for Rural Health Education in Victoria, Inc.).

Lawrence, G. (1987). *Capitalism and the countryside: The rural crisis in Australia.* Sydney, Australia: Pluto.

Lawrence, G., & Williams, C. (1990). The dynamics of decline: Implications for social welfare delivery in Australia. In T. Cullen, P. Dunn, & G. Lawrence (Eds.), *Rural health and welfare in Australia.* Wagga Wagga, Australia: Centre for Rural Welfare Research.

Martin, E. (1993). Constraint/restraint: Can we do anything about it? In Association for Australian Rural Nurses (Ed.), *Nursing the country: Conference proceedings of the Association for Australian Rural Nurses Inc.* (pp. 98-101). Warrnambool: Association for Australian Rural Nurses.

Martin, E. (1994). The Support Awareness Program for Nurses in southern Tasmania: A cooperative effort between city and rural health. In Association for Australian Rural Nurses (Ed.), *Windmills, wisdom and wonderment: Conference proceedings of the Association for Australian Rural Nurses Inc.* Roseworthy: Association for Australian Rural Nurses.

McMurray, A., St. John, W., Lucas, N., Donovan, A., Curry, A., & Hohnke, R. (1998). *Advanced nursing practice for rural and remote Australia: Report to the National Rural Health Alliance.* Gold Coast, Australia: Griffith University.

New South Wales Health. (1998). *Rural and remote nursing summit report.* North Sydney, Australia: Author.

Palmer, G., & Short, S. (1994). *Health care and public policy: An Australian analysis.* South Melbourne: Macmillan Education Australia.

Pearson, A. (1993). Expansion and extension of rural health workers' roles to increase access to health services in rural areas. In K. Malko (Ed.), *A fair go for rural health: Forward together* (pp. 213-218). Armidale, Australia: University of New England.

Rolley, F., & Humphreys, J. (1993). Rural welfare: The human face of Australia's countryside. In T. Sorensen & R. Epps (Eds.), *Prospects and policies for rural Australia* (pp. 241-257). Melbourne, Australia: Longman Cheshire.

Siegloff, L., & Hegney, D. (1996). Recognition for their role: The Nurse Practitioner Project, Wilcannia, New South Wales. In Association for Australian Rural Nurses (Ed.), *Windmills, wisdom and wonderment: Conference proceedings of the Association for Australian Rural Nurses Inc.* Roseworthy: Association for Australian Rural Nurses.

Sigsby, L. (1991). Crisis and ethical dilemmas: Who will care for the rural nurse? *Heart and Lung, 19,* 518-533.

Smith, C. (1996). *A vision for the recruitment and support of undergraduate students to rural nursing as a career.* Melbourne, Australia: CURHEV.

Spencer, J. (1997). Education for rural nurses. In L. Siegloff (Ed.), *Rural nursing in the Australian context* (pp. 59-76). Canberra: Royal College of Nursing Australia.

Stevens, R., & Allan, J. (1992). Professional Nursing Network: The reality of forming networks for rural nurses. In M. Courtney (Ed.), *Issues in rural nursing* (pp. 157-162). Armidale, Australia: University of New England.

Sturmey, R., & Edwards, R. (1991). *The survival skills training package: Community services and health workforce in rural and remote areas: Needs and recommendations study.* Canberra, Australia: Commonwealth Department of Community Services and Health.

Thornton, R. (1992). Rural nursing practice. In G. Gray & R. Pratt (Eds.), *Issues in Australian nursing 3* (pp. 121-132). Melbourne, Australia: Churchill Livingstone.

Titulaer, I., Trickett, P., & Bhatia, K. (1997). The health of Australians living in rural and remote areas: Preliminary results. In National Rural Health Alliance (Ed.), *Strengthening health partnerships in your rural community: National Rural Public Health Forum* (p. 61). Canberra: National Rural Health Alliance.

Tonna, A. (1991). Specialised services: Some issues. In M. Craig (Ed.), *A fair go for rural health* (pp. 61-67). Canberra, Australia: Department of Health, Housing and Community Service.

Walmsley, D. (1993) The policy environment. In T. Sorensen & R. Epps (Eds.), *Prospects and policies for rural Australia* (pp. 32-56). Melbourne, Australia: Longman Cheshire.

Western Australian Department of Health. (1994). *Decentralisation of rural health: Management reforms in the rural health sector.* Perth: Author.

Chapter 15

Rural Nursing in Canada

Donna C. Rennie
Kathryn Baird-Crooks
Gail Remus
Joyce Engel

KEY TERMS

➢ Province
➢ Ministry of Health
➢ Regional health administration
➢ Inuit
➢ Aboriginal
➢ Rural remote
➢ Rural isolated
➢ Rural nursing
➢ Extended practice

OBJECTIVES

After completing this chapter, you will be able to

➢ Describe the Canadian health care system and the nature of health services for rural residents.
➢ Identify important contributions of nursing to rural health of Canadians.
➢ Examine four issues that affect the practice of nurses in rural areas of Canada.
➢ Discuss practice, educational, and research issues of rural nursing in Canada.

ESSENTIAL POINTS TO REMEMBER

> ➤ The Canada Health Act of 1978 provided for publicly administrated, comprehensive, universal, accessible, and portable health services for all citizens of Canada. The current health care system in Canada is publicly funded and privately delivered. Although nurses deliver services to residents in remote and isolated areas, generally in other parts of Canada services are primarily delivered by physicians.

> ➤ There are limited data on the health of rural Canadians, and most are collected and reported in smaller provincial or regional studies. The health concerns of rural populations include injury and chronic conditions such as respiratory disease, cancer, cardiovascular disease, and diabetes. Rates of fatal and hospitalized injury are known to be higher among rural dwellers.

OVERVIEW

This chapter describes rural nursing in Canada. Political, social, cultural, and economic factors are examined that affect nurses' practice, education, recruitment, and retention in rural areas.

BACKGROUND

Canada, one of the largest nations in the Western Hemisphere, is composed of 10 provinces and two northern territories. The topography is diverse, with large areas of mountains on the Pacific West Coast, flat prairie landscapes of the Central West, rock and lakes of the Great Canadian Shield, northern wilderness, and Arctic tundra. A large part of the Canadian population of close to 29 million (Statistics Canada, 1998) is located in the southern part of the country, distributed between the Atlantic and Pacific shores in close proximity to the Canada–United States border (Figure 15.1). Vast areas of the country are unpopulated, whereas nearly two thirds of the population lives in Ontario and Quebec (Statistics Canada, 1999a). As of the 1996 Canada Census, 22.3 % of Canadians lived in rural regions and small towns with populations of less than 10,000. This is a decline of 12% since 1976. Approximately 68% of those living in rural and small-town regions live in rural areas of less than 1,000 population (Statistics Canada, 1999b). Newfoundland is the only province where more than 50% of the population lives in rural or small-town areas (Mendelson & Bollman, 1998). The major industries in rural areas include farming, fishing, logging, and mining (see Figure 15.1).

The out-migration of youth in search of employment is a continuing problem for rural development. The highest mobility is seen with individuals 20 to 24 years of age, and of those who move, more are likely to participate in education or employment activities. Those who return are between the ages of 25 and 29 and are also more likely to be well educated and participate in the labor force. Compared with urban residents, rural residents are half as likely to have university degrees and are more likely to have Grade 9 as

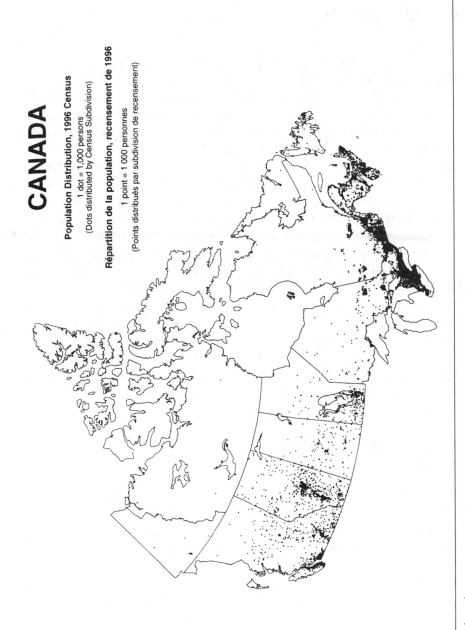

Figure 15.1. Map of Canada

SOURCE: Statistics Canada (1997).

their highest level of education. Though rural residents are less likely to own computers, they are more likely to be employed in small businesses (Felligi, 1996).

THE CANADIAN HEALTH CARE SYSTEM

Under the terms of the British North America Act of 1869, which established the Confederation of the Dominion of Canada, responsibility for health, education, and social services was delegated to the provinces. Vollman and Tenove (1997) noted that "this division of powers was maintained in the 1982 Constitution Act and reflects the beliefs of Canadians that government has a responsibility to provide services to all people and special assistance to those in need" (p. 24). The Canada Health Act of 1978 provided for publicly administered, comprehensive, universal, accessible, and portable health services for all citizens of Canada (Health Canada, 1997). Hence, the current health care system in Canada is publicly funded and privately delivered. Although nurses deliver services to residents in remote and isolated areas, generally in other parts of Canada services are primarily delivered by physicians (Health Canada, 1997). The health care system is under the jurisdiction of provincial and territorial governments, and partial funding for the program comes from the federal government through transfer of payments to provinces. Both cash contributions and tax points are considered when funds are transferred from the federal government to each province. There are some differences in the health care plans offered by provinces, particularly in financial support of plans. Generally, provincial tax revenues are used to fund provincial programs, although in two provinces residents pay a yearly premium. Health care costs for Native or aboriginal Canadians do not fall under the jurisdiction of provincial health care plans but are administered directly by the federal government.

HEALTH OF RURAL DWELLERS IN CANADA

There has been little national-level study of the health risks of rural Canadians. Much of the information on health of rural dwellers is reported in smaller provincial or regional studies. Identified health concerns of rural populations include injury and chronic conditions such as respiratory disease, cancer, cardiovascular disease, and diabetes. Rates of fatal and hospitalized injury are known to be higher among rural dwellers. In a study by Hader and Seliske (1993), rural residents who lived outside of the nine major cities in Saskatchewan had rates of unintentional injuries that were twice those of urban dwellers. Injury categories included traffic injuries, injuries in the home, and community and occupational injuries. Males of 5 to 44 years of age were particularly at risk for falls and fire. In a study of seat belt use by Albertans, 68% of motor vehicle fatal injuries occurred in rural areas, compared to 31% for urban areas.(Thompson & Russel, 1994).

The male farming population, particularly farm operators/owners, are more likely to be injured than women and are usually between 20 and 59 years of age. Other factors associated with injury on the farm are farm experience of more than 20 years, full-time operation on farms, and beef farming. Higher commodity prices have been found to be associated with an increase in tractor fatalities in rural dwellers (Brison & Pickett, 1992, 1997; Gerberich & Gibson, 1995; Kelsey, 1992; Pahwa, Zazada, McDuffie, McNeil, & Dosman, 1995; Pickett, Brison, Niezgoda, & Chipman, 1995; Young, 1995).

In both male and female children under 15 years of age living in noncity crop-growing regions of Saskatchewan, the prevalence of respiratory illness requiring physician services was as great as in urban regions and greater than in noncropland regions (Dickinson, Denis, & Li, 1995). However, studies have shown that asthma prevalence in rural children living in areas of less than 1,000 population is slightly lower than in urban children (Rennie, 1996).

Canadian studies of pesticide use with farming populations have identified increased risk of some cancers for those exposed. Compared to general populations, rural populations of farmers appear to have excesses in risk for certain cancers, including non-Hodgkin's lymphoma and multiple myeloma (McDuffie, Towstego, & Pahwa, 1994). Adults have been observed to have an increased risk for Parkinson's disease with rural exposure to certain pesticides (Semchuk, 1991).

In the recent Canadian Heart Health Survey, cardiovascular disease burden, as measured by health services utilization factors, appeared to be greater for rural than for urban populations, although differences in specific risk factors such as high blood pressure were not seen (Chen, Reeder, Young, MacDonald, & Gelskey, 1995). In a study of rural and urban populations in Alberta, rural residents were noted to engage in healthier behaviors, including sleeping 7 or more hours per day, eating three meals, and limiting alcohol use (Johnson, Ratner, & Bottorff, 1995). Within rural populations, the Hutterite population and Anabaptist sects who live an agrarian-communal lifestyle in the prairie provinces appear to have a higher risk for cardiovascular disease than their rural counterparts (Brunt, Reeder, Stephenson, Love, & Chen, 1995). Morbidity and mortality rates are higher among Native and Inuit infants than among all Canadian infants (Macmillian, Macmillian, Orford, & Dingle, 1996). Inuit children from the ages of 6 to 13 were shown to have low rates of atopy (5.3%). Though asthma and atopy were low in this population, there was evidence of chronic airflow obstruction (7%) and high prevalence of passive and neonatal smoke exposure (Hemmelgarn & Ernst, 1997). Compared with the general population, specific Native populations are more likely to be at risk for death due to alcohol, pneumonia, suicide, and homicide. Diabetes has become a major concern with Native populations. The prevalence of diabetes in aboriginal adults is 6% compared with 2% in all Canadian adults (Macmillian et al., 1996). Although certain health problems appear to be more common in aboriginal populations compared with all populations, few of these studies considered the effect of poverty on the findings.

HEALTH SERVICES IN RURAL AREAS

In trying to be more responsive to the health care needs of all Canadians, the health care system has gone through considerable change in the 1990s. Several western provinces have engaged in funding and delivery reform of institutional services. This reform has direct effects for rural residents. Beginning in 1993, the government of Saskatchewan eliminated all hospital, nursing home, and public health boards and placed these institutions under the control of regional health authorities (RHAs). Each RHA was made jointly responsible for planning and providing hospital care, home care, nursing home care, and public health services. Many of the smaller boards were not represented on the newer, larger boards, and travel to regional board meetings became more difficult. Thus, the input from smaller, remote communities into decisions about services was less direct. Furthermore, certain services that were once locally available are now situated in central locations. In some areas, hospitals closed and community health centers were established. However, regionalization has had some positive effects too. For instance, RHAs have more autonomy over decisions regarding services that would meet the specific health needs of groups of residents within the region (Saskatchewan Health, 1996).

Other provinces have begun initiatives similar to the reforms in Saskatchewan. Since 1995, Alberta has consolidated 120 hospital boards into 17 regional health authorities. Thompson and O'Neil (1996) indicated that the budgets given to the new regional boards for the 1995-96 fiscal year led to the loss of a significant number of rural acute care beds and the closure of some rural hospitals. Newfoundland has restructured its health care boards and reduced the number from 31 to 8, with some of the rural facilities downgraded to ambulatory services with holding beds (O'Maonaigh, 1997). Three provinces, British Columbia, Manitoba, and Ontario, have conducted task forces or undergone reorganization specifically for rural and northern health care delivery (British Columbia Ministry of Health, 1995; Manitoba Health, 1997; Ontario Ministry of Health, 1998).

Because of large federal and provincial debts, there has been a decrease in funding to health and social programs. This trend threatens the quality and quantity of services provided to rural and urban Canadians. The consequences of decreased funding for rural residents have been many (Vollman & Tenove, 1997). Changes in how services are provided or decreases in funding for services can result in poorly coordinated planning and limited public policy related to health care. Health promotion activities may be put on hold as more immediate pressing needs are met. To address decreases in funding, some services formerly offered by the government are being offered by the private sector. Consequently, there has been increased competition between these professional provider groups for the limited resource dollars. Changes in service delivery can result in the misuse or inappropriate use of the system by clients and providers until the change has stabilized. When funds are limited and services are cut, rural populations may not be able to retain physicians, who go elsewhere for better working conditions and higher salaries. Fluctuating changes in federal and provincial governments can limit long-term planning by provinces as well. As a result, many rural areas that are experiencing remoteness and low population densities could face further disintegration of the health and well-being of their residents.

The increasing number of elderly individuals and couples choosing to live in rural areas has implications for the types of services that will be required. As a population ages, there is a need for more health care services. Providing long-term care and extended-care services for elderly rural residents will be a priority for health care providers. For certain provinces, such as Manitoba and Saskatchewan, the share of the population that is of aboriginal background will increase dramatically in the future. In Manitoba, aboriginals represent 5% of the population over 65 years and 26% of the population under 15 years of age (Felligi, 1996). Services will be required to meet the unique health care demands of these groups.

DEFINING *RURAL* AND *RURAL NURSING* IN THE CANADIAN CONTEXT

At present, there is no consistent, single definition of what constitutes a rural setting or rural nursing. *Rural* is occasionally defined for what it is not or in terms of its being nonmetropolitan (Rourke, 1997). Yawn (1994) suggested that rather than defining *rural* as anything outside of a large population cluster, it might be more accurate to consider it in terms of economics, demographics, social structure, or health care needs. Typically, in Canada, for example, the term *rural* might be seen as referring to areas where access to health care services is limited by distance and a lack of qualified care providers, particularly physicians (Alberta Physicians Resources Planning Group, 1997). MacLeod, Browne, and Leipert (1998) noted that definitions of rural and remote practice tend to reflect the skills and expertise needed by practitioners who work in areas where distance, weather, limited resources, and little backup shape the character of their lives and professional practice.

Many definitions of *rural* depend on population density or distance from major resources. Statistics Canada (1993) defined rural areas in national census reports as places having populations of less than 1,000 and a density of less than 400 persons per square kilometer (km). The Rural Committee of the Canadian Association of Emergency Physicians (Canadian Association, 1997) defined *rural remote* as rural communities about 80 to 400 km or from 1 to 4 hours' transport in good weather from a major regional hospital. *Rural isolated* refers to rural communities more than about 400 km away or about 4 hours' transport in good weather from a major regional hospital. Research definitions of *rural* vary between the more general definition of *rural* as nonurban to the more specific definition based on the particular size of a community or group of communities.

Berlan-Darque and Collomb (1990) noted that because definitions of *rural* are not consistent among all nations, the compilation of world statistics is an almost impossible task. Comparisons between countries become difficult as well. Deavers (1992) identified the importance of appropriately defining the concept of *rural* to formulate and implement rural policy. Weinert and Boik (1995) suggested that the lack of a definition for *rural* inhibits the ability to forge cohesive political coalitions, to describe the distinctive health care needs of rural populations, and to search for solutions to the problems of rural dwellers. An evidence-based definition of *rural* is crucial if we are to better understand rural nursing and provide the appropriate support for nurses working in rural areas.

Neither Statistics Canada nor the Canadian Nurses Association (1998) is able to generate data sufficiently specific to rural nursing. That deficit hinders reliably interpreting and discussing rural-urban migration patterns as they relate to nursing or identifying the inputs and outflows within the rural health workforce. Leduc (1997) suggested a preliminary model to measure levels of rural practice, called the Canadian General Practice Rurality Index (GPRI). This model includes six weighted variables: remoteness from a basic referral center, population, number of general practitioners, number of specialists, and presence of an acute care hospital. The model requires further study to determine its validity and reliability.

At present, there is no consistent definition of rural nursing for Canadian practice. The issue of defining rural nursing is significant because it affects nursing care, preparation of nurses, and nursing work-life issues. Whether rural nursing is a distinct specialization influences theory development, research generation, and development of appropriate curricula.

At this point in the evolution of rural nursing in Canada, it is critical to ask whether the rural nurse is a specialist with particular skills and knowledge that are peculiar to the rural setting or a generalist who performs a broad range of typical nursing care within a more isolated setting. Gregory (1992) suggested that the former is more accurate and pointed to the broad knowledge base required for rural practice. The ability to function autonomously and the ability to adapt nursing interventions to a low-tech environment are historically characteristic of rural nursing practice in Canada.

HISTORY OF RURAL NURSING IN CANADA

The history of nursing in rural Canada is as long as the history of Canada. The predominance of agriculture, fur trading, mining, and the timber industry facilitated the development of sporadic urban areas surrounded by isolated rural areas (Allemang, 1985). Trusted spinster or widowed women often assumed charge of the hospitals, which also emerged in the city. In underdeveloped rural regions, nursing services were delivered by Grey Nuns and other religious orders and by untrained lay women who traveled by foot, cart, and any other transportation that was available. As settlement progressed and rural areas became less predominant, services in these communities were often delivered by women who were designated as nurses. These women were widely respected for their knowledge and remedies derived from everyday experience and for their devotion to the sick within their community. Unlike the women in the urban settings, these caregivers were well-known women in the community. They rose to a position of respect and courage by virtue of their caring, insight, and ability to use knowledge meaningfully to assist neighbors and friends.

By the beginning of the 20th century, nurses in Canada had firmly established themselves as essential components of institutional and home-based sick care. Throughout the rural West, nurses emerged as significant care providers, offering hospital care and district nursing services. District nurses acted as midwives; provided school health and infectious disease services; delivered home-based, basic nursing services; and trained homemakers (Allemang, 1985; Cashman, 1966). Middleton (cited in Storch, 1985) asserted that the work of the physician and the work of the nurse were so closely aligned that it was difficult to speak of one without referring to the other. Although this viewpoint reflects the nondifferentiation of nursing from medicine, it may also reflect the status accorded nurses and the high regard in which they were held at that time.

By 1966, the district nurse, who had walked, ridden, or driven to deliver babies, cared for seriously ill individuals, and prescribed medicines, had all but disappeared. District nurses from this era express regret for the loss of relationships with their clients, which were characterized by low technology, shared experiences, and the challenges of their joint community context (Cashman, 1966). They further grieve the loss of a highly connected relationship with the client and their ability to make clinical decisions within the context of this relationship.

RURAL NURSING DEMOGRAPHICS

There are 264,305 registered nurses in Canada. Of these, 61.3% work in hospital settings that are publicly funded (Canadian Nurses Association, 1998). The remainder may be self-employed or employed by public health, home care, physicians' offices, industry, or various publicly funded community agencies. Information concerning the number of nurses employed or living in rural environments could not be located. The Canadian Nurses Association (1997) predicted that by the year 2011, Canada will experience a critical shortage of registered nurses. This anticipated shortage is the result of the "graying" of the nursing population, which, according to statistics from the province of Alberta, is approaching a mean age of 45 years (Alberta Association of Registered Nurses, 1998).

SCOPE OF NURSING PRACTICE

Nurses in rural areas can function in a variety of roles, but their roles in hospitals tend to be more generalized than those of their urban counterparts. Though some rural nurses may continue work in smaller hospital settings, many practice situations are now more community based. With the continued restructuring of health care, many rural hospitals have disappeared and are being replaced by community health centers that focus on emergency services, outpatient services, and health promotion activities. Many of the activities in health promotion require that the nurse be familiar with new health strategies, including health public policy, program evaluation, and community assessment activities that include participatory research and needs assessments. With other types of health care workers (home care aides, extended-care workers, emergency response workers) becoming more common in rural settings, the nurse is expected to provide education and leadership to these groups, as well as to be a member of a multidisciplinary team that plans for community health care within the region.

Whereas community health nurses in southern Canada primarily focus on health promotion and prevention activities, community health nurses employed in frontier nursing stations have a much broader scope of practice. Services such as treatment of common medical disorders, treatment of pediatric problems, low-risk obstetrical care, including delivery, and acute emergency care are all expected functions of a practice that also includes well-child care and delivery of a variety of community health programs (Graham, 1994). As a result of cutbacks in funding, a few Canadian nurses are developing independent businesses to provide nursing services. For example, home care services and extended-care needs are being determined by nurses to meet the demands of a rural aging population who prefer to remain in their home community.

FACTORS AFFECTING RURAL NURSING PRACTICE

Extended Nursing Practice

The Alberta Physicians Resources Planning Group's (1997) report cited arduous working conditions, isolation, and inadequate compensation as deterrents to recruitment and retention of rural physicians. Thus, many rural areas are underserved by medical practitioners (Baird-Crooks, Graham, & Bushy, 1998), and access to reasonable care is jeopardized. In such a climate, extended or advanced nursing practice that includes more primary care skills becomes an acceptable and viable alternative to physician-directed services. In 1995, the province of Ontario was the first to provide appropriate legislation for nurses in advanced practice (MacLeod et al., 1998). Recently, legislation under the Public Health Act of Alberta has enabled rural nurses to prescribe medication and perform assessments beyond the usual practice of nurses in urban areas. Further, the Alberta Association of Registered Nurses has recently approved a separate registry for nurses who are able to meet the established criteria for extended practice. Rural nurses who up to this time have worked in less independent settings need to be aware that these extended functions require appropriate preparation for the skills. Because the demand for extended care nurses exceeds the current supply, there may be a tendency to have nurses functioning in these positions who are not properly prepared to meet all the demands of such a practice. Though nurses with extended practice skills or those in independent practice may provide alternative or additional service to physicians who are overworked or in short supply in rural areas, failure of provincial insurance plans to directly reimburse nurses limits expansion of such services in rural areas. Failing to reimburse these practitioners could result in reduced accessibility to services for those residing in rural areas and could discourage nurses from work with these vulnerable groups.

Nursing Shortage

The current nursing shortage has certain implications for nursing care in rural areas. Bigbee (1993) noted that although rural nurses tend to be even older than the average nurse in other areas of practice, they also tend to retire earlier. Complicating the probability of an older and retirement-ready rural nursing workforce is the probability that the influx of younger practitioners will be slow and insufficient to compensate for attrition through retirement. Historically, rural nurses tend to arrive in communities by virtue of either having returned to practice in the communities from which they came or having moved into the area as a result of friendship or marriage. Those who come for reasons other than the reestablishment or establishment of roots tend to remain only long enough to gain the generalist experience available in rural practice. The slowness and uncertainty of inward migration and the rapid escalation of retirement create an even more critical shortage than that anticipated in the urban environment.

Isolation and Remoteness

Approximately 6% of the Canadian population live in the northern part of the country in settlements of varying size. Nurses provide primary care in these areas to largely Native and Inuit populations. According to the Canadian Nurses Association (M. Ippersiel, personal communication, 1998), as of 1996, there were 91 nurses employed in remote nursing stations across Canada's vast north regions. At this juncture, it must be pointed out that rural nursing and nursing in the far north (remote nursing) are distinct from one another. Although the two share similarities, nurses employed by the Medical Services Branch of Health and Welfare Canada, in remote northern nursing stations, currently work in an advanced practice capacity. This rarely is the case for their more southerly counterparts. This situation has been a cause of some dissent between groups of nurses and physicians. The argument has been raised that nurses are capable of functioning in an extended practice mode in northern climates but seem to lose this ability once they proceed south of the 60th parallel. At this point, the argument is ongoing.

Education

In 1982, the Canadian Nurses Association passed a resolution that supports baccalaureate education as the minimum requirement for entry into the practice of nursing by the year 2000 (Sherwood & Henderson, 1991). Although each curriculum must be approved by the provincial regulating body, there remain many differences in the foci of each. In addition, much of the practice experience that undergraduate students acquire occurs in large urban settings, with an occasional sojourn to more remote nonurban settings. Graduate education that is specific to the rural environment is in its infancy. There are long-established outpost nursing programs in Canada to prepare nurses to work in the remote north (MacLeod et al., 1998). At present, few postgraduate programs specific to rural nursing are available. Although rural nursing is now seen to be a unique practice environment that calls for "innovative graduate and undergraduate educational programming to promote the recruitment and retention of the best prepared nurses to rural areas" (Bigbee, 1993, p. 140), there has been limited initiative to promote such programs.

Recruitment and Retention

The inclusion of rural content and practice in nursing education is promising in that it is anticipated that exposure to work in rural communities will assist in recruitment to these settings. Baird-Crooks and Graham (1996) found that students were amazed at the variety of knowledge and skills required to work in rural areas and showed a desire to gain experience in various rural areas once they graduated. Retaining these nurses, however, will continue to be problematic unless they are educationally and psychologically prepared to work in conditions that can be rigorous and isolated. The preparation of skilled nurse managers and the creation of professional development opportunities that address the needs and issues of nurses in rural areas are key to providing incentives, rewards, and ongoing development for these nurses. With a nursing shortage anticipated, it becomes essential that various levels of government and nursing schools address the problems of recruitment and retention. Government and education must work together to provide programming and mentorship in addressing the educational and leadership concerns inherent in rural nursing.

Continuing Education

Canadian rural nurses face the challenge of retaining the generalist function with a scarcity of technological and human resources compounded by distance and transportation difficulties. Isolation can make it difficult for nurses to maintain current knowledge and skills. The Internet and other types of communication technology are making it possible for many nurses to further their education, despite being thousands of miles from an educational institution. However, because nursing is a scientific and skill-based profession, retaining proficiency can be problematic unless the nurse is willing to relocate for periods of time to take classes. This option can pose problems for a family as well as for a health care facility in a rural area already experiencing a nursing shortage.

Lack of Anonymity

Upon entering a rural practice setting, the nurse may experience a period of being less well known while community members develop trusting relationships with the newcomer. However, Canadian rural nurses also confront the difficulty of lack of anonymity and of being recognized and utilized as the local nurse. Recognition can continue long after official retirement from a paid position. For example, it is not unusual for a nurse married to a local farmer to be called upon at all hours of the day or night to minister to a neighbor who may be many miles away. Registered nurses are often members of emergency response teams that assess, stabilize, and transport victims. As an emergency team member, the nurse may be on call around the clock without financial remuneration.

SUMMARY

This chapter examined the role and scope of nursing practice in rural Canada. Often these nurses undervalue their abilities because they see themselves as being "jacks of all trades" and not specialized. It is imperative that the various levels of government be made aware of the vital role nurses have in a rural community and the importance of supporting nursing education and practice to meet the health care demands associated with the rural way of life.

DISCUSSION QUESTIONS

> ➤ What concepts should be considered in a definition of rural nursing for Canada? Why? Discuss the effect that changing demands for health care could have on the future of extended or advanced nursing practice in Canada.
> ➤ What is the significance of a "rural definition of health" for policy development and service delivery actions with rural populations? What strategies might be employed to educate nurses for rural practice? What informal support systems are available or are used by rural nurses in your area? How do these systems influence the delivery of nursing care?

SUGGESTED RESEARCH ACTIVITIES

Little research is available on rural nursing in Canada. Most of the existing information about rural populations and their health related needs emanates from the United States and Australia. Therefore, the areas for rural Canadian research are limitless. Salient topics and questions for future nursing studies include

> ➤ Identification and validation of definitions of *rural* and *rural nursing*
> ➤ Assessment of the supply and demand for rural nurses, including those factors that enhance recruitment and retention
> ➤ Characteristics of the nurse-client relationship that support nurse retention
> ➤ The role of the rural nurse with other members of a multidisciplinary team in providing comprehensive health care for rural residents
> ➤ The factors that enhance collegial support for nurses in remote practice settings
> ➤ The specific educational needs of rural nurses

REFERENCES

Alberta Association of Registered Nurses. (1998, July). *Nursing shortage* [News release]. Edmonton, Alberta: Author.

Alberta Physicians Resources Planning Group. (1997). *Alberta Physicians Resources Planning Group report.* Edmonton, Alberta: Author.

Allemang, M. A. (1985). Development of community health nursing in Canada. In J. Stewart, J. Innes, S. Searl, & C. Smillie (Eds.), *Community health nursing in Canada* (pp. 3-29). Toronto, Ontario: Gage Educational Publishing.

Baird-Crooks, K., & Graham, E. (1996). [The experience of baccalaureate nursing students in the rural setting]. Unpublished raw data.

Baird-Crooks, K., Graham, E., & Bushy, A. (1998). Implementing a rural nursing course in a Canadian province. *Nurse Educator, 23*(6), 33-37.

Berlan-Darque, M., & Collomb, P. (1990). Rural population—rural vitality. *Sociologia Ruralis, 31,* 252-261.

Bigbee, J. L. (1993). The uniqueness of rural nursing. *Nursing Clinics of North America, 28,* 199-207.

Brison, R. J., & Pickett, W. (1992). Non-fatal farm injuries in eastern Ontario beef and dairy farms: A one-year study. *American Journal of Industrial Medicine, 21,* 623-636.

Brison, R. J., & Pickett, W. (Eds.). (1997). *Fatal farm injuries in Canada, 1991-1995: A report from the Canadian Agricultural Injury Surveillance Program.* Kingston, Ontario: Canadian Agricultural Injury Surveillance Program.

British Columbia Ministry of Health. (1995). *Report of the Northern and Rural Health Task Force.* Victoria, British Columbia: Author.

Brunt, H., Reeder, B., Stephenson, P., Love, E., & Chen, Y. (1995). The Hutterite and rural Saskatchewan heart health surveys: A comparison of physical and laboratory measures. In H. H. McDuffie, J. A. Dosman, K. M. Semchuk, S. A. Olenchuk, & A. Senthilselvan (Eds.), *Agricultural health and safety: Workplace, environment, sustainability* (pp. 513-520). Boca Raton, FL: CRC Press.

Canadian Association of Emergency Physicians, Rural Committee. (1997). *Recommendations for the management of rural, remote and isolated emergency health care facilities in Canada.* Ottawa, Ontario: Author.

Canadian Nurses Association. (1997, November). *Major nursing shortage looming* [News release]. Ottawa, Ontario: Author.

Canadian Nurses Association. (1998). Direct access to nursing services: About choice and access. *Nursing Now: Issues and Trends in Canadian Nursing,* No. 4 [On-line serial]. Available: http//www.cna-nurses.ca/english/

Cashman, T. (1966). *Heritage of service: The history of nursing in Alberta.* Edmonton: Alberta Association of Registered Nurses.

Chen, Y., Reeder, B. A., Young, T. K., MacDonald, S., & Gelskey, D. (1995). Cardiovascular risk factors in rural and urban residents of the Canadian prairies. In H. H. McDuffie, J. A. Dosman, K. M. Semchuk, S. A. Olenchuk, & A. Senthilselvan (Eds.), *Agricultural health and safety: Workplace, environment, sustainability* (pp. 521-524). Boca Raton, FL: CRC Press.

Deavers, K. (1992). What is rural? *Policy Studies Journal, 20,* 184-189.

Dickinson, H., Denis, W., & Li, P. S. (1995). Respiratory disease in Saskatchewan: Selected regional and social variations. In H. H. McDuffie, J. A. Dosman, K. M. Semchuk, S. A. Olenchuk, & A. Senthilselvan (Eds.), *Agricultural health and safety: Workplace, environment, sustainability* (pp. 87-90). Boca Raton, FL: CRC Press.

Felligi, I. P. (1996, September). *Understanding rural Canada: Structure and trends* [On-line]. Available: http://www.statcan.ca:80/english/freepub/21F0016XIE/rural96.html [1999, January 13].

Gerberich, S., & Gibson, R. W. (1995). Regional rural injury study: A population based effort. In H. H. McDuffie, J. A. Dosman, K. M. Semchuk, S. A. Olenchuk, A. Senthilselvan (Eds.), *Agricultural health and safety: Workplace, environment, sustainability* (pp. 249-256). Boca Raton, FL: CRC Press.

Graham, K. (1994). Inservice education for northern nurses. *Canadian Nurse, 90*(3), 33-36.

Gregory, D. M. (1992). Nursing practice in native communities. In A. J. Baumgart & J. Larsen (Eds.), *Canadian nursing faces the future* (2nd ed., pp. 181-198). Toronto, Ontario: C. V. Mosby.

Hader, J., & Seliske, P. (1993). *Injuries in Saskatchewan.* Saskatoon: University of Saskatchewan, Department of Epidemiology, Health Status Research Unit.

Health Canada. (1997). *Canada's health system* [On-line]. Available: http://www.hwc.ca

Hemmelgarn, B., & Ernst, P. (1997). Airway function among Inuit primary school children in far northern Quebec. *American Journal of Respiratory and Critical Care Medicine, 156,* 1870-1875.

Johnson, J. L., Ratner, P. A., & Bottorff, J. L. (1995). Urban-rural differences in health promoting behaviours of Albertans. *Canadian Journal of Public Health, 86,* 103-108.

Kelsey, T. (1992). Farm product prices and agricultural safety: Connections and consequences. *Journal of Rural Health, 8,* 52-59.

Leduc, L. (1997). Defining rurality: A general practice rurality index for Canada. *Canadian Journal of Rural Medicine, 2,* 125-131.

MacLeod, M., Browne, A. J., & Leipert, B. (1998). Issues for nurses in rural and remote Canada. *Australian Journal of Rural Health, 6,* 72-78.

Macmillian, H. L., Macmillian, A. B., Orford, D. R., & Dingle, J. L. (1996). Aboriginal health. *Canadian Medical Association Journal, 155,* 1569-1578.

Manitoba Health. (1997). *Annual report: Rural and northern operations* [On-line]. Available: http://www.gov.mb.ca/health/ann/3-am7.html

McDuffie, H. H., Towstego, L., & Pahwa, P. (1994). In H. H. McDuffie, J. A. Dosman, K. M. Semchuk, S. A. Olenchuk, & A. Senthilselvan (Eds.), *Supplement to "Agricultural health and safety: Workplace, environment, sustainability."* Chelsea, MI: Lewis.

Mendelson, R., & Bollman, R. (Eds.). (1998). *Rural and Small Town Analysis Bulletin, 1*(1) [On-line serial], Doc. No. 21-006-XPB. Available: www.statcan.ca

O'Maonaigh, C. (1997). Focus on Newfoundland and Labrador. *Canadian Journal of Rural Medicine, 2,* 73-75.

Ontario Ministry of Health. (1998). *Access to quality health care in rural and northern Ontario* [On-line]. Available: http://www.gov.on.ca:80/MOH/english/pub/ministry/ruralca.html

Pahwa, P., Zazada, M., McDuffie, H. H., McNeil, G., & Dosman, J. A. (1995). Results of a survey on farm accidents in Saskatchewan. In H. H. McDuffie, J. A. Dosman, K. M. Semchuk, S. A. Olenchuk, & A. Senthilselvan (Eds.), *Agricultural health and safety: Workplace, environment, sustainability* (pp. 275-282). Boca Raton, FL: CRC Press.

Pickett, W., Brison, R. J., Niezgoda, H., & Chipman, M. L. (1995). Non-fatal farm injuries in Ontario: A population based survey. *Accident Analysis and Prevention, 27,* 425-433.

Rennie, D. C. (1996). *A population based study of asthma and wheezing in school age children.* Unpublished doctoral dissertation, University of Saskatchewan, Saskatoon.

Rourke, J. (1997). In search of a definition of "rural." *Canadian Journal of Rural Medicine, 2,* 113-115.

Saskatchewan Health. (1996). *Health renewal is working: Progress report, October, 1996.* Regina, Saskatchewan: Author.

Semchuk, K. M. (1991). Parkinson's disease and exposure to rural environmental factors: A population based case-control study. *Canadian Journal of Neurological Sciences, 18,* 279-286.

Sherwood, J., & Henderson, E. (1991). Our history: A proud heritage 1980-1991. *AARN Newsletter, 47*(11), 12-14.

Statistics Canada. (1993). *Census of agriculture: Selected data for Saskatchewan rural municipalities.* Ottawa, Ontario: Government of Canada.

Statistics Canada. (1997). *A national overview: 1996 census of Canada* (Catalogue No. 93-357-XPB). Ottawa, Ontario: Industry Canada.

Statistics Canada. (1998, November 30). Population by selected age groups and sex for Canada, provinces and territories, 1996 census: 100% data [On-line]. Available: http//www.statcan.ca/english/census96

Statistics Canada. (1999a). *The 1999 Canada yearbook.* Ottawa, Ontario: Author.

Statistics Canada, Agriculture Division. (1999b). [Population of rural and small town areas and in larger urban centres]. Unpublished tabular data.

Storch, J. L. (1985). The Canadian health care delivery system: Policies, programs, services. In J. Stewart, J. Innes, S. Searl, & C. Smillie (Eds.), *Community health nursing in Canada* (pp. 33-48). Toronto, Ontario: Gage Educational Publishing.

Thompson, E. J., & Russel, M. L. (1994). Risk-factors for non-use of seatbelts in rural and urban Alberta. *Canadian Journal of Public Health, 85,* 304-305.

Thompson, J., & O'Neil, D. (1996). Focus on Alberta. *Canadian Journal of Rural Medicine, 1,* 87-89.

Vollman, A. R., & Tenove, S. C. (1997), Canadian health care delivery system. In P. A. Potter, A. G. Perry, J. R. Kerr, & M. K. Sirtnik (Eds.), *Canadian fundamentals of nursing* (pp. 21-43). St. Louis, MO: C. V. Mosby.

Weinert, C., & Boik, R. J. (1995). MSU Rurality Index: Development and evaluation. *Research Nursing and Health, 18,* 453-464.

Yawn, B. P. (1994). Rural medical practice: Present and future. In B. P. Yawn, A. Bushy, & R. A. Yawn (Eds.), *Exploring rural medicine: Current issues and concepts* (pp. 1-16). Thousand Oaks, CA: Sage.

Young, S. C. (1995). Agriculture related injuries in the parkland region of Manitoba. *Canadian Family Physician, 41,* 1190-1197.

CHAPTER 16

Analysis of Rural Nursing

Australia, Canada, United States

KEY TERMS

- ➤ Global village
- ➤ Global economy
- ➤ Privatization
- ➤ Population density
- ➤ Remoteness
- ➤ Communication infrastructures
- ➤ Economic diversity
- ➤ Telehealth/telemedicine

OBJECTIVES

After reading this chapter, you will be able to

- ➤ Describe commonalities among nursing practice in rural environments in three highly industrialized nations: the United States, Australia, and Canada.
- ➤ Discuss the common themes that permeate the discussion in this book and how these fit at an international level.
- ➤ Propose potential areas for nursing research with an international partner.

ESSENTIAL POINTS TO REMEMBER

- ➤ Declining national health care resources are a concern shared by all three nations. There is increasing competition among national and international market forces. Rapidly emerging is an interdependent global economy that does not allow for national isolationism.
- ➤ Worldwide, efforts are underway to increase economic diversity in rural areas. Correspondingly, the health problems of the people who live in rural areas are affected by the predominant industry in a given region. As for nursing care

needs, these vary with and depend on the particular population mix within a given community.

➢ An obstacle for describing rural nursing in Canada, Australia, and the United States is the imprecise definition of what constitutes a rural or an urban area. Inherent features of ruralness across nations are greater distances between services and providers, geographic remoteness, lower population density, and scarce resources.

OVERVIEW

This chapter presents an analysis and synthesis of the three previous chapters that focus on rural nursing in the United States (Chapter 13), Australia (Chapter 14), and Canada (Chapter 15). Common themes are highlighted as these relate to rural nursing theory, practice, and research.

BACKGROUND

As we enter the new millennium, all three nations are experiencing relocation and dislocation among many of their people. These changes are posing enormous opportunities and some challenges for nurses and the health care system in the United States, Australia, and Canada. What seemingly is chaotic, confusing, and conflicting change really is a realignment of purposes, processes, and people. During the transition, the familiar is being altered—sometimes for the better and sometimes for the worse. The recurrent themes in rural nursing that are listed in Chapter 1 of this book are present in Australia and Canada as well as the United States. These themes also provide a context in which rural nurses must deliver care, examine the rural phenomenon, and develop the theoretical foundations for practice in the rural environment: specifically,

➢ Imprecise definitions for *rural* and *urban*
➢ Incomplete and conflicting data on the health status of rural populations
➢ Few(er) people living in large(er) and more remote geographical regions
➢ Inadequate public utilities, transportation, and communication infrastructures
➢ Managed health care, cost containment, and access to services
➢ Sparse resources
➢ Recruitment, retention, and education of health professionals
➢ Access to and use of biomedical, telecommunications, and information technology
➢ Quality assurance and measurement of health outcomes
➢ Need for the rural perspective in policy making and health planning
➢ Partnership models
➢ Ethical issues

The remainder of this chapter summarizes other similarities and differences for rural nursing among the three highly industrialized nations. By no means is the discussion comprehensive. Rather, the intent is to evoke interest among nurses in the global village.

Hopefully, nurses will collaborate to study, develop, and refine the foundations of rural practice at an international level.

REFORMING HEALTH CARE DELIVERY SYSTEMS

Common macro forces in health care delivery are elaborated on in the next few paragraphs. To begin, all three chapters emphasize that declining national health care resources are a concern shared by all three nations. There is increasing competition among national and international market forces that respond to consumer demands. In all three nations, the goals of health care reform are to reduce cost, improve access, and ensure quality and consumer satisfaction. Changes are occurring in how health care is financed too. In the United States, there is a trend toward less privatization and the expansion of large, and hopefully integrated, health care systems. In Australia and Canada, the trend seems to be for more privatization and less government management. Essentially, the health care delivery systems of the three nations are becoming more similar than different. In all three nations, there is a trend toward decentralization of financial control and management of health care resources. In the United States, decentralization is occurring from the federal government to the states; in Canada, from the national government to provincial governments; and in Australia, from the federal government to state and territory governments. Hence, state and provincial governments are forced to develop reform initiatives that meet the particular health care needs and preferences of their citizens.

The three nations are experiencing similar demographic changes. With improved health care and lifestyles, people are living longer; hence, there is a growing elderly population. There is increasing diversity, especially in the United States. But all three nations have increasing numbers of people who are vulnerable and have special health care needs. Among all three, the rural population is declining along with the number of acres of agricultural land as production methods are becoming more efficient. Worldwide, efforts are underway to increase economic diversity in rural areas. Correspondingly, the health problems of the people who live in rural areas are affected by the predominant industry in a given region. As for nursing care needs, these vary with and depend on the particular population mix within a given community.

Health care reform is also changing where care is delivered and what types of services are rendered to clients. More precisely, there is a shift from acute in-hospital care to community-based care. Illness care is being replaced by ambulatory care services, along with interventions promoting health and preventing illness in individuals and communities. Partnerships are the way of the future. Nurses are collaborating with clients, peers, health professionals from other disciplines, and those from outside the health care field when designing and implementing interventions. For nurses, this mandates learning skills that enable them to participate in social change and policy development, such as community development, advocacy, group facilitation, empowerment, and coalition building. Little is known about the effectiveness and outcomes of existing partnership interventions, offering a rich area for nurse researchers. These kind of studies from the international community are needed to build and refine the theoretical foundations for rural nursing too.

HOW TO DEFINE *RURAL*?

Perhaps the greatest obstacle to describing rural nursing in Canada, Australia, and the United States is imprecise definitions of *rural* and *urban*. Inherent features of ruralness identified by the authors of the three chapters are distance between services and providers, geographic remoteness, and lower population density. Likewise, the authors report varying degrees of remoteness, ranging from suburban, to rural, to remote rural areas (Canada, Australia) and frontier areas (United States). Internationally, the challenges are similar in delivering health care and nursing services. The challenges become more significant the further a client lives from an urban-based health care facility. There is great diversity within and among rural communities in their social, economic, and cultural patterns. Therefore, it is difficult to generalize about the health and nursing care needs of rural residents. Imprecise definitions also affect the manner in which data are collected, analyzed, and interpreted. Hence, how rurality is defined and perceived has implications for nurse scholars refining theoretical foundations for rural nursing.

FEATURES OF RURAL NURSING PRACTICE

The characteristics of nursing practice in rural environments are very similar in Canada, the United States, and Australia (Table 16.1). As a group, rural nurses have a strong historical heritage of resilience, resourcefulness, adaptability, and creativity. Their specialty area of practice is being a "generalist"! Perhaps they fit the criteria included in the emerging theory of hardiness described in Chapter 3. Their greatest attribute is knowing what resources are available in the community and how to access these for client systems. Nurses in rural practice settings care for clients across the life span with a variety of health conditions. On the one hand, they must be flexible and effective team players. On the other hand, because there are fewer of all types of health professionals, they often have opportunities to function more autonomously. In all three nations, the role of nursing is expanding.

Advanced practice nurses more often are assuming the role of primary health care providers in rural and medically underserved regions of the three nations. In fact, out of necessity, nurses have been involved in this kind of practice for decades in remote regions of the three nations. Internationally, their educational programs are designing curricula to prepare nurses to function in the expanded role. In the United States, the legal role and scope of APRNs seem somewhat better delineated than in Canada and Australia; however, there are significant variations between states. Hegney indicates that the APRN role is not fully legitimized in Australia. Rennie, Baird-Crooks, Remus, and Engel indicate that Canadian nursing organizations currently are addressing the issue. Both Canadian and Australian nurses are currently consulting with U.S. peers to develop

TABLE 16.1   Comparison of Rural and Urban Nursing Practice on Select
Characteristics

Feature	Rural	Urban
Clients	Of all ages and across the life span Personally acquainted with many of them Sense of connectedness to the community despite geographic distances	More likely to focus on one or two age groups Usually not personally acquainted
Scope of practice	Expected to wear many hats Interface with other disciplines Greater opportunity for expanded roles	More precise job description for each discipline
Roles	Generalist role Role overlap with other disciplines	More opportunities to specialize Disciplines have more clearly delineated roles
Resources (materials/other professionals/ technology/ fiscal and other)	Sometimes fewer formal services Greater flexibility in planning and delivering nursing care Informal networking facilitates continuum of caregiving	Usually have more (there always are some limitations) Greater structure in planning and delivering nursing care within an institution
Patient/client health conditions and diagnosis	Exposure to clients with wide range of health conditions and diagnoses Opportunities to become an "expert generalist"	Specialize; work with fewer types of conditions and diagnoses
Degree of autonomy	Greater Fewer peers with whom to consult	More limited Better access to peers and other professionals
Pace	Generally slower	Usually more intense; hurried
Public visibility	High public visibility—known by many locals Difficult to remain anonymous	Less visibility Easier to maintain anonymity
Discharge planning and client follow-up	Formal processes as mandated by regulatory agencies within health care facility Familiarity with clients means increased opportunities for nurse-client interaction outside of facility; continues informally after discharge (in community settings) Creativity encouraged to prevent fragmentation of care	Formal process as mandated by regulatory agencies, usually limited to within facility (hospital, clinic, agency) Formal referrals to other agencies and providers
Coordination of a continuum of care for clients	Extended family and familiarity among residents facilitate integration of informal services with formal services Flexibility in planning continuum of care with family system	Reduced access to informal networks Greater reliance on formal services

(Continued)

TABLE 16.1 Continued

Feature	Rural	Urban
Status in community	Nursing viewed as an occupation of status, usually highly esteemed Few nurses means high public visibility Acknowledged as a community health resource Well thought of by community (individual variations)	Denser population means less public visibility More nurses and other health professionals—recognition is dispersed among them
Community involvement (informal health education; local policy development)	Multiple roles in home and community social systems (church, school, civic groups, etc.) Plays many roles in health care facility that extend into community roles Little differentiation (less clear boundaries between work, home, and community)	Community activities/roles shared by more people having a particular interest in that activity
Confidentiality	Can be problematic due to familiarity among residents and the visibility of their actions to others	Less problematic because of less familiarity and public visibility but must always be a concern
Quality-of-life issues	Small-town atmosphere Family, recreation, and lifestyle opportunities differ from those of highly populated settings Regional variations—vary from community to community	Regional variations—vary from community to community

NOTE: There are wide variations among and between rural and urban communities and individuals. Therefore, these characteristics are experienced in varying degrees by individual residents in both settings.

legislation regarding APRNs' scope of practice in their nations. Again, there are many similarities among the three nations with regard to advanced practice nursing in rural and remote regions. Hence, nurses need to engage in collaborative international work to study the various nursing delivery modalities and their subsequent outcomes on the health of rural communities.

VISIBILITY VERSUS ANONYMITY

The rural lifestyle is similar regardless of where a small community is located on the globe. That is, because there are fewer people, they tend to be acquainted, and social dynamics differ from those in more populated urban areas. Informal social structures predominate, the pace of life seems to be less hectic, and there is a connectedness among the people who live in rural towns. These situational dynamics have advantages and disadvantages, depending on individual perspectives and preferences. On the one hand, local residents and extended kinship networks are there to assist and support a member in need. On the other hand, everyone who lives there knows what is going on with most of the other people who live in the community. Nurses have high public visibility and usually are highly esteemed by the community. This rural feature blurs the boundaries between nurses' professional work roles and their personal lives. For someone not familiar with rural community dynamics, this can be stress producing—for the nurse as well as his or her family. Conversely, for someone accustomed to informal face-to-face exchanges, the absence of such interaction can lead to a sense of social isolation. Community social and cultural dynamics need to be examined relative to nursing, as these are critical dimensions of how nurses are educated and how they practice in rural environments.

EDUCATION, RECRUITMENT, AND RETENTION ISSUES

Another recurrent theme in Canada, Australia, and the United States concerns issues surrounding the education, recruitment, and retention of nurses and other health professionals in rural parts of their nations. Innovative strategies using technology are being developed by universities and schools of nursing to deliver offerings to rural outreach sites. Likewise, nursing curricula finally are beginning to incorporate and coordinate clinical practica to expose nursing students to the rural practice environment. What is lacking is identification of the core content that is necessary to prepare students and graduates to effectively function in a rural community. Little is written on that topic, and it seems as if the educational needs are similar at an international level. Hopefully, this book will help to fill this information deficit. Partnership again emerges as a common theme in the three chapters: that is, partnering among nurse educators; among universities and rural communities; among faculty in urban-based educational facilities and nurses in rural clinical sites; and among all nurses with health professionals from other disciplines. Empirical data are critically needed about models that work and how these can improve the health outcomes of rural communities.

As for recruitment and retention of nurses in rural areas, a range of strategies are being tried by federal/national and state/provincial/territory governments. One is financial incentives to entice professionals to work in rural areas, especially with populations that are medically underserved. Exposure of students to the rural environment is another strategy that increasingly is being used by schools of nursing to help meet the health care needs of rural residents in their catchment region. The international authors concur that nurses who most likely will work in a rural area are those having a rural background. Regardless of the work setting, improved employee retention is highly dependent on effective recruitment strategies. With the increased use of APRNs in underserved rural areas, recruitment models are being developed to improve retention. Most of these models mandate community involvement rather than simply having a professional recruitment agency or "headhunter" find someone to go to work in a clinic or hospital in a rural town. Of critical importance in retention of nurses and other health professionals is the "fit" of the community with the personality and preferences of the provider who is recruited into a rural area. Obviously, the areas of education, recruitment, and retention related to rural nursing are wide-open fields for nurse researchers. That information also is an important aspect for nurse scholars who are developing the theoretical foundations if rural nursing is to be characterized as a specialty area of practice.

TECHNOLOGY AND THE GLOBAL VILLAGE

According to the authors of the three preceding chapters, the telecommunications and telehealth (telemedicine) industries continue to grow at a steady rate. Technology is helping to reduce the professional isolation that nurses and other health professionals sometimes experience in more remote rural practice sites. Telehealth is the use of tele-communications technologies to transmit diagnostic images and video to provide medical consultations and health-related service over long distances (i.e., when the two entities are not in the same room). Education and a range of health-related services are offered to rural communities using technology. In the literature, certain specialties dominate telehealth usage, specifically mental health, cardiology, orthopedics, radiology, and dermatology. In Canada, the United States, and Australia, the sites, programs, organization, technology, and applications used to deliver health-related services and educational offerings have expanded considerably in the last decade. Clients on the receiving end of that care are demographically varied in both urban and rural areas: Some are homebound, whereas others obtain services in mobile venues. With changing technology, there is a trend to deliver services directly into the home of a client, as well as into prisons, extended-care facilities, and schools. However, there is a need for nurses to be involved in identifying the health care needs at the state and provincial level for rural populations where telehealth and telecommunications technology can provide cost savings. The nursing perspective is a critical aspect for future industry growth. After all, it is nurses who will be using or teaching clients how to use much of that technology. Along with the increased use will be a corresponding increase in the number of legal, ethical, financial, and policy issues. Nurses must become actively involved in all of those discussions so that both nursing and rural perspectives are accurately represented (Association of Telemedicine Service Providers, 1999). That information must be disseminated in nursing literature so peers can learn from it, avoid similar pitfalls, and expedite the appropriate use of technology in rural areas.

RURAL NURSING AS A SPECIALTY AREA OF PRACTICE

The international authors agree that there currently is no theory to guide rural nursing practice. There is consensus that rural nurses need expert generalist skills, reinforced by the expanding body of international nursing research focusing on nurses in the rural environment. Progress is being made in concept development relative to rural practice

(Lee, 1998). However, there is a need for reflection after the studies have been completed to ensure that investigators have not overlooked vital clues relative to the core concepts in the metaparadigm of nursing (health, person, environment, nursing). Definitions of these concepts are of intrinsic importance in the development of nursing knowledge, practice, education, and research questions focusing on rural phenomena. Reflections on past studies can raise awareness of central issues surrounding the delivery of health care in rural communities as well. Existing evidence should be measured relative to the corresponding values of other clinicians in other kinds of rural communities. Clarification of the core nursing concepts is essential if nurses are to ensure that they remain the focus of nursing services in the future. Before assuming new roles or redefining practice, professional organizations must continue to consult with rural nurses to get their perspective.

SUMMARY

This chapter presents a summary of rural nursing in three highly industrialized nations—Canada, Australia, and the United States. The intent is to create interest among nurses at an international level. The future of rural nursing is dependent on the ability to define and defend core nursing concepts. As members of a global village enhanced by technology capabilities, nurses need to engage in international partnering to develop the theoretical foundations for evidence-based nursing practice in remote, less populated, and culturally diverse geographical regions.

DISCUSSION QUESTIONS

> ➤ Analyze common themes related to rural nursing in the United States, Australia, and Canada. Evaluate the similarities and differences among the three.

> ➤ Contact a nurse in rural practice in an international community. Using the information in Table 16.1, discuss nursing practice in rural communities. What are the similarities and differences?

SUGGESTED RESEARCH ACTIVITIES

> ➤ Complete an analysis using the nursing concept described in Chapter 3 (health, person, environment, nursing) for the content presented in Chapter 13 (United States), Chapter 14 (Australia), and Chapter 15 (Canada). Evaluate the fit of the information with Dunkin's framework (Chapter 5). Publish your findings.

> ➤ Partner with nurse(s) in another nation. Implement a study on a relevant rural phenomenon of common interest. Publish your findings.

REFERENCES

Association of Telemedicine Service Providers. (1999, January 8). *ATSP survey reports telemedicine growth in 1997; economic barriers remain a concern* [Press release]. Portland, OR: Author.

Lee, H. (1998). *Conceptual basis for rural nursing.* New York: Springer.

ADDITIONAL SUGGESTED READINGS

Federal Office of Rural Health Policy. (1998, January). *Rural health: A vision for 2010. Report from an invitational workshop.* Washington, DC: Author.

Ferguson, V. (1998). *Educating the 21st century nurse: Challenges and opportunities.* New York: National League for Nursing.

Helvie, C. (1998). *Advanced practice nursing in the community.* Thousand Oaks, CA: Sage.

Hickey, J., Ouimette, R., & Venegoni, C. (1999). *Advanced practice nursing: Changing roles and clinical application.* Philadelphia: J. B. Lippincott.

Kenney, J. (1999). *Philosophical and theoretical perspectives for advanced nursing practice.* Boston: Jones & Bartlett.

Keyzer, D. (1998). Reflections on practice: Defining rural nursing care. *Australian Journal of Rural Health, 6*(2), 100-104.

Lancaster, J. (1998). *Nursing issues in leading and managing change.* St. Louis, MO: C. V. Mosby.

Salmon, M. (1999). Thoughts on nursing: Where it has been and where it is going. *Nursing Health Care Perspectives, 20*(1), 20-25.

CHAPTER 17

Ethical Situations

What Nurses in Rural Practice Should Know

KEY TERMS

➢ Ethical situations
➢ Ethics committee
➢ Bioethical dilemma
➢ Kinship networks
➢ Advance directives
➢ Ethics principles
➢ Ethical norm
➢ Autonomy
➢ Paternalism
➢ Beneficence
➢ Justice
➢ Utility

OBJECTIVES

After reading this chapter, you will be able to

➢ Describe ethical conflicts that could present in rural health care settings.
➢ Discuss the role and scope of ethics committees in the rural health care delivery system.
➢ Examine nurses' roles on ethics committees.
➢ Discuss ethical situations that can occur in rural settings.

ESSENTIAL POINTS TO REMEMBER

➢ Ideally, with open and effective communication, bioethical dilemmas should never happen. However, when clinical ethical situations occur, rural nurses must be knowledgeable about available resources to deal with these situations.

> Selected dimensions of rural residency can play a role in ethical situations and how these are resolved. The most common of these are kinship networks and community social structures that can pose threats to confidentiality, which can affect prevention and resolution of ethical situations in rural settings.

> Ethical awareness among nurses begins with appraising one's own personal values regarding health, health care, death, and nursing practice and then comparing and contrasting them with the values stated in the Code of Ethics for Nurses.

> A health care facility should have a functioning ethics committee before an ethical situation presents. The membership will vary from one facility to another but will generally include a physician, a lawyer, an ethicist, and an administrator. Nurses *always* should be represented on an ethics committee and be able to participate effectively in those discussions.

OVERVIEW

This chapter discusses common ethical situations that can arise in rural health care settings. The purpose of the discussion is to create awareness among nurses about ethics and approaches to prevent and respond to ethical situations in the rural practice setting (Bushy & Rauh, 1995).

BACKGROUND AND RATIONALE

Rural nurses are not exempt from ethical conflicts! The accuracy of this statement is reinforced by the following true stories, all of which occurred in "typical" rural communities having fewer than 5,000 residents. The names, places, and outcomes have been modified to protect all who were involved. Even though these particular situations occurred in small towns, such cases are not unique to rural residency.

> Greg, a 25-year-old fisherman, was diagnosed as having a positive blood test for AIDS. He was not surprised, and he insisted that the physician not inform his wife of the lab results. The couple have been married for 8 years and have two school-age children. Greg's mandate is in direct conflict with the physician's belief regarding the right of a spouse to be informed when a patient has a positive HIV test.

> Lucy, 92 years old, suffered a severe heart attack 3 weeks ago. Since then, she has been comatose and fed through a gastric tube. Recently, her family demanded that tube feedings be discontinued to respect Lucy's verbal request "When the time comes, let me die in peace." The two daughters do not think that their mother has a living will. Several employees in the extended-care facility, as well as some community residents, perceive the family's request as tantamount to "starving Lucy to death."

> Steve, 57 years old, was transferred from a large VA hospital on the West Coast to a nursing home in his hometown in a southwestern state. He has not lived here for at least 30 years. The transfer orders indicate that he has advanced cancer of the pancreas. The community "rumor mill" attributes his emaciated condition to an advanced stage of AIDS. On the basis of information gleaned from the "community grapevine," two employees refuse to provide direct physical care to him. This 40-bed institution has no written policy regarding treatment protocols for residents with infectious diseases, specifically HIV/AIDS, hepatitis, or tuberculosis.

Most readers probably are able to corroborate that they have been involved in similar situations or know of other nurses who have (Bushy & Rauh, 1995; Combs, 1996). Ethical situations are not far-fetched; rather, they can occur every day wherever nurses practice.

RECOGNIZING ETHICAL SITUATIONS

These three examples show that rural as well as urban nurses encounter ethical situations—perhaps more often than they care to admit. Moreover, certain dimensions of residency can play a role in ethical situations and how these are resolved. For instance, rural residents sometimes are described as family oriented and have better access to extended kinship networks. This demographic feature can facilitate, and sometimes hinder, family consensus as to the most appropriate treatment option for their loved one. Confidentiality issues also may be a consideration in a small community, as in Lucy's situation. Health care providers must always take into consideration the values and beliefs of clients when dealing with ethical situations (Duncan, 1992; Erlen, 1998a, 1998b; Turner, 1996).

Most nurses have not had a formal ethics course in their program of study. Further, those in rural communities may not have access to continuing education programs to learn more on the topic. With today's biotechnological capabilities of prolonging life, and with declining resources, it is imperative that all nurses become familiar with basic ethics principles as well as preventing and responding to potential ethical situations. Nurses frequently are the first to become aware of potential and real dilemmas because they provide direct care to the client and interact at various levels with the family (Hockenberger, Jarr, Henderson, & Henley, 1998; Noland, 1998) (Table 17.1).

Awareness begins by becoming familiar with basic terminology and concepts for the discipline of ethics. Ethics content may seem rather esoteric to many health care providers, nurses in particular, unless it has clinical relevance. Thus, nurses must be exposed to basic theoretical content and take some time to reflect on its clinical relevance. Discussing the abstract information with peers can help them to develop clinical insights regarding bioethics. Ethical decision making is a nonlinear, systematic process. The nurse begins with the situation at hand, seeks and incorporates new information and other perspectives, and then identifies and modifies interventions. In many ways, this parallels the nursing process.

A fundamental component is learning about one's own personal values regarding health, illness, health care, death, dying, and nursing practice. Then the nurse is in a position to compare and contrast his or her perspectives with the Code of Ethics for Nurses, recognizing congruencies and differences between the two. Ultimately, the nurse should be able to ascertain how personal and professional values fit with the mission of a health care institution and whether he or she is willing to practice in it. A self-appraisal prepares nurses to more effectively recognize the potential for ethical conflicts with clients and their families and to intervene to prevent these from becoming an ethical dilemma. Then, if need be, nursing must be represented in interdisciplinary discussions to work through the case. Not every nurse will be able to be on the committee. However, nurses' perspec-

TABLE 17 1 Overview of the Ethical Decision-Making Process

Process	Actions
Promote and develop awareness	Complete self-appraisal of personal values and beliefs
	Educate health professionals and community
	Compare personal values and beliefs with nursing's professional code of ethics
	Assess congruence with an (employing) institution's philosophy and mission
	Recognize real or potential ethical situations and make appropriate referrals to institution's ethics committee
Assess situation and define problem	Determine if it is an ethical, legal, or medical situation or a combination thereof
	Seek expert consultation
	Identify the patient(s)
Collect and analyze data	Collect data (e.g., advance directives, legal statutes)
	Analyze case, using ethics principles
	Identify all options
	Consider all real and potential environmental influences for each treatment option (e.g., legal; values of client and his/her family; community standards)
	Appraise benefits and risks for each for client and his/her family, community, providers
Select and implement intervention	Identify the best or most appropriate intervention
	Implement action
Evaluate process and outcomes	Perform process evaluation (formative/ongoing evaluation of the process and system infrastructures)
	Perform summative (outcome) evaluation to determine appropriateness of action and the functionality of ethics committee
Educate professionals and the community	Educate health professionals, using this case to address deficits, prevention strategies, recognition of potential problems, ethics principles, etc., and to give a clinical frame of reference for abstract ethics concepts
	Educate the community on such topics as the need to complete advance directives and the process for doing it and realistic expectations from health care providers

tives must also be brought to the table by a peer who has the background and abilities to participate effectively in the process.

INSTITUTIONAL BIOETHICS COMMITTEES

An institutional bioethics committee is the arena for interdiscipline discussion regarding a real or potential ethical situation in the clinical setting. If the health care facility does not have one, as often is the case in very small facilities, nurses should be aware of nearby facilities that do. In several instances, nurses in a small hospital have had an instrumental role in implementing such a committee by facilitating ethical awareness among peers and in their community. It is prudent for an institution to have a functioning ethics committee in place before there is an urgent need for one. Membership varies from one facility to another, but the interdisciplinary committee usually includes a physician, a lawyer, an ethicist, an administrator, and, of course, at least one nurse (Jarr et al., 1998). When an ethical situation presents on the clinical unit, it should be referred to the bioethics committee according to the institution's policy and procedures. Subsequently, the committee must determine if the case has a medical, legal, or ethical dimension, but such boundaries can be imprecise. If the situation is determined to be a *true* ethical conflict versus a medical or legal conflict or a combination thereof, the committee members can proceed to analyze the issue. If there are legal or medical dimensions, expert consultation must be sought regarding those dimensions. For ethical problems, the case is carefully analyzed by the committee to identify all of the options to deal with the situation. Then the consequences of each potential option and/or medical intervention must be identified. The analysis includes identifying real and potential outcomes for each action or lack of action. Each of these options must be closely examined on the basis of an ethical norm that guides whether an action is appropriate.

Generally, undoing a treatment after it has been started can pose more problems than initially withholding it from someone who is near death. For instance, it may be less complicated to withhold inserting a feeding tube, starting intravenous chemotherapy, or placing a ventilator on a patient than to discontinue such treatment after it was started. Withholding treatment, therefore, also must be considered as an alternative (Feutz-Harter, 1998; Memel, 1987; Valente & Trainor, 1998). Therefore, early on, the physician or a nurse in an advanced practice role should attempt to determine the person's preferences. Before serious illness occurs, providers must work closely with the client to evaluate if the outcomes of an intervention will serve to increase or decrease patient and/or family suffering, improve their quality of life, postpone the patient's death, or be the proximate cause of death. Health care providers must always be sensitive to clients' beliefs about life and death. Awareness, sensitivity, and effective communication skills go a long way in preventing ethical conflicts from ever occurring.

For instance, extended family in the community may want to care for their loved one in the home or to have a certain spiritual leader present. Cultural beliefs influence not only preferences for care but also the manner in which the client and family define a "quality" life. Further, these views may not be congruent with those of a technologically oriented nurse or physician. Another important aspect of ethical decision making is to identify who is responsible for the person: for instance, for an adult who is mentally ill, a child, a victim of Alzheimer's disease, or a patient who has had sedating medication. Obviously, many ethical situations can be avoided or more easily resolved when the client has a living will or documented advance directives.

The complexity of most ethical situations requires that a number of individuals participate in the discussion. One or two people usually cannot anticipate the full legal, ethical, or medical ramifications of the situation. Further, the courts recommend that ethical decisions be made by medical experts as opposed to being resolved by the legal system. Still, legal ramifications impinge on many ethical decisions, and practitioners must always consider the consequences of their actions. The consequence, for instance, could be personal remorse, legal prosecution, revocation of a professional license, or even incarceration. Far-reaching ramifications of an ethical conflict reinforce the need for intradisciplinary (within nursing) and interdisciplinary discussion.

Ethics committees are the arena for ethical debates, and nurses have a responsibility to be informed and actively represented in those discussions. When a rural hospital is part of a larger health care system, this committee usually is located within the tertiary center and sometimes includes representatives from affiliating agencies. Generally, in very small hospitals, there is no formal ethics committee. However, because health care providers are personally acquainted with clients, there may be more opportunities for dialogue regarding patients' and families' expectations. Sometimes, health care facilities within a geographical area organize a regional committee to deal with ethical conflicts. Regardless of the structure, most committees also have an educational component. Their mission is to create ethical awareness and inform the community and health professionals about ethics topics (Bushy & Rauh, 1995; Dimmitt, 1994; Stark, 1996).

RECOMMENDATIONS

Ethical conflicts that arise between providers and clients and their families generally are not black-and-white situations. Usually, there are many shades of gray and no clear-cut answers. Nurses are in a position to recognize the potential for ethical situations because they directly interact with clients with greater frequency than other disciplines, especially in rural settings. Therefore, they must become informed about ethics theory, basic ethical principles, and commonly used terms in ethics, such as *ethical norm, autonomy, paternalism, beneficence, utility,* and *justice* (Table 17.2). An extensive discussion about ethics is beyond the scope of this chapter. Readers are advised to seek out textbooks on the topic and even enroll in an ethics course to learn more.

Rural nurses must become familiar with resources to help them when these events occur: for instance, an ethics committee or an ethicist who could be consulted if necessary. Likewise, advanced practice nurses should learn how to educate adults about advance directives when providing primary health care to adults. Nurse administrators should invite speakers to offer continuing education on ethics-related topics. Interdisciplinary discussion on ethical topics should occur *before* situations like Lucy's, Greg's, and Steve's exemplified at the beginning of this chapter. Such exchanges, accompanied by the systematic analysis of real and potential situations can promote ethical awareness and show clinical relevancy. Rural nurse administrators should make every effort to prepare staff nurses for these occurrences. Interdisciplinary analysis of hypothetical situations such as the cited examples is an effective strategy to educate health professionals on dealing with and resolving ethical situations. However, for a full and meaningful exchange to occur, the following guidelines must be adhered to by all involved in the dialogue:

> *All opinions have equal status.* Often it is the most unusual and unconventional idea that ends up being the most useful and prudent in developing collective wisdom.
> *All members in the group must listen to the satisfaction of the sender of the message.* It is absolutely essential to listen to the speaker and hear his or her intent. Respect each other as well as the speaker. Listen to learn! Listen nondefensively! Listen without discounting! Do not prepare your response while a speaker is speaking. Do not respond or interrupt until another has finished speaking. Hear the person out until the end of the comment.

TABLE 17.2 Ethics Terminology

Ethical norm	A statement (principle) that actions of a certain type ought (or ought not) to be done
Autonomy (principle)	Respect for individuals' right to act autonomously (not controlled by others) in making decisions that affect their lives
Paternalism	Limiting an individual's liberty when his/her actions might result in harm, or fail to produce an important benefit
Beneficence	Act(s) of kindness; an obligation of doing or promoting good for another
	Doing no harm; maximizing possible benefits and minimizing possible harm
Utility	The greatest good/happiness for the greatest number
Justice	Equals should be treated equally; those who are unequal should be treated differently according to their difference

➤ *All members respect the confidentiality of the group.* (This standard is self-explanatory!)

➤ *The group as a whole must directly address issues, concerns, or inappropriate action.* No gossip; use direct, specific disagreement. Avoid passive-aggressive behaviors at later times within the group or outside the setting.

➤ *Once the group reaches consensus, all will speak with one voice about the issue.* Avoid "behind the back" or "under the table" comments; there should be no undermining or second-guessing in public about the group's decision.

➤ *The group should strive for win-win solutions and use negotiation rather than confrontational approaches.* People generally are more satisfied receiving part of a request than nothing, as long as the decision is perceived as fair.

SUMMARY

Ethical issues can occur even in the smallest health care facilities. The purpose of this chapter is to create awareness among rural nurses about ethical situations and how these can be dealt with. Whether the setting is rural or urban, nurses must know about resources and how to access them when they encounter real and even potential ethical conflicts.

DISCUSSION QUESTIONS

➤ Identify an ethical situation that you have encountered or might encounter in a rural practice setting.

➤ Organize a discussion group with peers, and if possible invite an ethicist to participate.

> Systematically analyze the case by applying the basic ethics principles, such as autonomy, beneficence, justice, and utility (see Table 17.2).
> What legal, medical, and cultural factors affect the case?
> Learn about the ethics committee in your institution. If possible, interview one or more members.
> Is it a systemwide or locally focused committee?
> Who are the members?
> Is nursing represented on it?
> How are/were committee members selected?
> What educational preparation did they receive to effectively participate in these discussions?
> How are referrals made to the committee?
> What should nurses know about this process?
> How are decisions made?
> What initiatives (efforts) has this group implemented to educate local health professionals? The community?

SUGGESTED RESEARCH ACTIVITIES

Develop an ethical awareness continuing program for nurses and paraprofessionals in a particular rural health care facility.

> Implement the program.
> Evaluate the process and outcomes.
> Disseminate the findings by publishing an article in a nursing journal and presenting at a regional or national nursing conference.
> Design and implement a descriptive study to assess the nurses' knowledge about ethics.
> Examine nurses' attitudes regarding the most appropriate time to educate people in rural communities about advance directives.

REFERENCES

Bushy, A., & Rauh, J. (1995). Ethics dilemmas in rural practice. In B. Yawn, A. Bushy, & R. Yawn (Eds.), *Exploring rural medicine* (pp. 271-286). Newbury Park, CA: Sage.

Combs, E. (1996). Home health, AIDS, and refusal to care. *Home Healthcare Nurse, 14,* 188-194.

Dimmitt, J. (1994). Cases of conscience: Casuistic analysis of ethical dilemmas in expanded role settings. *Nursing Ethics, 1,* 200-207.

Duncan, S. (1992). Ethical challenge in community health nursing. *Journal of Advances in Nursing Science, 7,* 1035-1041.

Erlen, J. (1998a). Culture, ethics, and respect: The bottom line is understanding. *Orthopaedic Nursing, 17*(6), 79.

Erlen, J. (1998b). Treatment decision making: Who should decide? *Orthopaedic Nursing, 17*(4), 60.

Feutz-Harter, S. (1998). Legal issues in nursing practice. In J. Lancaster (Ed.), *Nursing issues in leading and managing change* (pp. 364-392). St. Louis, MO: C. V. Mosby.

Hockenberger, S. (1998). When is enough, enough? Caring for terminally ill patients. *Plastic Surgical Nursing, 18,* 207.

Jarr, S., Henderson, M., & Henley, C. (1998, August). The registered nurse: Perceptions about advance directives. *Journal of Nursing Care Quality, 12*(6), 26-36.

Memel, S. (1987). When do ethical issues become legal issues? *Health Executive, 2*(5), 46-49.

Noland, L. (1998). Ethical issues in nursing practice. In J. Lancaster (Ed.), *Nursing issues in leading and managing change* (pp. 337-364). St. Louis, MO: C. V. Mosby.

Stark, R. (1996). Ethical considerations in rural health nursing. *Medical Law, 15,* 277-282.

Turner, L. (1996). Rural nurse practitioners: Perceptions of ethical dilemmas. *Journal of the American Academy of Nurse Practitioners, 8,* 269-274.

Valente, S., & Trainor, D. (1998). Rational suicide among patients who are terminally ill. *AORN Journal, 68,* 252.

CHAPTER 18

Research

The Link Between Rural Theory and Evidence-Based Practice

KEY TERMS

- ➤ Program evaluation
- ➤ Formative evaluation
- ➤ Summative evaluation
- ➤ Research process
    - ➤ Implementation
    - ➤ Dissemination
    - ➤ Utilization
- ➤ Evidence-based practice
- ➤ Qualitative studies
- ➤ Quantitative studies
- ➤ Integrative literature review
- ➤ Continuous quality improvement (CQI)
- ➤ Triangulated data

OBJECTIVES

After reading this chapter, you will be able to

- ➤ Examine the need for research in developing a theory that can lead to evidence-based nursing practice in rural environments.
- ➤ Discuss methodologic adaptations that should be considered when developing and implementing nursing studies having a rural focus.
- ➤ Analyze the role of program evaluation, quality assessment, and client satisfaction in expanding the theoretical basis for rural nursing practice.
- ➤ Propose nursing research questions to study health conditions of rural clients across the life span and the health care continuum.

ESSENTIAL POINTS TO REMEMBER

➤ Knowledge about the research process is pivotal to the development of a theoretical base for nursing regardless of the setting, whether rural or urban, and across the continuum of care. Nurses must be able to read the literature critically and then implement relevant findings in their practice. Rural nursing administrators can create a culture that supports and nurtures nurses in the development of studies and utilization of findings.

➤ Even when the results of an investigation directly relate to rural practice, nurses in those settings tend not to use the findings. An often cited reason for this failure to apply findings is the unfamiliarity of terminology used in nursing research reports. Whether research findings are adopted into nursing practice protocols within an institution is highly dependent on the level of support for such adoption by nursing administrators.

OVERVIEW

In the preceding chapters of this book, research activities were suggested that could strengthen the profession's theoretical base. This chapter focuses on research issues that are relevant to the rural environment and the nurses who practice there (Bushy, 1991; Lee, 1998; Winstead-Fry, Tiffany, & Shippee-Rice, 1992).

BACKGROUND

Nursing has been gradually expanding its domain of knowledge since the time of Florence Nightingale, who carefully charted the progress of patients under her care. Nightingale established the core of information from which to instruct nurses for more than a century in caring for the sick and injured in another time and another place. Over the decades, nurses have built on her findings and have come to realize that practice must be based on research findings (evidence based) in this era of health care restructuring. If rural nursing is to be recognized as a true "profession," our practice must be built on a scientific foundation (Champagn, Tornquist, & Funk, 1997; Fitzpatrick, 1998; Lacey, 1994; Lee, 1998; McCarthy & Hegney, 1998; National Institute for Nursing Research [NINR], 1990, 1993a, 1993b, 1993c, 1994a, 1994b, 1995). A concern among many nurses in rural practice is that the health status and mortality rates of residents living and working in this environment are not equal to the rates of their urban counterparts. Because the disparity has persisted over time, nurses working to sustain the health of rural residents are asking some fundamental questions: What can we do? How can nursing systematically study what nurses do to ensure that their actions contribute to effective clinical outcomes, cost containment, and acceptability in rural environments? What is the most effective way to disseminate the findings to rural nurses who can use the information in their practice? What can be done to develop nurses in rural practice who have had limited exposure to research content so that they can critique the literature and then use relevant scientific findings in clinical practice? The next section addresses a few of those questions as they affect rural nursing (Funk, Champagn, & Tornquist, 1995).

WHY RURAL NURSING RESEARCH?

Knowledge about the research process is pivotal to the development of a theoretical base for nursing regardless of the setting, whether rural or urban, and across the continuum of care. Nurses should first be aware of the important role of research in clinical practice. Then they must possess the skills to read the research literature critically and distinguish when, and how, to implement evidence-based findings in their practice. To achieve this multifaceted goal, continuing education must be made available for nurses who have not been exposed to that particular content in their basic educational program. Typically, nurses practicing in rural areas tend to be older and to have fewer years of formal education than their urban counterparts. Overall, there are fewer rural nurses who have Bachelor of Science in Nursing (BSN) degrees, and only a few have completed Master's of Science in Nursing (MSN) degrees. A higher proportion have completed an associate degree (AD) or diploma program. Lower levels of education and less recent education make it less likely that rural nurses have been exposed to research in their program of study (American Association of Colleges of Nursing, 1998).

It is important to stress that baccalaureate-prepared nurses do not have the background to plan and implement studies. Rather, they are prepared to assist in data collection, critique research articles, and help to implement clinically pertinent findings. Ideally, the role of doctorally prepared nurses is to develop studies; the role of graduate-prepared nurses is to implement the findings; and the role of baccalaureate-prepared nurses is to assist the former two groups of nurses, identify problems for investigation, and collect data. Because there are very few nurses with advanced degrees, this ideal may not be realistic. Other barriers to implementing, disseminating, and utilizing nursing research in rural practice are related to personnel, access, cost, and cultural, educational, social, and economic factors (Table 18.1). Therefore, other means must be sought to carry out these activities, such as partnering of nurses in academic settings with those in rural health care facilities.

Rural nurses consistently request continuing education on a variety of research topics. Familiarity with the content also is essential for implementing continuous quality improvement (CQI) and quality assurance programs that are mandated by external regulatory agencies of health care institutions. Administrators of health care institutions should expect all of their employees to be involved in CQI activities. These activities are steeped in research methods. Research content can be difficult to assimilate by simply reading a text, and such a course lends itself to at least some direct instructor-student interactions. Alternative and complementary teaching strategies along with face-to-face instruction currently are being developed, such as Web-enhanced content (part of the content is obtained via the Internet) and self-directed learning modules (independent study with instructor guidelines). In designing a research course, regardless of the teaching strategies, faculty should incorporate assignments that are relevant to rural nursing practice, such as critiquing articles and developing evidenced-based protocols in a health care institution, specifically a rural health clinic or a critical access hospital.

External regulatory mandates and internal administrative expectations are an ideal opportunity for nursing faculty to collaborate with rural-based peers in research activi-

TABLE 18.1 Barriers to Implementing, Disseminating, and Utilizing Rural Nursing Research

Staff	Shortage of personnel
	High patient/nurse ratio
	Negative attitudes on the part of staff/administration
	Professional isolation/little peer support
	Not having educational preparation (fewer BSN- and MSN- prepared nurses
	Less familiarity with technology (i.e., computer literacy, comfort level with Internet resources)
	Poor cooperation by support staff/not understanding process or purpose
	Medical staff does not approve/support nursing project(s)
	Inexperience of researcher/interviewer
	Not possessing communication skills/resources to disseminate findings (oral/written word)
Resources	Employee time not dedicated to research-related activities (CQI)
	University resources and expert consultation not accessible to rural clinicians
	Limited/lack of space, research facilities, library resources, technologic support services
	No incentives/recognition for nurse pursuing research activities
Financial	Costs (indirect/indirect) of doing research to institution
	Lack of funds targeted for research-related activities
	Lack of resources designated for staff education to learn the process, implement the study, and disseminate findings
Other	Insufficient number of (available) subjects
	Problems in accessing subjects (distance/fear/illness/stress, etc.)
	Researcher/subject time constraints
	No Institutional Research Review Board (IRRB)
	IRRB not granting approval
	Incomplete/inaccurate documentation in records/record keeping
	Nonexistent/inadequate information systems to analyze data

ties. As partners, nurses in their various roles can collaborate to identify, investigate, and disseminate (publish and present) information about rural nursing phenomena. Together they can design, implement, and evaluate evidence-based nursing interventions. In rural health care facilities, collaborative efforts should extend to other disciplines, including physicians, social workers, economists, pharmacists, physical and nutritional therapists, sociologists, health planners, and informatics and telecommunications experts. Collaboration between, and among, other types of health professionals, nurse researchers, nurse clinicians, and nurse administrators can result in mutually beneficial outcomes. There also is the potential for making contributions to nursing's evolving theoretical base: in this instance, theory on practice in rural environments.

RURAL RESEARCH CONSIDERATIONS

The research process is systematically rigorous to ensure that data are valid and reliable and that they accurately reflect the phenomenon being investigated. That principle also

Research **257**

applies to nursing studies that focus on rural phenomena. Nurse scholars must therefore take into consideration some of the more unusual features of rural environments when designing studies, collecting and analyzing data, and implementing studies with that focus. A few of the more frequently encountered rural features that need to be considered are examined in this section (Barnsteiner, 1996; Bushy, 1991; Health Resources Services Administration [HRSA], 1998; McMurray, 1998).

Adapt Procedures

Nurse researchers focusing on a rural issue or studying a population living in a nonurban area must be aware that methodological adjustments may be needed. For instance, because there is a smaller population from which to select a sample, there may be a correspondingly lower number of subjects than for a similar study in a highly populated setting. Likewise, issues surrounding anonymity and confidentiality may need to be considered.

For example, residents in a small community usually are quite willing and eager to help out a "local girl" who is getting a "nursing degree." In many cases, accommodation extends to participating in the nursing student's research assignments. Ensuring confidentiality and anonymity can be a challenge, especially when the local grapevine is healthy and active among residents who are interested in what is happening in their community. Or study participants may fear that if their answers are not "right," the care they subsequently receive in the local clinic may not be as good. Hence, when designing a nursing study, modifications may be needed to ensure confidentiality and anonymity of subjects in a close-knit community. Of course, the approach will vary with the focus of the study and the setting.

Select Instruments

Selection of measurement instruments is another critical component of the research process. Regardless of the setting or the topic being investigated, careful consideration must be given to this activity. Because of space constraints, instrument development and selection will not be discussed in detail in this chapter. Readers having an interest in this topic are referred to research textbooks for detailed guidance. Essentially, when selecting an instrument, the researcher must consider

- ➤ The problem under investigation
- ➤ The reliability and validity of the tool
- ➤ The characteristics of the sample, such as subjects' age, ethnic and cultural background, income, education, level of anxiety, and reading, writing, and verbal communication skills
- ➤ The effectiveness of the instrument in communicating findings to a targeted audience

Nurses must be aware that even well-accepted and highly acclaimed instruments having strong validity and reliability may not be culturally appropriate for rural minorities or subgroups. In fact, some individuals who readily agree to participate in a "nurse's" study may not be able to read or understand words on a highly acclaimed and seemingly simple pencil-and-paper client satisfaction survey. It is prudent, therefore, to implement a pilot study to determine if the tool is culturally and linguistically appropriate for the sample. (*Cultural* and *linguistic appropriateness* means that subjects can understand what is written in the consent form and the data collection tools.) The investigator then can make the refinements to collect data that are culturally valid and reliable.

Protect Human Subjects

Protection of human subjects must be ensured in all types of research. However, rarely do institutional research review boards (IRRBs) exist in rural heath care facilities. Therefore, other approaches may be needed to obtain approval to implement the study and ensure protection of human subjects. For example, a nurse planning to implement a study in a very small hospital may need to obtain a letter of approval from the institution's chief executive officer (CEO) or nursing administrator or perhaps the board of directors. A letter of support may need to be written by the mayor or another formal leader, such as the tribal chairperson or a community planner (Chapter 7).

Design the Study

With respect to the most appropriate type of design, both qualitative and quantitative studies are necessary to enhance the theoretical base for nursing practice in rural settings. Subsequently, findings from the two kinds of studies must be triangulated (integrated) to yield a full picture of the phenomenon of interest. Nursing has long recognized the uniqueness of an individual's experiences and interactions (qualitative approaches) while simultaneously identifying commonalities from which to make predictions (quantitative approaches). Through integration of the two types of data, patterns can be identified, predictions made, and evidenced-based interventions developed for a particular human condition. Both approaches must be equally valued, and their unique contributions must be carefully weighed. These are but a few of the considerations that must go into a research design, but they are of particular importance when one is studying a nursing phenomenon in the rural practice environment. Essentially, the problem statement, along with what is known about the problem, preempts the methodology used in a study with a particular population.

Disseminate and Utilize Findings

Despite unprecedented growth in nursing research and even with the phenomenal expansion of communication capabilities, the greatest challenge that remains is dissemination of findings to clinicians. It is, after all, those who care for clients that can make the most use of that information. Once a study is completed, application of the findings to nursing practice may be immediate or, as often is the case, over a period of time. In the latter case, research findings may be linked to other previously completed studies or conceptualized in terms of related investigations. Regardless of the time needed to implement the findings, the goal of empirically based data is improving client care (McConnell, 1997).

Disseminating and utilizing nursing research findings in rural settings can be even more of a challenge where communications technology may not be as reliable and where opportunities for professional dialogue among nurses may be limited. One of the major limitations in disseminating empirical findings is that researchers are based primarily in institutions of higher learning. On the one hand, nurse scholars mostly are found in urban settings due to the cost associated with creating and funding research. Rural practitioners, on the other hand, tend to be more clinically oriented and service oriented than research focused. The two groups can be linked by dissemination of research findings to fit the needs of a particular audience—clinicians, scholars, or even consumers. Other challenges to nurses in rural practice are the cost, time, and distance to attend a research conference. Therefore, strategies must be developed by nurse scholars to deliver the information to peers who live and work in outlying catchment areas.

Clinical trials usually take place in larger urban health science centers. Nurses have conducted extensive clinical trials on wound care, symptom management, appropriate times for clients' focused health promotion education, and interventions to manage dementia. Yet even when the results of an investigation directly relate to rural practice, nurses in those settings tend not to use the findings. A number of reasons are offered, and the most often cited is terminology used in nursing research reports. Not being familiar with research-related terms hinders clinicians in understanding and implementing the findings. Although most nurses recognize the value of research, many are unsure of what actually constitutes research and which findings could, or should, be implemented in the practice setting. Recently, integrative research reviews focusing on a particular phenomenon, such as the management of elevated temperatures and pain and symptom management in patients with a particular diagnosis, have become available. For these reports, an author has analyzed, synthesized, and summarized findings from a cluster of nursing studies. Such reports can be useful to clinicians in developing clinical protocols and delineating parameters for CQI activities. However, the nurse must still be able to critique these to determine if the summary is applicable to a particular setting (Ingersoll, 1996; McCarthy & Hegney, 1998).

Language is perhaps the greatest obstacle in implementing relevant nursing findings. For example, scholarly reports often are verbose and written in research jargon. These reports are not readily understood by the "average" nurse who never had a research course or who was exposed to that particular content some years ago. Consequently, a staff nurse may conclude that the report is written for the benefit of other researchers rather than for use by clinicians. Statistics can be especially intimidating and easily misunderstood by a nurse who never has had a research course or by someone who took an undergraduate statistics course many years earlier. To deal with this chasm, research findings should be disseminated in both written and oral form and should target three separate audiences:

> ➢ Nurse researchers, so that they can analyze, replicate, refute, and refine the methods and findings
> ➢ Clinicians in various specialties, so that they can implement and utilize the findings in their practice
> ➢ Consumers of health care, so that they can become aware and, hopefully, be motivated to modify risky health behaviors

Unfortunately, among faculty in institutions of higher learning, greater value tends to be placed on disseminating information to the first audience, even though reaching the latter two groups may take greater skill. Prioritizing in this manner does little to disseminate research findings to those who can implement them in practice or to motivate clients to modify risky behaviors.

Evaluate Program Outcomes and Quality of Services

Evaluation research is another dimension of the implementation of quality assurance programs such as CQI programs. This type of study is valid and extremely important in this era of cost containment and managed care. However, it frequently is not taken seriously by nurse researchers. Evaluation studies, when designed with rigor and precision, can measure the effect of an intervention on one or more outcomes (summative evaluation). Such studies are appropriate to describe the processes (formative evaluation) that lead to successful, or unsuccessful, program implementation. These studies are critically needed for innovative models of health care delivery that mandate the use of advanced practice nurses, such as rural health clinics, federally qualified community health centers, and rural hospitals classified as critical access facilities. When community members participate in designing evaluation studies, the data may have greater validity and the findings may be better accepted. Active participation can empower residents to use the findings for decision making to address a particular community health-related concern. Evaluation studies, therefore, should not be underestimated by nurse researchers, as these are fundamental to designing, implementing, and evaluating evidence-based nursing interventions with rural clients.

Measure Client Satisfaction

Client satisfaction surveys are another important source of nursing research data and a component of intrainstitutional (within a facility) and interinstitutional (among facilities in an MCO) CQI programs. These kinds of studies have increased dramatically in the last 10 years with the expansion of managed care and the heightened public awareness of health care costs. The rationale for implementing satisfaction studies is that clients' adherence to recommended treatment protocols is directly linked to their satisfaction with rendered services and with providers. Another rationale, though often unwritten, for monitoring client satisfaction is that it can drive fiscal success in a competitive market—in this case, health care services. After all, the best marketing tool is a satisfied customer! This fundamental economic principle applies to nursing and evaluation of nursing services too. However, the tools to measure client satisfaction must be culturally valid and reliable. Space constraints in this chapter do not permit in-depth examination of the development of survey tools. Readers are referred to research texts for additional details on designing, implementing, and evaluating survey methods.

Even with a variety of real and potential barriers, a major influence on whether research findings are adopted into nursing practice is the degree of support and encouragement for such behaviors within an institution. In other words, the administrative infrastructure allows utilization of research findings and encourages nurses to incorporate evidence-based interventions in their practice. Creating such an atmosphere is highly dependent on the commitment of nurse administrators and managers to communicate relevant empirical findings to staff nurses. The trickle-down effect instills a spirit of inquiry among nurses. Ultimately, having a research culture is an important aspect of quality assessment, CQI, and ensuring client satisfaction. Education that instructs and motivates is key in encouraging clinicians to adopt evidence-based practice within an institution. Time must be allocated in the workload of nurses for research-related activities, particularly for nurses in advanced practice roles. The following are additional strategies that can promote a spirit of inquiry among nurses in rural health care settings (Agency for Health Care Policy Research, 1999; American Nurses Association, 1999; McSkirmming, 1996; Yuen & Towari, 1996):

➢ Assign a (research) mentor to work with advanced practice nurses, on a rotating basis, on areas of interest to them or their practice setting (research foci).
➢ Partner with a university-based nursing education program. Invite faculty members having an interest in rural issues to speak about research to their clinical peers. Request the speaker to provide condensed versions of research studies on a selected area of practice, or perhaps on a variety of topics. The information should be presented in language that is easily understood by staff nurses on a particular clinical unit. Encourage open dialogue between the speaker and the participants. Invite clinicians to identify research problems that could be developed into a nursing study.
➢ Access relevant resources on the research process or on a particular clinical situation. Make these materials readily available to nurses on a clinical unit to read; encourage discussion about the content and its clinical relevance.
➢ Coordinate journal clubs or "brown-bag lunches" for nurses to dialogue and learn about selected research topics. Critique research articles of common interest to the group. If appropriate, invite individuals from other health care disciplines to join in these activities.

Where nurse administrators and clinicians examine research together, there is a greater potential for implementing evidence-based interventions in that institution. Designing relevant studies should evolve from clinicians' feedback on the appropriateness and usefulness of empirical findings. A two-way feedback loop is at the heart of incremental theory development for rural nursing. To reiterate, nursing must have a coordinated research agenda that counters the proliferation of haphazard studies that all have a different focus. A haphazard approach, coupled with nurses' inclination to tack "bits and pieces of practical knowledge" onto data disseminated by other disciplines, has prevented nursing's theoretical base from gaining depth and reflecting the discipline's true practice domain.

Developing nurses' ability to analyze and critique studies is another way to promote a research culture and use empirically based findings. Nursing administrators should promote discussion, among interdisciplinary members of the health care team, of the body of research on a specific clinical topic. The group leader should be able to translate research jargon into useful clinical language. Even though increasing numbers of nurses have taken a basic research course, the ability to critique a research report is dependent on professional dialogue with peers about the topic. Ongoing exposure is particularly important with the proliferation of methodological approaches. Even nurses who recently completed a research course may not be familiar with evolving methods of analysis. Nor do most have the skill to combine data in order to expand clinical insights and determine the data's usefulness. Therefore, administrators must assess the knowledge level of nursing staff regarding their preparation and interest in the research process. Subsequently, efforts must be undertaken to develop skill and entice the interest of clinicians to implement evidence-based interventions that could improve outcomes.

DEVELOPING A THEORY FOR RURAL NURSING

The question often is raised as to whether rural nursing is a specialty area of practice. This book is an effort to synthesize and organize what is known about nursing and the rural context. In recent years, a great deal has been written on the topic of ruralness, some of which is highly relevant to the discipline of nursing and to nurses. Lee (1998), in her book *Conceptual Basis for Rural Nursing,* examined ruralness in relation to nursing in the Rocky Mountain region of the United States. This publication will be highly useful in examining nursing in other rural contexts. However, to develop a theory that can guide nurses in a variety of roles and diverse rural practice settings, a research agenda must be put forth to focus efforts of nurse scholars (Bushy, 2000; HRSA, 1998; National Institute of Occupational Safety and Health [NIOSH], 1998; NINR, 1990, 1993a, 1993b, 1993c, 1994a, 1994b, 1995). The twofold purpose of such an agenda is developing a spirit of inquiry among rural nurses and suggesting research topics for nurse scholars.

SUMMARY

Research is the vital link between developing a theory for rural nursing and implementing evidence-based nursing interventions. It is my hope that the information in this book can motivate researchers, educators, and clinicians to address the information deficit. Perhaps, in the near future, rural nursing will be acknowledged as a specialty area of practice, performed by an expert generalist who functions as a resource broker between formal and informal caregivers within the community. Collaboration among scholars and clinicians will lead to development of evidence-based nursing interventions that are appropriate for diverse clients in diverse rural environments. In turn, this knowledge base will expand the theoretical foundation for rural nursing, ultimately improving the health status of America's rural communities.

DISCUSSION QUESTIONS

➤ Explain the relationship between research, theory, and practice. Give examples of how the three dimensions interface for nursing in the rural environment.

➤ Identify common themes in the research agendas but forth by NIOSH and NINR. How can these two agendas guide the development of a theoretical framework for nursing practice in the rural environment?

SUGGESTED RESEARCH ACTIVITIES

➤ Develop a research problem statement for one (or more) of the minority health disparities described in *Healthy People 2010* (U.S. Department of Health and Human Services [USDHHS], 1999). How does your problem fit the nursing research agenda put forth by NINR? The National Occupational Research Agenda (NIOSH, 1998)?

➤ Complete a literature review and write an integrative review on rural occupational health and safety issues (e.g., children and farm accidents; morbidity and mortality in the fishing industry; tractor accidents among farmers; animal-related farm injuries; depression among injured miners; exposure of children of migrant workers to agricultural chemicals). What is known? What are the information deficits?

➤ Partner with the community to develop a health promotion nursing intervention that targets a vulnerable population that is at particular risk for those injuries. Plan and execute the intervention. Develop evaluation tools to monitor the outcomes. List short-term as well as long-range outcomes. How could each of these be measured? What are potential funding sources to implement the proposed intervention?

REFERENCES

Agency for Health Care Policy Research. (1999). *National Guideline Clearinghouse (NGC) Project* [On-line; Internet clearinghouse for clinical practice guidelines]. Available: www.guideline.gov

American Association of Colleges of Nursing. (1998, November 30). *Position statement on nursing research.* Washington, DC: Author. Available: www.aacn.nche.edu

American Nurses Association. (1999). *Competencies for telehealth technologies in nursing.* Washington, DC: Author.

Barnsteiner, J. (1996). Research-based practice. *Nursing Administration Quarterly, 20,* 52-58.

Bushy, A. (1991). Meeting the challenges of rural nursing research. In A. Bushy (Ed.), *Rural nursing* (Vol. 2, pp. 304-318). Newbury Park, CA: Sage.

Bushy, A. (Ed.). (In press). *Rural minority health in the 21st century: Eliminating disparities. Conference proceedings for the Fourth Annual NRHA Rural Minority Conference.* Kansas City, MO: National Rural Health Association.

Champagn, M., Tornquist, E., & Funk, S. (1997). Achieving research-based practice. *American Journal of Nursing, 97*(5), 16AAA-16DDD.

Fitzpatrick, J. (1998). *Encyclopedia of nursing research.* New York: Springer.

Funk, S., Champagn, M., & Tornquist, E. (1995). Barriers and facilitators of research utilization. *Research Utilization, 30,* 395-407.

Health Resources Services Administration. (1998). *Rural health research in progress.* Rockville, MD: Author.

Ingersoll, G. (1996). Evaluation research. *Nursing Administration Quarterly, 20,* 28-40.

Lacey, E. (1994). Research utilization in nursing practice: A pilot study. *Journal of Advanced Nursing, 19,* 606-610.

Lee, H. (1998). *Conceptual basis for rural nursing.* New York: Springer.

McCarthy, A., & Hegney, D. (1998). Evidenced-based practice and rural nursing: A literature review. *Australian Journal of Rural Health, 6,* 96-99.

McConnell, E. (1997). Giving an outstanding presentation. *American Journal of Nursing, 97*(12), 62-63.

McMurray, A. (1998). Undertaking research for the benefit of the rural community. *Australian Journal of Rural Health, 6,* 89-95.

McSkirmming, S. (1996). Creating a cultural norm for research and research utilization in a clinical agency. *Western Journal of Nursing Research, 18,* 606-610.

National Institute for Nursing Research. (1990). *HIV patient infection: Prevention research and care directions.* Bethesda, MD: Author.

National Institute for Nursing Research. (1993a). *Developing knowledge for practice: Challenges and opportunities.* Bethesda, MD: Author.

National Institute for Nursing Research. (1993b). *Nursing informatics: Enhancing patient care.* Bethesda, MD: Author.

National Institute for Nursing Research. (1993c). *Physical activity and cardiovascular health promotion for older children and adolescents.* Bethesda, MD: Author.

National Institute for Nursing Research. (1994a). *Long-term care for older adults.* Bethesda, MD: Author.

National Institute for Nursing Research. (1994b). *Symptom management: Acute pain studies in children and adolescents to prevent cardiovascular disease.* Bethesda, MD: Author.

National Institute for Nursing Research. (1995). *Community-based health care: Nursing strategies.* Bethesda, MD: Author.

National Institute of Occupational Safety and Health. (1998). The National Occupational Research Agenda: A model of broad stakeholder input into priority setting. *American Journal of Public Health, 88,* 353-356.

U.S. Department of Health and Human Services. (1999). *Healthy people 2010: National health promotion and disease prevention objectives.* Washington, DC: Government Printing Office.

Winstead-Fry, P., Tiffany, J., & Shippee-Rice, R. (1992). *Rural health nursing: Stories of creativity, commitment, and connectedness* (NLN Pub. No. 21-2408). New York: National League for Nursing.

Yuen, F., & Towari, A. (1996). Scholarly research activities in nursing administration: Some issues. *Journal of Nursing Management, 4,* 301-305.

APPENDIX A

Hypertext Links to Access Internet Sites Related to Rural Nursing

Hypertext links can provide additional information related to at-risk and vulnerable populations. Because URL addresses change frequently, the reader may need to access these sites through other addresses. These are starting points to additional information for designing and providing health services for special populations.

Site Name and URL	Type of Information
Agency for Health Care Policy and Research http://www.ahcpr.gov	Research, clinical, and preventive guidelines
Alternative medicine http://www.altmedicine.com	Complementary and holistic health care
American Public Health Association http://www.apha.org	Public health, vulnerable populations
Association of Community Health Nursing Educators http://www.health.uncc.edu/achne	Links to other sites and information on community health nursing issues, practice, and education
Association of Telemedicine Service Providers http://www.atsp.org	Telemedicine-related news and resources; on-line journal
Bureau of Primary Health Care http://www.bphc.hrsa.dhhs.gov	Health promotion and disease prevention
Bureau of the Census www.census.gov	Census data, maps, research links
Center for Patient Advocacy http://www.patientadvocacy.org	Managed care information
Centers for Disease Control and Prevention http://www.cdc.gov	Data, prevention and control of disease; links to federal and state resources
Children's Health Insurance Program (CHIP) http://www.hcfa.gov/init/children.htm	State activities for children's financial access to health services
Community Campus Partnerships for Health http://futurehealth.ucsf.edu/ccph.html	Academic-community models for special populations

| Consumer Information Center
http://www.pueblo.gsa.gov	Consumer information
Council of Ethical Organizations
http://www.ethicsandcompliance.com	Ethics resources
Environmental Protection Agency
http://www.epa.gov	Information on environmental issues
Families USA
http://www.familiesusa.org	Managed care information
Food and Drug Administration (FDA)
http://www.fda/gov/fadhomepage.htm	Food, nutrition, and drug information
Health Care Financing Administration (HCFA)
http://www.hcfa.gov	Health care delivery system issues and resources
Health Care for the Homeless Information Resource Center
http://www.prainc.com/hch	Clinical information and resources, recommendations for policy and practice, Web-based study modules on special issues in health care of homeless
Health Resources Services Administration
http://www.hrsa.dhhs.gov	Links to managed care information related to special populations
Health United States
http://www.cdc.gov/nchswww	Data on income, education, and health status of U.S. communities
Healthy People: 2010
http://web.health.gov/healthypeople
http://www.cdc.gov/nchs | National goals and strategies for promoting health and reducing illness; emphasis on high-risk populations |
| Indian Health Service
http://www.ihs.gov | American Indians and Alaskan Natives |
| International Healthy Cities Foundation
http://www.healthycities.org | Objectives, strategies for healthy communities movement |
| Medicaid
http://www.hcfa.gov/medicaid/medicaid.htm | Data, program, and policy information |
| Medicare
http://www.hcfa.gov/medicare/medicare.htm | Data, program, and policy information |
| National Cancer Institute
http://www.nci.nih.gov | Cancer information |
| National Clearinghouse for Alcohol and Drugs
http://www.health.org | Information on alcohol, drugs, substance abuse |
| National Clearinghouse on Child Abuse
http://www.calib.com/nccanch | Domestic violence and neglect |
| National Coalition for the Homeless
http://nch.ari.net | On-line library, links to organizations |

National Committee for Quality Assurance http://www.ncqa.org	Agency accreditation; consumer issues
National Health Information Center http://nhic-nt.health.org	Health-related information
National Health Service Corps http://www.bphc.hrsa.dhhs.gov/nhsc	Preparation, recruitment, and retention of community-responsive primary care clinicians
National Institute for Nursing Research http://www.nih.gov/ninr	News, Priority Expert Panel reports on health care issues, diversity programs, and resources
National Institute of Mental Health (NIMH) http://www.nimh.nih.gov	News on mental health issues, research fact sheets, statistics, and reports, patient education materials
National Institute of Occupational Safety and Health http://www.cdc.gov/niosh	Workplace safety issues, programs
National Institute on Aging Information Center http://www.nih.gov.nia	Aging and gerontology
National League for Nursing (NLN) http://www.nln.org	Nursing education research priorities and disseminating strategies, identified by the NLN's panel
National Library for the Blind and Handicapped http://www.lcweb.local.gov/nls	Resources for the blind and physically handicapped
National Maternal Child Health Clearinghouse http://www.cirrcsol.com/mch	Maternal child health
National Rural Health Association http://www.nrharural.org	Rural health issues and minority health disparities
National Rural Nurses Organization http://www.nro.org	Information and links for rural nursing
Newsletters on Line http://www.newslettersonline.com	Links to health-related publications
Nursing Center http://www.nursingcenter.com	Links to numerous nursing journals' articles; forum discussions; means to earn CE credits on line
Office of Disease Prevention and Health Promotion http://odphp.osophs.dhhs.gov	Information on income, education, and health status
Office of Minority Health Resources Center http://www.omhrc.gov	Minority health issues/cites
Office of Rural Health Policy (USDA) http://www.nal.usda.gov/orhp	Programs, research, publications, links, and an information service on rural health care
Parish Nursing http://lewis.up.edu/nrs/parishnurse	Resources to work with a faith community

Policy Research Associates, Inc.
http://www.prainc.com

Has information resource center on health care for homeless

President's Initiative on Race
http://aspe.os.dhhs.gov/race

Health disparities among racial and ethnic groups; DHHS goals and plans

Primary Care Clinical Practice Guidelines
http://medicine.uscf.edu/resources/guidelines

Resources for primary care providers, including evidence-based guidelines

PubMed and Grateful Med
http://www.ncbi.nlm.nih.gov/PubMed/news.html
http://www.ncbi.nlm.nih. gov/PubMed/news.html

MEDLINE, the National Library of Medicine's database, search and link capabilities

Rural Information Center (USDA)
http://www.nal.usda.gov/ric

A service offering information and referrals for rural communities, officials, organizations, and citizens

Sheps Center for Health Services Research
http://www.shepscenter.unc.edu

Oldest and largest health services research center. Has numerous links to other rural sites

Substance Abuse and Mental Health Services
http://www.samhsa.gov

Preventing and treating substance abuse and mental health problems

U.S. Department of Agriculture
http://www.usda.gov

Agroeconomic and related health issues

U.S. Department of Health and Human Services
http://www.os.dhhs.gov

Programs for special populations

APPENDIX B

Nonmetropolitan Counties, 1997

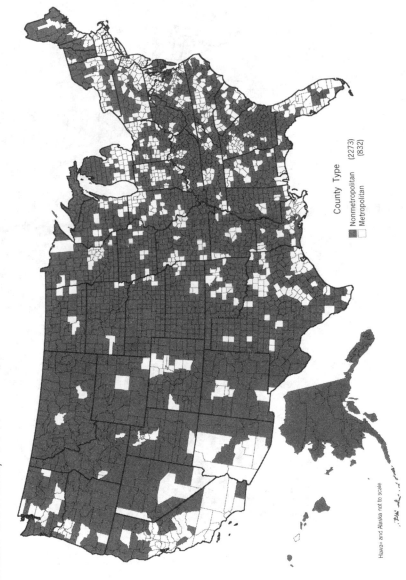

County Type

Nonmetropolitan (2273)
Metropolitan (832)

Hawaii and Alaska not to scale

Appendix C

Frontier Counties, 1994

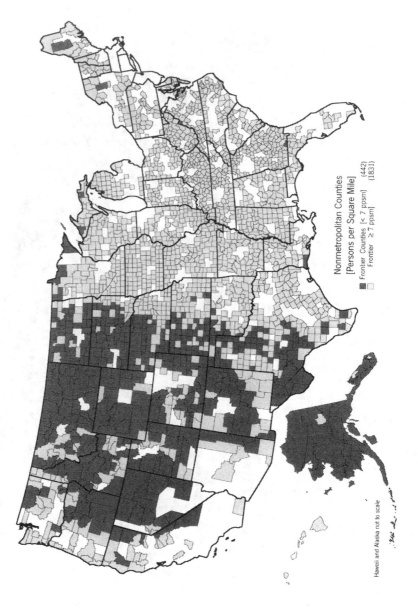

Nonmetropolitan Counties
[Persons per Square Mile]

Frontier Counties [< 7 ppsm] (442)

Frontier ≥ 7 ppsm] (1831)

Hawaii and Alaska not to scale

APPENDIX D

Legislation Affecting Rural Health Care

Year	Legislation	Intent and Provisions
1948	Hill-Burton Act	Provided for construction of health care facilities where these were lacking. Many rural communities built hospitals with these funds. A number of these hospitals currently are experiencing economic problems and are on the verge of closing.
1954	Transfer Act	Provided that all functions, responsibilities, authorities, and duties related to the maintenance and operation of hospitals and health facilities and the conservation of Indian health be administered by the Surgeon General of the U.S. Public Health Service.
1957	Indian Health Assistance Act	Provided for construction of health facilities for Native Americans.
1962	Migrant Health Act	Authorized federal aid for clinics serving migratory agricultural workers and their families.
1964	Economic Opportunity Act	Provided a legal framework for the antipoverty program.
1968	Neighborhood Health Centers	Extended grant to migrant health services.
1970	Health Training Improvement Act	Provided expanded aid to allied health professionals.
1971	Comprehensive Health Manpower Training Act	Increased federal programs for development of health care workers.
1972	Health Service Corps Act	Encouraged health professionals to practice in areas designated as HPSAs.
1973	Health Maintenance Organization and National Health Planning and Resource Development Act	Increased health insurance coverage for the rural population.
1975	Indian Self-Determination Act	Gave tribes the option of staffing and managing Indian Health Service programs in their communities and provided for funding for improvement for tribal capability to contract for health care services.
1976	National Consumer Health Information Act	Provided medical services in areas with an insufficient number of physicians.

1976	Indian Health Care Improvement Act	Intended to elevate the health status of Native Americans and Alaska Natives to a level equal to that of the general population by authorizing a higher budget for the Indian Health Service.
1977	Rural Health Clinics Service Act	Provided medical services in areas with an insufficient number of physicians.
1981	Planned Approach to Community Health (PATCH)	Provided funding to states for delivery of preventive care and health promotion to rural communities.
1981	Omnibus Budget Reconciliation Act (OBRA)	Consolidated categorical grant programs into block grants that served to increase state discretionary use of federal monies (block grants for maternal and child health, services for disabled and other children with special health care needs, Supplemental Security Income services for disabled children, hemophilia treatment centers, and other programs aimed at specific groups or health problems).
1991	NIOSH Agricultural Health Initiative	In recognition of the high morbidity and mortality rates in this industry, focused efforts to address the problems of health and safety in the industry.
1996	Welfare to Work Act	Intended to reduce number of welfare recipients, increase productivity of dependent members of society, and reduce intergenerational dependency.
1997	Rural Hospital Flexibility Program (Sec. 4201 of the Balanced Budget Act)	Created options for struggling small rural hospitals with designation of "critical access hospital"
1986-2000	Decentralized (state) control over health care programs	Added amendments to existing federal health care legislation to revise policies.

Health Professional Shortage Areas (HPSAs), 1997

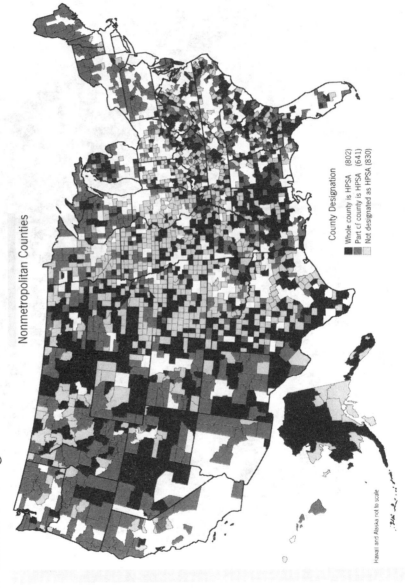

Nonmetropolitan Counties

County Designation

Whole county is HPSA (802)
Part of county is HPSA (641)
Not designated as HPSA (830)

Hawaii and Alaska not to scale

APPENDIX F

USDA County Type: Persistent Poverty, 1989

Nonmetropolitan Counties

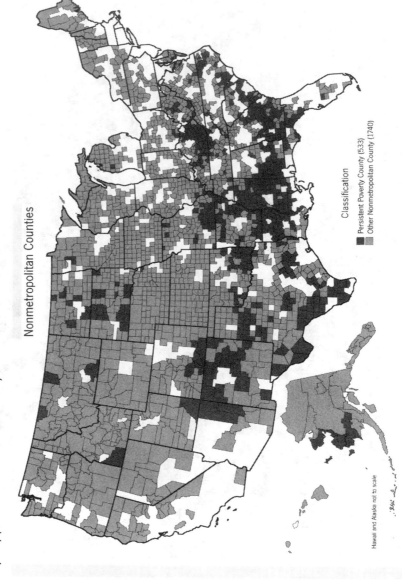

Classification

■ Persistent Poverty County (533)
▦ Other Nonmetropolitan County (1740)

Hawaii and Alaska not to scale

INDEX

ABOUT THE AUTHOR

Angeline Bushy, PhD, RN, CS, holds the Bert Fish Endowed Chair at the University of Central Florida, School of Nursing, where she is a professor. She holds a BSN. from the University of Mary at Bismarck, North Dakota; an MN in Rural Community Health Nursing from Montana State University; an MEd in Adult Education from Northern Montana College; and a PhD in Nursing from the University of Texas at Austin. A clinical specialist in community health nursing, she has lived and worked in rural facilities located in the north central and intermountain states. She has published and presented internationally and nationally an various rural nursing and rural health issues. She has edited the textbooks *Rural Nursing: Volume I & Volume II* and coauthored *Exploring Rural Medicine: Current Issues and Concepts* and *Special Populations in the Community: Advances in Reducing Health Disparities*. Her research focus is on the health care needs of rural populations and the education, role, and scope of rural nursing practice. She is actively involved with Web-based distance education and is a lieutenant colonel in the U.S. Army Reserve. Angie and her husband Jack, a social worker have one daughter, Andrea Dacyl, who is also a social worker.

About the Contributing Authors

Kathryn Baird-Crooks, MEd, RN, has been an instructor in the Division of Health Studies at Medicine Hat College for the past ten years. She has had a varied career in nursing, primarily in rural acute care. She developed one of the first rural nursing courses in Canada. She has published and presented papers in the area of rural nursing nationally as well as internationally.

Jeri Dunkin, PhD, RN, is Associate Professor and holds the Saxon Endowed Chair in Rural Nursing at Capstone College of Nursing, The University of Alabama, Tuscaloosa. She has been involved with rural health care for many years and is editor of the *Online Journal of Rural Nursing and Health Care*. Her research focus is in the area of health promotion of rural populations, particularly with respect to environmental factors and asthma. She is actively involved in distance learning using technology and the Internet. Jeri and her husband are very proud of their seven grandchildren and enjoy touring on their Goldwing motorcycle.

Joyce Engel, PhD, RN, is Dean in the Division of Health Studies at Medicine Hat College. She has been proactive for rural nursing education and was instrumental in offering one of the first such courses in Canada. She has published and presented papers nationally and internationally in the area of rural nursing.

Desley Hegney, PhD, is Professor of Rural Nursing at the University of Southern Queensland and the Cunningham Center, Toowoomba Health Services, Toowoomba, Queensland, Australia. She is the editor of the *Australian Journal of Rural Health* and currently is president of the Queensland Branch of the Association for Australian Rural Nurses Inc. She has had many years of experience in rural nursing and is recognized internationally as an expert on rural practice issues.

Gail Remus, RN, MN, is Associate Professor and Co-ordinator of the Post Registration Nursing program at the College of Nursing, University of Saskatchewan. Prior to coming to the University of Saskatchewan in the mid-1980s she worked as a community health nurse and a home care co-ordinator in a rural community within that province. She and her husband continue to be actively involved in farming; they have two children and four grandchildren.

Donna C. Rennie, PhD, RN, is Associate Professor in the College of Nursing and in the Centre for Agricultural Medicine, College of Medicine, University of Saskatchewan. The focus of her research is respiratory epidemiology, in which she holds a doctorate. She teaches a rural nursing course offered by distance to registered nurses enrolled in a post-diploma nursing program at the University of Saskatchewan. She grew up in rural Manitoba and spent many years as a nurse in northern Manitoba.